PRAISE FOR
eating for pregnancy

"A food-friendly guide to pregnancy and beyond…. The more than 150 recipes in the book are presented in categories that fit with contemporary lifestyles…. It's a realistic approach at a time when more and more meals take place outside the home."

—*The Washington Post*

"As an obstetrician this is a welcome resource for our patients. We often wish we had more time during prenatal visits to review healthy eating and recommendations for adequate nutrition. This book is a welcome addition!"

—DIANE SNYDER, M.D.

"*Eating for Pregnancy* has features that distinguish it from other books in the pregnancy category, including a family approach to eating and cooking during pregnancy, diabetic exchanges, an extensive chapter on vegetarian cooking, and tips for coping with morning sickness. It's a book for motherhood in the 21st century."

—*Pittsburgh Tribune-Review*

"This book is full of information that is vital to maintaining a healthy pregnancy. The recipes are creatively delicious and make eating nutritiously an exciting and achievable goal."

—DIANE FORLEY, *chef-owner of Verbena Restaurant, New York City*

"From an overview on nutrition and pregnancy through the recipes…this book is a must-have. The recipes reflect an appealing fresh and light approach."

—*ForeWord Magazine*

"Delicately balancing optimum and unnecessary weight gain…simple yet flavorful dishes…an overwhelming amount of information."

—*Publishers Weekly*

"Whether you want to get pregnant, are pregnant or adopting a baby, I encourage you to buy this book because it is full of simple, delicious recipes and lots of sound advice on how to eat better and enjoy a healthier lifestyle."

—CINDY PAWLCYN, *chef and restaurateur*

"Every pregnant woman knows that what she eats impacts the health of her baby. But coming up with healthy menus day in and day out can be as daunting as delivery itself. For well-meaning moms everywhere, the simple solution is *Eating for Pregnancy*…. If your idea of the perfect meal is equal parts easy, delicious and nutritious, this book is for you."

—*New Parents Magazine*

"Finally…a cookbook for mothers-to-be…. A new cookbook that offers nutrition guidelines for moms-to-be and includes recipes the entire family will enjoy."

—*Saginaw News*

"Everything in the book is intended to be not only easy to prepare, but also healthy and appealing to every member of the family."

—*Monadnock Ledger*

"A must for mothers-to-be."

—*Cape Gazette*

CATHERINE JONES, a graduate of La Varenne Culinary School in France, worked for the late Jean-Louis Palladin, both in his kitchen and on his book *Jean-Louis: Cooking with the Seasons* (Thomasson-Grant, 1989). The daughter of a retired diplomat and the wife of a Foreign Service officer, Jones has seen much of the world. Her previous book, *A Year of Russian Feasts* (Jellyroll Press, 2002), brings Russian traditions and food to America. She is the mother of a five-year-old daughter and a two-year-old son. Jones and her family live in Bethesda, Maryland.

ROSE ANN HUDSON, R.D., L.D., a perinatal nutritionist and registered dietitian, served on the staff of the Columbia Hospital for Women in Washington, D.C., for twelve years. She has been on the staff of Inova Fairfax Hospital in Fairfax, Virginia, for seven years, and she has a private practice. She counsels both high-risk patients and women experiencing healthy pregnancies. She is the mother of two daughters, ages thirteen and eleven. Hudson and her family live in Rockville, Maryland.

catherine jones WITH rose ann hudson, R.D., L.D.

eating for pregnancy

AN ESSENTIAL GUIDE

TO NUTRITION

WITH RECIPES

FOR THE WHOLE FAMILY

marlowe & company
new york

Published by
Marlowe & Company
An Imprint of Avalon Publishing Group Incorporated
245 West 17th Street, 11th Floor
New York, NY 10011

Library of Congress Cataloging-in-Publication Data

Jones, Catherine Cheremeteff.
Eating for pregnancy : a practical, healthy, up-to-date approach to cooking and eating during
pregnancy that works great for the entire family / Catherine Jones, with Rose Ann Hudson.
p. cm.
Includes bibliographical references and index.
ISBN 1-56924-511-8
1. Pregnancy—Nutritional aspects. 2. Prenatal care. I. Hudson, Rose Ann. II. Title.
RG559 .J665 2003
618.2'4—dc21   2002038688

9 8 7 6 5 4 3

Designed by Pauline Neuwirth, Neuwirth & Associates

Printed in the United States of America
Distributed by Publishers Group West

for all mothers-to-be
and their families

CONTENTS

Red Bell Pepper Sauce ▪ Sautéed Salmon on a Bed of Greens with
Citrus Vinaigrette ▪ Roasted Salmon with Papaya Salsa ▪ Tilapia
Mediterranean-Style

Peach and Blackberry Cobbler ▪ Apple-Blueberry Granola Crisp ▪
Strawberry Whole Wheat Shortcake ▪ No-Bake Fresh Strawberry-
Raspberry Pie ▪ Low-Fat Frozen Raspberry Pie ▪ Reduced-Fat Ricotta
Cheesecake ▪ Pumpkin Pie ▪ Carrot Cake with Cream Cheese
Frosting ▪ Angel Food Cake with Lemon Drizzle ▪ Vanilla Flan with
Fresh Berries ▪ Orange, Blueberry, and Date Salad with Frozen Yogurt
▪ Patricia Terry's Pumpkin Bread ▪ Fruit-Filled Granola ▪ Rhubarb
Sauce

Body Mass Index Chart ▪ Recommended Weight Gain for Pregnant
Women Using the Body Mass Index ▪ Calorie and Protein Require-
ments for Pregnant Women with a Normal Body Mass Index ▪ Food
Groups and Serving Sizes for Pregnant Women ▪ Vitamin A and C
Fruit and Vegetable Sources ▪ Protein Sources ▪ Dairy Calcium
Sources ▪ Nondairy Calcium Sources ▪ Iron Sources ▪ Fiber Sources ▪
Folic Acid Sources ▪ Breakfast Cereals That Contain 100 Percent of
the Daily Value of Folic Acid ▪ Cereals That Contain 100 Percent of
the Daily Value of Vitamin B_{12} ▪ Well-Done Temperature Guide ▪
Food Safety Tips on Meat, Poultry, and Seafood ▪ Barbecue Food
Safety Tips ▪ Slow Cooker Safety Tips ▪ Safe Cooking in the
Microwave Oven ▪ Tips for Cleaning Fresh Produce ▪ Tips for Wash-
ing and Storing Greens ▪ Tips to Help Keep Your Kitchen Workspace
Clean

a few words from catherine jones

THERE IS NOTHING like a positive pregnancy test to focus your attention on your lifestyle and eating habits. Suddenly you realize that everything you eat, drink, or do with your body can directly affect the new life you are carrying. Do I have to give up my coffee or diet soda? What is a healthy lunch, snack, or dinner? What nutrients do I need, what foods can harm my baby, what foods are good for my baby? *Eating for Pregnancy* answers all of these questions and more.

A difficult first pregnancy inspired me to write this book. I needed nutritional advice and realistic ways to use that advice. My equally challenging second pregnancy, combined with my preschooler's picky eating, focused me on quick, tasty, and family-friendly recipes.

I've made a point to explain each recipe fully and clearly—so clearly that even novice cooks, other family members, or a friend or helper could prepare the recipes if the mother-to-be is on bed rest or on the go. I've included tips for variations, advance preparation, timesaving shortcuts, cooking techniques, and slow cooker preparation to make life easier in the kitchen. Busy moms with little ones tugging at their legs tested every recipe to guarantee that they will work for you.

Nothing beats a home-cooked meal, but restaurant dining, fast food, frozen dinners, and semi-prepared and convenience foods are realities in our busy lives. At the same time we worry that these alternatives may not be healthy for our families. *Eating for Pregnancy* takes all of these realities and concerns into account and offers practical advice on how to meet the nutritional needs of pregnancy whether you are dining out or eating at home.

Feeding young children can be a real challenge. *Eating for Pregnancy* offers suggestions on getting youngsters to try healthy foods. After talking to many moms and experimenting at home, I have a few of my own mantras. First, don't dismiss a recipe out of hand as something your child would never eat. Kids' tastes change monthly, daily, or even from moment to moment. If a friend likes green vegetables, hummus, salmon, or other healthy foods, suddenly your child may too. Second, keep introducing your children to new foods, and reintroduce previously rejected foods in new ways. Always feel free to adjust recipes to suit your family's tastes, even if they may lose some of their nutritional value. And finally, children eat more and a better variety of foods when they are sitting down at the table with an adult, a parent, or care-giver who is also eating.

Pregnancy brings incomparable rewards—and a lot of stress. I hope the advice and tips in this book make eating for pregnancy a little easier, and that the recipes inspire you to cook and eat well during your pregnancy, and for years afterward.

a few words from
rose ann hudson

⌒

GREW UP in an Italian family where food was the center of life. Sunday meals and holidays revolved around fun, laughter, arguments, and lots of delicious healthy food. Every Sunday morning, my three sisters and I awoke to the aroma of spaghetti sauce bubbling on the stove. Often the kitchen chairs were draped with homemade pasta hung out to dry. My grandparents, Phillip and Alma Perroots, who lived close by, had an enormous vegetable garden. Almost every day all summer long there was a basket of just-picked produce on our doorstep—fresh tomatoes, beans, broccoli, lettuce, and corn. My father, Thomas Angotti, who is an amateur chef, still makes fresh bread, pasta, and Italian feasts for his whole family.

These childhood memories had a big impact on my love of cooking and my decision to become a dietitian. I get tremendous satisfaction helping people improve their diets and maintain good health through the foods they eat. I particularly enjoy working with pregnant women, and the first thing I tell expectant mothers is that pregnancy is a very special time in their lives, and that since they might go through it only once it is important to enjoy these months as best they can.

From my twenty years of experience with perinatal nutrition, I have found that the biggest challenge for pregnant women is knowing what foods to eat and how much. When Catherine Jones approached me with the idea of coauthoring this book, I immediately envisioned the book that my clients have been asking me for over the years. *Eating for Pregnancy* gives you all the nutritional information you need as well as delicious family-friendly recipes. Some features unique to the recipes are "What's in this for baby and me?," which highlights the nutritional value of a dish; Complete Meal Ideas, which offers suggestions on how to create a balanced meal; and information for diabetics, including American Diabetic Association (ADA) exchange values as part of the nutritional break-downs, and tips on how to modify recipes to be more diabetic-friendly.

Making healthy lifestyle changes during pregnancy can last a lifetime and can be one of the greatest gifts you give yourself and your family. I have instilled in my two teenage daughters the importance of eating in moderation and making healthy food choices. While

I try to recreate the fun Italian dinners I grew up with as often as possible, simple meals with my family, home-cooked or not, bring a sense of security and connection to everyone.

Enjoy your pregnancy, eat the best foods you can before, during, and after pregnancy, keep up healthy eating habits, and pass them on.

nutrition and pregnancy: an overview

⌒

Congratulations! You're pregnant! What lies ahead may be the most joyous, yet tumultuous experience of your life. Countless women have gone before you, and countless will follow, but every pregnancy is special and wondrous, and this one is uniquely yours.

Whether your pregnancy was meticulously planned, medically coaxed, or happened by surprise, one thing is certain—your life will never be the same. You will soon learn to share your body and your life with another human being who is totally dependent on you. If you have been pregnant before, you know much about what lies ahead, but, as you have probably been told, every pregnancy is different.

Eating for Pregnancy was not written to make you feel guilty about buying prepared or frozen foods, eating dinner out, or not meeting your daily calcium requirements. It was written to inform you of your nutritional needs during pregnancy, and to give you ideas of how to meet them, whether you are eating out, cooking at home, dining at your desk, or confined to your bed on bed rest. With any luck, some of the healthy eating and lifestyle habits you develop during pregnancy will stay with you and your family long after the baby is born.

This overview contains basic nutritional advice that serves as the foundation for the recipes and the information throughout the text of the book. If you are trying to get pregnant or think you may be pregnant, following are some key points to bear in mind.

SOME BASIC ADVICE

■ Start taking a folic acid supplement at least one month *before* pregnancy. Because half of all pregnancies are unplanned, a daily folic acid supplement of at least 400 mcg (micrograms) is advisable for *all* women of child-bearing age, especially for women who are trying to conceive (see Folic Acid Before Conception, page 12).

■ If you are planning to start a family, get early prenatal care, even *before* you are pregnant.

- Consult your doctor, health-care provider, or midwife immediately if you think you may be pregnant or if your home pregnancy test result is positive.
- Quit smoking, stop drinking alcohol and caffeinated beverages (including coffee, tea, and soft drinks), and inform your doctor of any prescription, over-the-counter, and/or illicit drugs you are taking.
- Reevaluate your eating habits. Do you skip breakfast, eat fast food for lunch, and graze on junk food for dinner? Follow a well-balanced diet designed for pregnant women. Learn what foods are good for you and try to incorporate them into your diet.
- Get moving. A little exercise will help reduce stress, gas, heartburn, and constipation (see Exercise Tips: Fitness for Two, page 288).
- Eliminate as much stress as possible from your work and home environment. This will help you cope with the intense fatigue of pregnancy and will help keep you emotionally stable when your hormones play tricks on you. Try to let go and relax.
- Get plenty of rest. Your body needs the extra sleep for a reason—so don't fight it. Try to get eight hours of sleep at night, and take short naps with your legs elevated during the day.
- Avoid X rays, hot tubs, and saunas.
- Avoid all rare and undercooked meat, poultry, and seafood.
- Pregnant women should be aware of certain dangerous food-borne illnesses and take precautions to avoid them. These include listeriosis (Listeriosis Warning, page 107), toxoplasmosis (Toxoplasmosis Warning, page 229), E. coli (E. Coli Warning, page 217), salmonellosis (Salmonellosis Warning, page 257, and Eggs and *Salmonella Enteritidis*, page 54).
- Pregnant women should limit their consumption of certain large fish that contain high levels of methylmercury, such as swordfish and shark (see Limitations of Certain Fish Consumption, page 247).

quit smoking before you get pregnant

Smoking deprives the fetus and placenta of oxygen, causing extreme harm to the developing baby.

Three Good Reasons to Quit Smoking

1. **Increased risk for premature birth, babies with low birth weight, stillbirth, and miscarriage.**

2. **Increased risk for intellectual deficiencies, learning disabilities, and behavioral problems later in childhood.**

3. **Increased risk for breathing problems and other health problems, including SIDS (sudden infant death syndrome).**

Good Eating Habits
and Gradual Weight Gain

A healthy diet helps make a healthy baby. During pregnancy, good eating habits are more important than ever. It is not the time to skip meals, eat junk food, or load up on empty calories for quick energy. The foods you eat have a direct effect on the development of your baby from conception to birth. It is important to strike a balance between healthy weight gain and nutritional intake. Try to keep in mind that you are not eating for two, you are eating carefully for one.

It is critical to learn about the nutritional value of the foods you eat and to select your diet with care. Selecting a *variety* of nutrient-rich foods versus calorie-rich foods will help prevent excessive weight gain, which can put you at risk for high blood pressure, gestational diabetes, and permanent obesity. Conversely, a diet too restricted in calories can be inadequate in protein, vitamins, and minerals. Insufficient calorie intake can result in the breakdown of stored fat (or ketones) in the mother's blood and urine, which can be harmful for the fetus.

So, what is the *ideal diet?* The ideal diet is the diet that fits into your lifestyle and at the same time meets all the nutritional requirements of your pregnancy. Your goal should be to follow a well-balanced meal plan that ensures optimal weight gain. A pregnant woman should increase her caloric intake by about 300 calories per day above her prepregnant state, assuming that her prior caloric intake was adequate. Certain factors may increase the nutritional requirements above the estimated demands of pregnancy. Some of these factors include poor nutritional status, obesity, young maternal age (teenage pregnancy), multiple pregnancy, closely spaced births, breastfeeding one or more children while pregnant, continued high level of physical activity, certain disease states (such as diabetes), and use of cigarettes, alcohol, and legal or illegal drugs.[1] Women who fit into any of these categories or who are experiencing a high-risk pregnancy should consult a registered dietitian for customized nutritional advice.

A pregnant woman should consume between 1,800 and 3,000 calories per day, depending on her prepregnant height and weight, and whether her nutritional needs are compromised by any of the factors mentioned above. For example, assuming prepregnant weight is within the "normal range" according to the Body Mass Index (see Body Mass Index Table, page 291), a woman who is 5'3" would require approximately 1,900 to 2,400 calories and at least 60 grams of protein per day, while a woman who is 5'7" would require approximately 2,100 to 2,700 calories and 70 grams of protein per day.

make your 300 extra calories count

Be wise about your 300-calorie additional intake. Choose to eat a sandwich with a glass of milk instead of candy bars and high-calorie sodas and soft drinks.

Just as important as the total number of pounds gained is the *rate* at which the weight is gained. The rate of weight gain

your prepregnant weight
and expected weight gain

WEIGHT GAIN	PREPREGNANT WEIGHT/CONDITION
25 to 35 lbs	average prepregnant weight (within ideal body weight range)
28 to 40 lbs	underweight prepregnant weight (10% below ideal body weight)
15 to 25 lbs	overweight prepregnant weight (20% above ideal body weight)
40 to 45 lbs	woman carrying twins

should be 2 to 5 pounds for the first trimester (fourteen weeks) and 3.5 pounds per month for the remainder of the pregnancy (fourteen to forty weeks). Ideally, the *total* weight gain during pregnancy should be between 25 and 35 pounds, if you were at an appropriate prepregnant body weight. Women with special nutritional requirements will need a customized weight-gain plan.

Don't become obsessed with your weight gain—feel free to put away your scale. Your weight will be closely monitored by your doctor during each office visit. A trend of excessive or inadequate weight gain in more than one month (a gain of more than 5 pounds and less than 2 pounds) indicates that your dietary intake may need to be evaluated. If the rate at which you put on weight is excessive and on an upward trend overall, take an inventory of your food intake to pinpoint problem areas. Try cutting down on fried or fatty foods, fast foods and convenience foods, and highly sweetened desserts and soft drinks. Also, monitor your portion sizes more closely.

PRODUCTS OF CONCEPTION[2]

NUMBER OF POUNDS	SOURCE OF WEIGHT GAIN
4–6	Maternal stores (fat, protein, and other nutrients)
2–3	Increased fluid volume
3–4	Increased blood volume
1–2	Breast enlargement
2	Uterus
6–8	Baby
2	Amniotic fluid
1.5	Placenta (tissue connecting mother and baby that brings nourishment and takes away waste)

If inadequate weight gain or weight loss is a trend, evaluate your exercise plan (especially if you exercise very frequently), because you may be burning off essential calories and not replacing them. Also, try increasing the amount of protein- and calcium-rich foods in your diet. Adding nonfat dry milk powder to milk, milk shakes, smoothies, hot cereals, dips, and soups is a way of getting extra protein, calcium, and calories. One-third cup of pasteurized instant nonfat dry milk provides 80 calories and 8 grams of protein. Keep in mind that it is not unusual to have a large one-month weight gain sometime in the second trimester. This may be attributed to a 25 percent increase in blood and fluid volume for the mother.

Planning a Healthy, Well-Balanced Diet

Planning a healthy, well-balanced diet to meet your pregnancy needs does not have to be difficult or time-consuming. Following is a Food Groups Guide for Pregnancy. For a list of foods and serving sizes that fit into these food categories, see Food Groups and Serving Sizes for Pregnant Women, page 293. A Vegetarian Food Groups Guide for Pregnancy is located in Chapter Four: Vegetarian Delights, on page 152.

FOOD GROUPS GUIDE FOR PREGNANCY[3]

Milk and dairy = 3 to 4 servings per day

Meat, poultry, fish, dried beans, eggs, and nuts = 2 to 3 servings per day

Bread, cereal, rice, and pasta = 6 to 11 servings per day

Vegetables = 3 to 5 servings per day

Fruits = 2 to 4 servings per day

It is helpful to understand some of the most important nutrients and their role in your baby's development. The Extra Daily Nutrient Allowances for Pregnancy table below illustrates some of the extra nutrients pregnant women need. Pregnant teens should consult a dietitian to determine the best intakes for their growing bodies and developing babies. Other conditions during pregnancy, such as multiples and diabetes, may also require special nutrient allowances.

Prenatal vitamins act as a safety net to your diet during pregnancy, and they should be taken as directed by your doctor. Keep in mind that they do *not* replace real food. During the first trimester, morning sickness can be exacerbated by certain prenatal vitamins. If you suspect this, try taking your vitamin with food, before bedtime, or ask your doctor to switch vitamin brands. If you stop taking your vitamin for any reason, you should continue to take a folic acid supplement throughout pregnancy.

Nutrient	Nonpregnant Women (25–50 years old)	Pregnant	Increase
Protein* (g)	50	60	10
Calcium* (mg)	800	1200	400
Iron* (mg)	15	30	15
Zinc* (mg)	12	15	3
Phosphorus (mg)	700	700	0
Vitamin A* (IU)	800	800	0
Folic Acid* (mcg)	400	800	400
Thiamine (B_1) (mg)	1.1	1.4	0.3
Riboflavin (B_2) (mg)	1.1	1.4	0.3
Niacin (mg)	14	18	4
Vitamin (B_6) (mg)	1.3	1.9	0.6
Vitamin (B_{12}) (mg)	2.4	2.6	0.2
Vitamin C (mg)	75	85	10
Vitamin D (IU)	200	200	0
Vitamin E (mg)	15	15	0

*Recommended Daily Allowances (RDAs) value. All unmarked nutrients reflect Adequate Intakes (AIs). RDAs and AIs may both be used as goals for individual intakes.

▶ *Protein*

During pregnancy extra protein is needed to help with fetal brain development and with muscle and tissue formation. Inadequate amounts of dietary protein can impair the development of the placenta and fetus, resulting in low birth weight and intrauterine growth retardation. For the mother, protein is essential for the increase in maternal blood volume and for the formation of amniotic fluid. During labor, delivery, and lactation, protein storage reserves are tapped, making it vital to have an excess amount. You will want to take in about 20 percent more protein than before pregnancy, raising the 50 grams required by the average normal nonpregnant woman to 60 grams per day (see Calorie and Protein Requirements for Pregnant Women with a Normal Body Mass Index, page 290). Some good sources of proteins include: chicken, lean red meats, fish, cottage cheese, pasteurized cheese, yogurt, eggs, and milk. Samples of vegetable protein sources include: tofu, tempeh, beans, legumes, nut butters, nuts, and seeds (see Protein Sources, page 295, for a more complete list).

▶ *Carbohydrates*

Carbohydrates provide your body with energy. Adequate intake of carbohydrates is necessary to allow protein that would otherwise be tapped for energy to be used for muscle building and tissue formation in the fetus. Complex carbohydrates, such as whole grains, pasta, rice, fruits, and vegetables, are a main source of vitamins (particularly the B complex vitamins), iron (in iron-fortified products), and fiber. While simple sugars, such as candy and sodas, may give you a temporary energy boost, they are sources of empty calories and should never be substituted for nutrient-rich foods.

▶ *Fats*

Pregnancy is the wrong time to start counting fat grams. Don't even dream about dieting, which can prevent you from meeting your nutritional requirements, *but* don't use your pregnancy as an excuse to pig out either. Fat plays a vital role in cell formation and fetal brain development, and therefore should not be restricted during pregnancy. Fats are the main source of the fat-soluble vitamins A, D, E, and K.

The type of fat you eat is not the main focus; however it is always wise to choose heart healthy, unsaturated fats (such as canola oil and olive oil) over saturated fats (such as butter, bacon, whole milk, and fatty meats). When preparing meats always use lean cuts and trim any visible fat. The recipes in *Eating for Pregnancy* are designed to be moderately low in fat and appropriate for the entire family.

The Essential Minerals

▶ *Calcium*

Calcium is an essential element for bone and teeth construction for the mother and her baby. Calcium intake should increase from about 800 milligrams to 1200 milligrams per day during pregnancy, and more for women carrying multiples or pregnant adolescents. The bones contain 99 percent of the calcium in the body and the remaining 1 percent is contained in the blood. If calcium intake is not adequate enough to meet the baby's needs (especially during the third trimester to accommodate the rapid skeletal growth in the fetus), the calcium reserves of the mother's bones are tapped, resulting in calcium depletion for the mother. Calcium in the bloodstream is very important, especially for pregnant women during labor. It is needed to maintain proper heartbeat, muscle contractions, nerve transmissions, and for the maintenance of connective tissue and blood clotting.

Consuming calcium through proper diet and supplements is only one phase of building and maintaining healthy bones (see Dairy Calcium Sources, page 296, and Nondairy Calcium Sources, page 297). In order for the body to absorb calcium, the calcium must be combined with vitamin D. The body can manufacture vitamin D with the help of sunlight (15 minutes to 1 hour per day of midday sunshine). For those who cannot be outdoors, fortified milk, whole or skim, and vitamin D-fortified cereals are good sources of vitamin D, as well as other nutrients (see Vitamin D, page 10). To prevent interference with iron absorption, calcium supplements should not be taken with a prenatal vitamin, and preferably between meals.

Lactose intolerance, or the inability to digest milk sugar contained in dairy products due to a deficiency of the enzyme lactase, is one of the major reasons women cannot meet their calcium goal. One option is to try yogurt made with live or active cultures whose bacteria releases lactose-digesting enzymes (see The Power of Yogurt, page 10). Or, you might consider Lactaid drops or pills, lactose-free milk products (which range from 70 percent to 100 percent lactose-free), or non-dairy beverages such as soy, almond, rice, and oat milks (choose fortified products whenever possible). Read labels carefully to select the brands that offer the most calcium, protein, and vitamins.

calcium and osteoporosis

Pregnancy does not have to drain your bones of calcium. If your daily calcium consumption is adequate to meet your needs as well as those of your developing baby, pregnancy can actually help preserve bone mass. The high levels of estrogen during pregnancy stimulate the activation of vitamin D (which promotes calcium absorption), and increase the production of calcitonin, which inhibits bone breakdown. While menopause may seem light-years away at this point in your life, maintaining a high calcium intake from pregnancy is a good habit to continue.

▶ *Iron*

Any woman who does not get a sufficient amount of iron during her pregnancy, or who starts her pregnancy with low iron stores, is at risk for iron deficiency anemia (see Iron Deficiency Anemia, page 14). Because it is impossible to meet your daily iron requirements through food sources alone, a prenatal vitamin that contains iron is recommended.

Iron is essential for the formation of hemoglobin, which carries oxygen in the blood. During pregnancy the increase in maternal blood volume is approximately 25 percent, or 4 pints. An iron intake of 30 milligrams is recommended for most healthy pregnancies, while pregnant women suffering from anemia may need additional supplementation. Adequate maternal iron stores are vital in protecting the mother from complications due to blood loss during pregnancy. Also, a three- to four-month supply of iron is stored in the liver of the fetus for use after birth, before food stores of iron are added to the baby's diet.

Heme iron from animal sources is more easily absorbed by the body than non-heme iron from plant sources. One easy way to increase the absorption of iron is to consume high-iron foods with a source of vitamin C. While it is true that some of the highest sources of iron (such as beef and eggs) are also high in cholesterol and fat, a low-cholesterol, low-fat diet is not recommended during a normal pregnancy without complications. Cholesterol levels may rise slightly during the second half of pregnancy, but usually they resume to normal levels within the six-month postpartum period. A woman with an elevated cholesterol level *prior* to pregnancy should consult her doctor or dietitian for dietary fat and cholesterol restrictions. (See Iron Sources, page 298.)

Vital Vitamins

Increased amounts of vitamins A, B, C, D, and E are recommended and are routinely prescribed by doctors in the form of a prenatal supplement. However, mega doses of certain vitamins and minerals can be extremely dangerous. For instance, excess intake of vitamins A and D can cause fetal malformation during the first trimester. It is very important to check with your doctor before taking any additional vitamin or mineral supplements.

▶ *Vitamin A*

Vitamin A is vital in promoting cell, bone, and tooth formation, normal vision, and healthy skin in the fetus. Pregnant women require 800 international units of vitamin A daily. Excessive intake of vitamin A (more than 5,000 IU in the form of retinol, not beta carotene) can increase the risk of birth defects, such as malformation of the head, brain, heart, or spinal cord. There is some concern about consuming too much liver, which is extremely rich in vitamin A, during pregnancy. Pregnant women should minimize their consumption of liver, if not eliminate it entirely from their diets.[6] Fruit and vegetable sources of vitamin A, such as mango, cantaloupe, tangerines, sweet potatoes, carrots, broccoli, and asparagus, are *not* toxic in large doses. They contain beta carotene, which the body converts to vitamin A based on need. Other good sources of vitamin A include egg yolks, pasteurized cheese, fortified dairy products, and butter (see Vitamin A Sources, page 294, for a more complete list).

the power of yogurt

Yogurt is made by heating milk and then adding culture. This fermentation process results in the breakdown of casein, or milk protein, one of the most difficult proteins to digest. Culturing, the process following fermentation, restores many of the enzymes destroyed during pasteurization, including lactase. Lactase is the enzyme that breaks down lactose (milk sugar) into glucose and galactose, and it is this breakdown that allows some people who are otherwise lactose intolerant to consume cultured yogurt without side effects (check yogurt labels for active cultures). One last bit of good news about yogurt–nonfat plain yogurt is so high in calcium that just 6 ounces provide as much calcium as 8 ounces of reduced-fat (1% or 2%) milk.

▶ *Vitamin C*

Vitamin C (also known as ascorbic acid) is essential for wound healing, healthy teeth and gums, maintaining resistance to infection, and iron absorption. A daily increase to 85 milligrams is recommended during pregnancy. However, don't overdo it. Excessive intake of vitamin C supplements could cause the newborn to have increased requirements for vitamin C, possibly leading to a deficiency syndrome called rebound scurvy. Pregnant women can fulfill their daily requirements of vitamin C by eating additional citrus fruits, berries, cantaloupe, tomatoes, broccoli, Brussels sprouts, and red bell peppers (see Vitamin C Sources, page 294, for a more complete list).

▶ *Vitamin D*

Vitamin D is manufactured by the body after exposure to the sun. It is necessary to promote the utilization of calcium and phosphorus by the body. Pregnant women

water-soluble and fat-soluble vitamins

Vitamins fall into two categories, water soluble and fat soluble.

▶ *Water-soluble vitamins* (all the B vitamins and C) dissolve in water and are not stored in your body. Your body uses the vitamins it needs and eliminates the rest.

▶ *Fat-soluble vitamins* (A, D, E, and K) are dissolved in fat and therefore can be stored in the body (specifically in the liver).

Keep in mind that any vitamin taken in extremely large doses can potentially be harmful. Vitamins A and D are extremely toxic if taken in large doses.

need 200 IU of vitamin D per day. A healthy, nonpregnant woman usually gets adequate vitamin D from exposure to sunlight. Be aware that vitamin D through supplements can be toxic in doses larger than 1,000 IU. Good sources of vitamin D include egg yolks, butter, milk products (all milk pasteurized in the U.S. is fortified with vitamin D), vitamin D-fortified cereals, sardines, salmon, herring, and mackerel.

▶ The B Vitamins

FOLIC ACID

Folic acid (also called folacin and folate) is essential for cell division and manufacturing DNA and RNA, the molecules that transfer genetic information and translate it into tissue production. Increased amounts of folic acid are valuable in preventing neural tube defects, such as spina bifida and anencephaly. Spina bifida is caused by an incomplete closing of the bony casing around the spinal cord, which results in partial paralysis. Anencephaly is a fatal defect in which a major part of the brain never develops. Approximately 2,500 infants suffering from spina bifida are born in the U.S. each year. The latest research also shows that folic acid can also help prevent oral and facial birth defects, such as cleft palate.[7]

Pregnant women should consume 800 micrograms of folic acid daily. Women carrying multiples and obese pregnant women may be prescribed additional folic acid. Some natural sources of folic acid include lentils, romaine lettuce, asparagus, chickpeas, beans, green leafy vegetables, citrus fruits, wheat germ, and brewer's yeast. Enriched breads and fortified breakfast cereals are also excellent sources of folate (see Folic Acid Sources, page 300, for a more complete list).

VITAMIN B₁₂

Vitamin B_{12} is essential in the formation of red blood cells and a healthy nervous system. It can be found only in animal products, vitamin B_{12}–fortified cereals, and yeast. The recommended dose of 2.6 milligrams of vitamin B_{12} during pregnancy is usually met through food sources; therefore supplements are not needed, except perhaps for strict vegetarians or vegans. (For more information on vegetarian diets and vitamin B_{12} supplements, see Chapter Four: Vegetarian Delights, page 152. Also see the list of Cereals that Contain 100 percent of the Daily Value of Vitamin B_{12}, page 302.)

Vitamin B_6

Vitamin B_6 assists in the formation of red blood cells and the metabolism of protein and fats. The extra protein allowance for pregnancy should be accompanied by an increase in vitamin B_6—a total intake of 1.9 milligrams per day. Good sources of vitamin B_6 include poultry, fish, pork, eggs, whole wheat products, and nuts (peanuts and walnuts).

Thiamine (B_1)

Thiamine helps the body convert carbohydrates into energy. It is also necessary for healthy functioning of the heart and brain, and for healthy nerve cells. Pregnant women should consume 1.4 milligrams of thiamine per day. Some good sources include unrefined cereal, brewer's yeast, lean pork, legumes, nuts, and seeds.

Riboflavin (B_2)

Riboflavin is important for body growth and cell reproduction. It is necessary for breaking down amino acids and releasing energy from carbohydrates. Pregnant women should consume 1.4 milligrams of riboflavin per day. Some good sources include meat, poultry, dairy products, grain products, and green vegetables such as broccoli, turnip greens, collard greens, asparagus, and spinach.

Niacin

Niacin assists with cell production. Pregnant women should consume 18 milligrams of niacin per day. Some good sources include poultry, meat, tuna, eggs, whole grains, nuts, legumes, and enriched breads and cereals.

PHOSPHORUS

Phosphorus is an essential component of bone mineral. It is present in nearly all foods, but the major food sources are protein-rich foods, milk and dairy products, rice, cereals and grains, poultry, and fish. Pregnant women should consume 700 milligrams of phosphorus per day.

ZINC

Zinc is essential for maintaining immunity, and for wound healing, fat metabolism, and sexual function. Zinc deficiency can cause poor fetal growth. Dietary sources of zinc include seafood, meat, eggs, dairy products, zinc-fortified cereals, legumes, and whole grains. Pregnant women should consume 15 miligrams of zinc.

High-Risk Pregnancies

Certain preexisting conditions or pregnancy-related complications require extra care and attention. For these high-risk pregnancies, women usually require a closely monitored, customized medical care plan, and some conditions may call for special nutrition guidelines. Following are some of the most common high-risk conditions.

▶ Obese Pregnant Women

Pregnant women who are overweight (defined as 20% above ideal body weight, or having a prepregnant body mass index greater than 26—see Body Mass Index Table, page 291) run a higher risk of high blood pressure and gestational diabetes during pregnancy. In general, overweight women should gain an average of 15 to 25 pounds during pregnancy. An obese pregnant woman (defined as having a prepregnant body mass index greater than 29), needs to gain weight, but at a very slow rate. The total weight gain recommended for an obese pregnant woman is about 15 pounds. It is advisable for an obese woman considering pregnancy to follow a healthy meal plan to lose weight *before* getting pregnant. No matter how overweight you are, dieting is *not* recommended during pregnancy. Also, women who are obese at conception may be prescribed additional folic acid to help prevent neural tube defects. If you are obese, consult your doctor and dietitian for an appropriate folic acid increase and a customized nutritional plan.

▶ High Blood Pressure During Pregnancy

Contrary to popular belief, when high blood pressure develops during pregnancy (particularly in women with no previous history of high blood pressure) following a *strict* low-sodium diet is usually not recommended. Instead, increasing protein and calcium seems to be most beneficial. Pregnant women with high blood pressure (also known as pregnancy-induced hypertension [PIH], or gestational hypertension) should try to avoid high-sodium foods such as bacon, sausage, processed foods, fast foods, and canned soups (see

High-Sodium Foods, page 239). For early detection of elevated blood pressure, blood pressure checks should be done on a regular basis (at least once a month) throughout pregnancy. Following are some of the most common warning symptoms of hypertension. Call your doctor right away if you notice any of them.

- Severe or constant headaches
- Swelling, especially in the face
- Blurred vision and sensitivity to light
- Pain in the upper right part of the abdomen
- Sudden weight gain of more than 1 pound per day

Sometimes pregnancy-induced hypertension can lead to a condition called preeclampsia, which can affect the placenta, and the mother's kidney, liver, and brain. When preeclampsia causes seizures, the condition becomes eclampsia, which can result in fetal complications, low birth weight, premature birth, stillbirth, and serious health risks for the mother. At greatest risk for preeclampsia are:[8]

- Women with chronic hypertension or high blood pressure levels before becoming pregnant
- Women who developed high blood pressure or preeclampsia during a previous pregnancy, especially if these conditions occurred early on
- Women who are obese prior to pregnancy
- Pregnant women under the age of twenty or over the age of forty
- Pregnant women carrying multiples
- Pregnant women with diabetes, kidney disease, rheumatoid arthritis, lupus, or scleroderma

▶ Iron Deficiency Anemia

Iron deficiency anemia is most commonly caused by low iron stores prior to pregnancy, or from blood loss during pregnancy. Certain preexisting, inherited medical conditions can increase the risk of iron deficiency during pregnancy. The most common are sickle cell anemia, an inherited form of anemia occurring primarily in African-Americans and women from South and Central America, and thalassemia, an inherited form of anemia, occurring mostly in people of Mediterranean origin and some women of Asian origin.

Pregnant women suffering from iron deficiency anemia can experience fatigue, shortness of breath, paleness, dizziness, light-headedness, or heart palpitations. Anemia can also lead to infection, premature labor, and a decreased ability to tolerate blood loss during childbirth. Increased iron supplementation and a high-iron diet (see Iron Sources, page 298) may be prescribed by a doctor. Be sure to take all iron supplements with citrus juice, *not* milk, as calcium can interfere with iron absorption. Leaf tea, coffee, and high-phytate foods also limit iron absorption. (For more information on iron absorption and phytate foods, see Chapter Four, Vegetarian Delights, page 152.)

▶ Teenage Pregnancy

Pregnant teenagers, eighteen years old or younger, have more nutritional requirements than pregnant adults. Teens have to meet their own increased nutritional needs for growth as well as the needs of the developing fetus. Generally, in addition to all of the standard nutrient intake requirements for pregnant women (see Extra Daily Nutrient Allowances for Pregnancy, page 6), a pregnant teenager requires 75 to 85 grams of protein, 1,300 milligrams of calcium, 1,250 milligrams of phosphorus, and approximately 400 additional calories. A pregnant adolescent should be counseled by her doctor, nurse, or dietitian for a meal plan that addresses all of her needs. Meal frequency should be evaluated, as teens may skip meals due to school and other activities. Also, the importance of adequate weight gain should be stressed to pregnant teens who may be hesitant to gain weight for fear of becoming fat.

▶ Multiple Pregnancies

Pregnant women carrying twins, triplets, or more have a particular challenge meeting increased nutritional needs. The calorie and weight gain requirements are *not* double or triple that of a single pregnancy. Generally, on top of the normal pregnancy requirements, a woman carrying twins needs an additional 300 calories per day, and a woman carrying triplets needs an additional 600 calories per day. The total weight gain for a woman with twins is about 40 to 45 pounds, and 50 to 55 pounds for a woman with triplets. Protein, calcium, iron, and folic acid requirements increase as well, and a doctor should be consulted for specific recommendations. A woman pregnant with multiples needs to consult a registered dietitian for a customized meal plan appropriate for her situation.

▶ Diabetes During Pregnancy

While some women have diabetes before becoming pregnant, others develop gestational diabetes, usually during the third trimester of pregnancy. Gestational diabetes occurs when a pregnant woman cannot produce enough insulin, or her body tissues

drugs: side effects and safety

Be sure your doctor is aware of any prescription medications or over-the-counter drugs you are taking if you are trying to get pregnant or are pregnant. All medications, including hemorrhoid treatments and cold remedies, should be cleared with your doctor or nurse if you are pregnant. Illegal drugs, such as cocaine, crack, and marijuana, may lead to premature delivery and contribute to low birth weight, fetal distress, neonatal addiction, and death. Infants born to substance abusers can suffer from withdrawal symptoms at birth, and they run the risk of sudden infant death.

do not properly utilize the insulin she produces, resulting in an excess amount of glucose (blood sugar) in the blood. Gestational diabetes is usually caused by changes in a pregnant woman's metabolism and hormone production and usually goes away after the birth of the baby. However, women with gestational diabetes are at increased risk of developing diabetes in the future and of developing gestational diabetes in any later pregnancies. Women most at risk for gestational diabetes usually fit into one of the following categories:[9]

- Women over the age of thirty
- Women obese prior to pregnancy
- Women with a family history of diabetes
- Women with a previous delivery of a 9.5-pound (or larger) baby, or a stillborn

All pregnant women should be tested for gestational diabetes using the glucose control test (GCT) between the twenty-fourth and twenty-eighth weeks of pregnancy. If diabetes is detected, your doctor, a diabetes nurse practitioner, and a registered dietitian will work closely with you to monitor your diet and exercise, your baby's weight gain, and your blood sugar level. Your doctor will also discuss possible complications during pregnancy and delivery, and potential problems with newborns. Any type of diabetes requires special nutritional attention in the form of a diabetic diet customized for pregnancy. The diabetic diet is based on the Exchange System created by the American Diabetic Association. Recipes in *Eating for Pregnancy* provide ADA exchange values and can be incorporated into a gestational diabetic diet.

If you have diabetes prior to pregnancy, it is *critical* that you plan ahead for your pregnancy. The American Diabetes Association suggests that a diabetic woman considering pregnancy should try to maintain good blood glucose control for *three to six months before she plans to get pregnant*. The first few weeks of pregnancy, when many women don't even know they are pregnant, is a crucial time for the development of vital organs, and tight blood glucose control is essential in order to prevent birth defects.[10]

▶ **General Recommendations for Pregnant Women with Gestational Diabetes**

- Consult a registered dietitian for an appropriate meal plan for optimal blood glucose control.
- Avoid sugar, honey, molasses, syrup, fruits canned in syrup, all sodas, sweetened beverages, candies, jams, jellies, cookies, cakes, pies, doughnuts, gum, frosted cereals, candy bars, ice cream, hot chocolate—you get the picture!
- Avoid fruit juices.
- Avoid alcohol.
- Try to eat your meals and snacks at the same time every day.
- Measure your food after it is cooked, for accurate portion sizes.

- Try to include all servings in each meal.
- Do not eat anything for two hours after you finish your meals.
- Do not skip meals or snacks.
- Remember that you are on a customized diet to control your blood sugar and not to lose weight.

Basic Guidelines for Nutrition After Delivery and Breastfeeding

Believe it or not, soon you will deliver a beautiful baby, you will be on your way home from the hospital, and you will start a new chapter in your life. If you are wondering what to do with all of the healthy eating habits you developed during pregnancy—continue them! If you plan to breastfeed your baby, you will need to follow certain general nutritional guidelines. These include:

- Continue to take all of your prenatal vitamins and any supplements as prescribed by your doctor.
- Follow a well-balanced diet that includes healthy snacks.
- Consume 500 extra calories per day (approximately 2,700 calories), or 200 calories above your pregnancy caloric intake, for the first twelve months. Calorie needs should be adjusted based on milk production, rate of weight loss, and special situations (see below). Also, consume about 65 grams of protein (possibly more if feeding more than one infant) and 280 micrograms of folic acid during the first six months of breastfeeding. You will also need approximately 1,200 milligrams of calcium and 15 milligrams of iron while breastfeeding.[11] For a specific meal plan to meet of all these nutritional needs, consult a registered dietitian.
- Avoid alcohol, smoking, and caffeine, and do not take any medications (prescription or over-the-counter) without your doctor's approval.
- Drink 8 fluid ounces of water each time you breastfeed, or at least six to eight eight-ounce glasses of water per day.
- Contact a lactation consultant for special situations including: mothers nursing multiples or tandem nursing (breastfeeding while pregnant); nursing mothers who are diabetic or who have had breast surgery; teenage nursing mothers; underweight nursing mothers; or mothers nursing babies born with a cleft palate, premature babies, hospitalized babies, or any other babies with special needs.
- Contact a lactation consultant, or your doctor, with questions about breastfeeding.

If you will be using formula to feed your baby, you will not need to maintain your pregnancy caloric intake, although crash dieting immediately after delivery is not advisable.

Whether breastfeeding or bottle feeding, let your body heal at its own pace. Ease into exercise slowly according to your doctor's recommendations, and continue to eat nutritious foods. Remember to stay well hydrated, rest when you can, accept help when it comes your way, and do something special for yourself from time to time. Enjoy your new family!

UNDERSTANDING THE NUTRITIONAL BREAKDOWNS OF THE RECIPES

EATING FOR PREGNANCY was created to be as user-friendly as possible, providing clear information about each recipe's nutritional value. To this end, each recipe asks the basic question, *"What's in this for baby and me?"* The answers that follow list nutrients that include 20 percent or more of the Daily Value per serving based on a 2,000 calorie nonpregnancy diet. You may want to go one step further to figure out exactly how these percentages compare with your pregnancy requirements. To do this you will need to review the values in the Approximate Nutritional Information at the bottom of each recipe and compare them to the Extra Daily Nutrient Allowances for Pregnancy on page 6.

The recipe headnote descriptions "excellent source of," "high in," or "rich in," preceding certain nutrients in boldface contain 20 percent or more of the Daily Values per serving and they correspond to the answers to *"What's in this for baby and me?"* Other nutrients listed as a "good source of," provide 10 percent to 19 percent of the Daily Values per serving. (Both these percentage figures are based on a 2,000 calorie nonpregnancy diet.) This wording was carefully chosen to comply with the 1990 Food and Drug Administration labeling system to describe ranges of nutrient content in foods.

All the nutritional values (unless otherwise stated) were calculated using Nutritionist Pro software from First DataBank (2002 First DataBank, Inc.). All ingredients in each recipe (except optional toppings) were included in the calculations for the Approximate Nutritional Information.

Every recipe in *Eating for Pregnancy* contains the following breakdowns: calories (cals.), protein (grams), carbohydrates (grams), fat (grams), fiber (grams), sodium (milligrams), and diabetic exchanges (based on the American Diabetic Association—ADA—exchange system). Vitamins and minerals are also listed if a recipe provides 20 percent or more of the Daily Value per serving. The B vitamins—thiamine, riboflavin, and niacin—were viewed as a group. Each of their individual nutritional values had to meet the 10 percent or 20 percent of the Daily Value criteria for the food or recipe to be considered a good or an excellent source. In some recipes you will notice that the portion size listed next to the ADA exchange value was reduced to be more diabetic friendly. These smaller portions reflect only the diabetic exchange values of the recipe, not the rest of the nutritional information. The word FREE mentioned in some of the ADA exchanges indicate foods with relatively few calories, less than twenty calories per serving. It is advisable for diabetics to limit FREE foods to a total of fifty to sixty calories per day, divided between meals and snacks. Also, the ▼ symbol following some of the recipe titles at the beginning of each chapter indicates that the dish is suitable for vegan diets.

The Complete Meal Ideas that follow most of the recipes offer menu suggestions. The serving sizes of these meal suggestions depend on your individual nutritional requirements and your daily meal plan. These complete meal ideas are not intended for diabetics. As a final word, *Eating for Pregnancy* does not endorse any products, food or other, even though they may be mentioned in the text or the recipes.

no more boring breakfasts

~

URING PREGNANCY you will quickly realize that you won't get very far without something in your stomach—especially if you are suffering from morning sickness. Health professionals have long considered breakfast the most important meal of the day. A nutritious breakfast provides the protein, energy, and vitamins needed to get you through the morning and the rest of the day. Admittedly, it can be hard to find the time for breakfast, especially if you have young, demanding children to dress and feed, and a deadline to get yourself out the front door. While everyone's morning routine varies, working in breakfast will become essential during the months ahead. Here are a few tips to help get your day off to a healthy start.

SOME BASIC ADVICE

- Make breakfast a habit. You'll be surprised at how quickly it becomes a good habit for the entire family.
- Wake up fifteen minutes earlier to be able to sit down for breakfast and try to eat slowly. This is understandably difficult if you have a tight work schedule or other children who need to get off to school or daycare. Sitting down to breakfast and all meals will reduce indigestion during pregnancy.
- Start your day with a piece of fresh fruit or fruit juice, or a glass of water.
- Try to get something warm in your stomach. Warm cereal, eggs, decaffeinated coffee or tea, or just plain hot water will warm your engines.
- Plan a week's worth of breakfasts so you are not faced with empty cabinets in the morning. Always try to have oranges, or any other fresh fruits, a box of fortified cereal or bread, enriched pancake mix, eggs, and muffins on hand, and waffles in the freezer.
- Use the weekends to make breakfast treats you can refrigerate or freeze to enjoy during the week.

- Women on the go or on bed rest can get a lot of mileage from muffins, particularly low-fat varieties, which can be refrigerated or frozen. Topped with peanut butter, or any nut butter—such as almond, cashew, or soy nut butter—muffins can provide a good dose of fiber and protein.

So, what is a healthy breakfast for pregnant women? A healthy breakfast should include protein, complex carbohydrates, milk or yogurt, fruit or fruit juice, and fat. A well-balanced breakfast, containing one-fourth of the daily calorie and protein requirements, includes about 550 calories and 20 grams of protein, depending on your height and weight. (See the Calorie and Protein Requirements During Pregnancy, page 290).

Good protein sources for breakfast are eggs, cheese, and nut butters. Eggs can be prepared almost any way you wish as long as the white and yolk are *completely* cooked. Adding a bit of cheese or tofu to your omelet can give you a double-protein fix. Hard-boiled eggs are ideal. They make a portable breakfast for women on the go, an easy breakfast for women on bed rest, and a great snack any time of day. As tempting as they may be, try to avoid high fat, salty breakfast meats such as bacon and sausage. Some health and whole foods stores carry soy breakfast strips or sausages that contain no nitrites, nitrates, or MSG, a healthier (though perhaps less satisfying) alternative to bacon.

Complex carbohydrates in the form of high-iron cereals, granola, whole grain muffins, waffles, and whole wheat toast provide essential B vitamins and energy. Look for cereals fortified with 100 percent of the daily value of folic acid and iron (see Cereals that Contain 100 Percent of the Daily Value of Folic Acid, page 301). Vegetarians, particularly vegans, should choose cereals fortified with 100 percent of the daily value of vitamin B_{12}, especially if there is concern about meeting daily requirements (see Cereals that Contain 100 Percent of the Daily Value of Vitamin B_{12}, page 302). Raisins and dried fruit increase your fiber intake, which helps fight constipation; but if you need to watch your sugar intake, it is best to avoid cereals with dried fruit.

A source of calcium—such as milk, yogurt, or low-fat cottage cheese—is recommended at every meal, particularly breakfast. For some women, milk and other dairy products are not easily tolerated in the morning, especially during the first trimester. If this is true for you, try consuming dairy products later in the day with a snack or with another meal. Calcium-enriched products, from fruit juices to breads, are a real bonus for pregnant women. Read labels to see which products might work best for you. Many of the breakfast recipes give the option of a Calcium Boost by adding pasteurized instant nonfat dry milk to pancake and waffle batters, fruit smoothies, and other dishes. Experiment with your favorite recipes and store-bought products to see how powdered milk can add extra calcium to your diet.

Fruit, preferably fresh, or packed in its natural juices (avoid fruits in heavy syrup), has essential vitamins and calories for a quick pick-me-up in the morning. A cut-up orange or half a grapefruit is the ideal breakfast fruit because it provides vitamins and fiber. Any fresh fruit is generally a better choice than fruit juice because whole fruits contain more fiber and are metabolized more slowly. Freeze-dried fruits, such as raspberries, bananas, and mangoes (many are high in vitamin C or A, iron, or potassium) can be added to muffin, pancake, or waffle batters, hot or cold cereals, and fruit salads. They are an easy and tasty way to increase your vitamin intake.

Fat is recommended for breakfast and at every meal. However, this does not give you the liberty to drown your whole wheat bagel in butter, or to make your waffles soggy with margarine. It simply means that *if* the other components of your breakfast are completely fat-free, spread 1 teaspoon of butter or margarine on your toast. A small amount of fat is necessary at every meal to provide calories for energy, and as a source of the fat-soluble vitamins A, D, E, and K.

MORNING SICKNESS AND TIPS FOR COPING

SOME DEGREE of nausea and vomiting occurs in about 50 percent of all pregnancies. It usually starts around the second month of pregnancy and lasts until about the fourth. It is called morning sickness because it commonly occurs in the morning, but it can occur anytime and it can last all day. It is generally believed that pregnancy hormones are the culprits of morning sickness. Why some women are affected by the increased hormonal levels and others are not remains a medical mystery. There is no cure for morning sickness. Listen to your body and figure out what works best for you. Eating small, frequent, low-fat meals generally improves food tolerance.

If you are suffering from morning sickness it is vital that you keep your body hydrated and get in as much nourishment as possible to avoid weight loss and dehydration. If vomiting becomes severe or persistent contact your physician immediately. Following are a few tips to help you get through the morning and the rest of the day.

Tips for Coping with Morning Sickness

- Before you get out of bed in the morning eat dry toast, crackers, or cookies—whatever works best. Allow about 10 minutes for the food to settle before rising.
- Move slowly upon waking—allow yourself a few extra minutes when getting out of bed to balance your body and your brain.
- Keep dry crackers with you at all times to satisfy sudden hunger and to quell nausea.
- Have breakfast items on hand so you don't have to go rummaging through your cupboards or refrigerator. See page 27 for a list of breakfast items to have on hand throughout pregnancy.
- Avoid sudden movement after eating or drinking.
- Don't let your stomach go empty—eat small frequent meals. Small meals are easier to digest than large ones.
- Try to include protein in your meals, especially dinner.
- Drink plenty of fluids, particularly if you are losing fluids through vomiting. Try to eat fruits and vegetables with a high water content, such as melons, citrus fruits, and salads.
- Don't mix liquids and solids—eat and then wait twenty minutes before drinking.
- Avoid greasy or fatty fried foods, especially fast food.
- Avoid highly seasoned foods.
- Avoid caffeinated beverages.
- Eat popsicles, fruit ice, or sherbet between meals. Chew ice or suck on an ice cube. Sip cold Gatorade or ginger ale.
- When you cook, open windows to eliminate cooking odors.
- Get plenty of rest. Physical and emotional fatigue can exacerbate nausea.
- Get plenty of fresh air. Go for a walk in the middle of the day. Make sure your workspace is well-ventilated and not too hot. Take deep breaths of fresh air from time to time.
- Take your prenatal vitamins at night. Consult your doctor to change brands if your vitamin makes you nauseous (some brands are more easily tolerated). Continue taking a folic acid supplement *even if* you stop taking a prenatal vitamin.
- Do *not* take any medication for nausea or vomiting unless prescribed by your doctor.

no more boring breakfasts

Breakfast Pizza Pancake

Whole Wheat Pecan Waffles

French Toast Banana Sandwich

Yogurt-Vanilla Pancakes

Diabetic-Friendly Strawberry-Raspberry Syrup

Whole Wheat Popovers

Ricotta Cheese Pancakes with Quick Blueberry Sauce

Cheese Omelet with Breakfast Chili

Brunch Casserole with Spinach and Red Bell Peppers

Banana Muffins with Walnuts and Wheat Germ

Bran Muffins with Dried Cranberries, Walnuts, and Candied Ginger

Summer Fruit Salad ▼

Winter Fruit Salad

Super Fruit Smoothies

▼ Vegan recipe

RECIPE NOTES

ALMOST ANYONE—pregnant or not—will agree that the early-morning hours are a difficult time to cook. The recipes included in this chapter are intended for when you feel like eating something homemade for breakfast, when you have a craving for pancakes or waffles and want a recipe that tastes good and works, or when your dietary requirements call for increased protein or calcium and you need some ideas to help make that happen.

These recipes are designed to be as family-friendly as possible. Anyone with young children knows that picky eating goes with the territory. Despite their finicky palates, it is important to continuously offer children a range of healthy foods, especially for breakfast. If you invest some time and energy into making homemade breakfast treats, you may soon hear your children (and others) asking for your special waffles, the big pizza pancake, your star-shaped French toast, or your yummy banana muffins.

Some notes about the recipes in this chapter:

- To avoid food-borne illnesses, be sure to thoroughly cook the yolks and whites of eggs and to follow egg safety guidelines (see Eggs and *Salmonella Enteritidis*, page 54).
- Use only eggs in their shell or egg products. Avoid farm-fresh eggs.
- All egg dishes (such as egg-based casseroles, quiches, flans, etc.) should be cooked to 160°F, as shown on an instant-read thermometer inserted into the center of the dish.
- The reduced-fat 2% milk called for in recipes can be replaced by whole milk or a soy beverage.
- All-purpose flour should, ideally, be enriched and unbleached.
- Unsalted butter is preferred, as the salt content varies and can interfere with taste.
- Canola oil and canola oil cooking spray can be replaced by vegetable or corn oil.
- Don't be afraid to experiment and modify the recipes to suit your family's needs and tastes.

pantry items for no more boring breakfasts

Fresh Produce
Baby spinach
Bananas
Blueberries
Cantaloupe
Fresh herbs: cilantro and dill
Kiwi
Lemons
Oranges
Raspberries
Scallions
Strawberries

Dairy and Soy Products
Extra-firm tofu
Grade A large eggs
Grated sharp cheddar cheese
Low-fat or fat-free plain yogurt
Nonfat buttermilk
Part-skim ricotta cheese
Reduced-fat 2% milk
Unsalted butter
Whole milk

Dry Staples
All-Bran cereal
Baking powder
Baking soda
Calcium-enriched bread (such as Cal-
    cium Rich Roman Meal)
Confectioners' sugar
Dried cranberries
Enriched all-purpose flour (preferably
    unbleached)
French or Italian baguette
Light or dark brown sugar
Nuts: pecans, sliced almonds,
    and walnuts

Pasteurized instant nonfat dry milk
Wheat germ
Whole wheat flour

Canned, Bottled, and Jarred Staples
Black beans
Canola oil
Canola oil cooking spray
Honey
Jams (any kind)
Maple syrup
Molasses
Orange marmalade
Peeled and diced tomatoes
(14.5-ounce can)
Roasted red bell peppers

Spices and Flavorings
Candied ginger
Chili powder
Ground cinnamon
Ground cumin
Ground ginger
Pure vanilla extract

Frozen Staples
Apple juice concentrate
Blueberries
Chopped spinach (10-ounce package)
Raspberries
Strawberries

From the Salad Bar
Assorted fresh fruit

breakfast staples to have on hand

▶ Any whole grain cereal fortified with 100 percent folic acid and 100 percent iron that is also low in fat and sugar (less than 3 grams of sugar per ounce)

▶ Whole grain fresh or frozen bread, muffins, bagels, or whole wheat English muffins

▶ Whole grain breads fortified with calcium and folic acid

▶ Cereal bars

▶ Quick-cooking oatmeal or Cream of Wheat cereal

▶ Frozen whole wheat calcium- or folic acid-fortified waffles

▶ Yogurt, preferably low-fat or nonfat

▶ Reduced-fat 2% milk, whole milk, or soy beverages

▶ Dried fruits (such as raisins, apricots, dates, or prunes) and freeze-dried fruits

▶ Fresh fruit, sliced fruit, or fruit cups packed in natural juices or light syrup; and no-sugar-added, calcium-fortified fruit juices

▶ Grade A large eggs, or a protein source such as pasteurized cheese (cottage or ricotta cheese) or nut butters

▶ Instant breakfast drinks

▶ Milk fruit shakes, smoothies, and yogurt drinks

four sample breakfast menus using breakfast staples

⌒

¾ cup fortified dry cereal with 8 ounces reduced-fat 2% milk
1 medium fresh fruit or 8 ounces fruit juice
2 slices whole grain toast with 2 tablespoons peanut butter

▦

Whole wheat bagel with ¼ cup part-skim ricotta cheese
1 medium fresh fruit or 8 ounces fruit juice
8 ounces reduced-fat 2% milk or 8 ounces plain low-fat yogurt

▦

2 frozen whole wheat waffles
1 medium fresh fruit or 8 ounces fruit juice
8 ounces reduced-fat 2% milk or 8 ounces plain low-fat yogurt

▦

¾ cup oatmeal
½ whole wheat English muffin
2 tablespoons peanut butter
1 medium fresh fruit or 8 ounces fruit juice
8 ounces reduced-fat 2% milk or 8 ounces plain low-fat yogurt

PLANNING AHEAD FOR NO MORE
BORING BREAKFASTS

▶ *Can be made the same day:*
   Breakfast Pizza Pancake
   French Toast Banana Sandwich
   Whole Wheat Popovers
   Ricotta Cheese Pancakes with Quick Blueberry Sauce
   Cheese Omelet with Breakfast Chili
   Super Fruit Smoothies
   Summer Fruit Salad
   Winter Fruit Salad

▶ *Can be made the night before:*
   Yogurt-Vanilla Pancakes (batter)
   Whole Wheat Pecan Waffles (batter)
   Summer Fruit Salad
   Winter Fruit Salad
   Diabetic-Friendly Strawberry-Raspberry Syrup
   Quick Blueberry Sauce
   Banana Muffins with Walnuts and Wheat Germ
   Bran Muffins with Dried Cranberries, Walnuts, and Candied Ginger
   Brunch Casserole with Spinach and Red Bell Peppers (make casserole)

▶ *Can be refrigerated for up to 3 days:*
   Banana Muffins with Walnuts and Wheat Germ
   Yogurt-Vanilla Pancakes
   Bran Muffins with Dried Cranberries, Walnuts, and Candied Ginger
   Breakfast Chili
   Diabetic-Friendly Strawberry-Raspberry Syrup
   Quick Blueberry Sauce

▶ *Can be frozen for up to 1 month:*
   Whole Wheat Pecan Waffles
   Banana Muffins with Walnuts and Wheat Germ
   Bran Muffins with Dried Cranberries, Walnuts, and Candied Ginger
   Light and Airy Whole Wheat Popovers

breakfast pizza pancake

～

What's in this for baby and me? Protein and folic acid.

TOPPED WITH A thin layer of your family's favorite jam and fresh berries, such as raspberries, blueberries, or strawberries, this pancake, high in **protein** and **folic acid**, turns into a scrumptious breakfast pizza. It is equally tasty (and surprisingly low-calorie) sprinkled with confectioners' sugar and fresh lemon juice. Or, for a real treat, top it with Diabetic-Friendly Strawberry Raspberry Syrup (page 38).

Getting your little one to watch this pancake pizza bubble and rise might convince him or her to try a bite. Allowing your child to sprinkle some confectioners' sugar on his or her slice might also work. Apart from the nutritional benefits (this pancake is also a good source of calcium, iron, and B vitamins), the best thing about this pizza pancake is that you don't have to stand over the stove to cook it. Notes for a **Calcium Boost** follow the recipe.

serves 2

½ cup reduced-fat 2% milk	**Optional Toppings**
2 large eggs	**3 tablespoons confectioners' sugar, or to**
½ cup all-purpose flour	**taste**
Dash of ground cinnamon or nutmeg	**Juice of ½ lemon, or to taste**
(optional)	**Jam**
1 tablespoon unsalted butter	**Fresh berries, washed, and sliced if large**

1. Preheat the oven to 425°F.
2. Whisk the milk and eggs in a bowl until well combined. Add the flour and cinnamon and whisk until smooth.
3. Melt the butter in a large (11- or 12-inch) **ovenproof** seasoned cast-iron skillet or nonstick skillet over high heat. Pour the batter into the skillet and cook over high heat for 1 minute. Transfer the skillet to the oven and bake for 15 minutes, or until puffed and golden brown.
4. Remove the pancake from the oven. Sprinkle generously with confectioners' sugar and a squeeze of lemon juice, if desired. Serve immediately. Pass extra confectioners' sugar at the table. Or, if you are making a breakfast pizza, spread a thin layer of jam over the pancake, then top with fresh berries.

▶ *Calcium Boost:* In a measuring cup, combine ¾ cup milk (instead of the ½ cup listed) with 3 level tablespoons of pasteurized instant nonfat dry milk. Mix until the milk powder has dissolved, then follow the directions in Step 2. Pancakes made with powdered milk tend to be slightly denser and to rise less, but they taste just as good.

marmite and folic acid

The name Marmite comes from the French word *la marmite,* or stew pot, which is the shape of the distinctive yellow-capped brown jar this 100 percent vegetarian enriched yeast extract comes in. Produced only in the United Kingdom, this salty brown spread is extremely high in folic acid and other B vitamins. Generally speaking, you either love marmite and become addicted to it, or you can't stand it. If you've never tried it, the content of folic acid, B_{12}, and other B vitamins might convince you to take the plunge, especially if you are a vegetarian. It is traditionally eaten thinly spread on buttered toast (or a bagel) or on crisp bread with cottage cheese. According to the nutrition label on the jar, the percentage of daily values (based on a 2,000-calorie diet) in ½ teaspoon (4 grams) of Marmite are as follows:

> 25% folic acid
> 15% thiamine
> 15% riboflavin
> 30% niacin
> 10% Vitamin B_{12}
> 2 grams protein

▶ *Cooking Tip:* The order in which you mix these ingredients is *very* important. The wet ingredients should be mixed before adding the dry ingredients. A seasoned cast-iron skillet works best and allows you to cut the pancake in the pan without damaging a nonstick finish. If you use an ovenproof skillet with a nonstick finish, slice gingerly or transfer the pancake to a large plate before cutting it.

▶ *Diabetic Tip:* Instead of confectioners' sugar, use a low-sugar jam (such as Polaner All Fruit; 2 teaspoons are FREE), or top your pancake with 2 teaspoons (also FREE) Diabetic-Friendly Strawberry Raspberry Syrup (page 38).

▶ *Complete Meal Ideas:* Serve this breakfast pizza pancake with:
Fresh fruit or juice of your choice
Reduced-fat 2% milk or low-fat yogurt

APPROXIMATE NUTRITIONAL INFORMATION: Serving size: ½ breakfast pizza pancake (without any topping); Calories: 273 cals; Protein: 11 g; Carbohydrates: 27 g; Fat: 13 g; Fiber: .84 g; Sodium: 95 mg; Folic Acid: .75 mcg; Diabetic Exchange: Bread/Starch 2, Fat 2, Meat (Medium Fat) 1

whole wheat pecan waffles

What's in this for baby and me? Protein and calcium.

AN EXCELLENT SOURCE of **protein** and **calcium**, and a good source of iron, fiber, B vitamins, and vitamin A, these pecan waffles are a weekend special that can be frozen for weekday breakfast bliss. Diabetic-Friendly Strawberry Raspberry Syrup (page 38), honey, maple syrup, molasses, and fresh berries are all fabulous toppings. Freeze any left-over waffles, or make an extra batch to freeze. If you're on the go, try a waffle sandwich made with peanut butter, or any other nut butter, and some jam, or a waffle sprinkled with confectioners' sugar for a snack. Notes for a **Calcium Boost** follow the recipe.

makes about eighteen 5½ x 2¼-inch waffles

¾ cup whole wheat flour

1 cup all-purpose flour

1 tablespoon baking powder

1 tablespoon sugar

½ teaspoon salt

2 large eggs plus 1 large egg white

6 tablespoons unsalted butter, melted

2 cups reduced-fat 2% milk

½ cup chopped pecans

Canola oil cooking spray, for greasing the waffle iron

1. Place the dry ingredients in a large bowl and whisk together.
2. In a second bowl or large measuring cup, whisk together the eggs, egg white, melted butter, and milk.
3. Add the wet ingredients to the dry ingredients and whisk together until well blended. Stir in the nuts.
4. Preheat the waffle iron. Spray the waffle grids with cooking spray. Spoon some batter onto the hot iron and spread to within ¼ inch of the edge of the grids. Close the lid and cook until the waffles are golden brown. Serve immediately.

▶ *Cooking Tip #1:* To prevent cooked waffles from getting soggy, if you are not serving them immediately, place them on a plate lined with a paper towel, or lean them up against each other in a tent-like position to allow the steam to escape. If they do get soggy or cold, toast them briefly in a toaster or place them directly on the rack of a 350°F oven for a few minutes.

▶ *Cooking Tip #2:* A Belgian waffle iron can be used to make these waffles. The yield will be about fourteen 4½ × 4-inch waffles.

▶ *Calcium Boost:* In a measuring cup, combine ⅓ cup pasteurized instant nonfat dry milk with the milk. Mix until the milk powder has dissolved, then follow the directions in Step 2. Waffles made with instant nonfat dry milk tend to be a little heavier.

▶ *Variation:* If you do not have whole wheat flour, you can use 1¾ cups all-purpose flour.

▶ *Storage Tip:* To freeze, cool the waffles, place them in a zip-lock bag, and freeze. To reheat, place the frozen waffles directly on the oven rack or on a piece of foil in a 350°F oven until heated through, about 7 minutes, or reheat them in a toaster. The waffles will keep for about one month in the freezer.

▶ *Diabetic Tip:* Reduce the unsalted butter to 4 tablespoons and omit the pecans. Use a low-sugar jam (such as Polaner All Fruit; 2 teaspoons are FREE), or top your pancake with 2 teaspoons (also FREE) Quick Diabetic-Friendly Strawberry Raspberry Syrup (page 38).

waffles unlimited

Frozen "designer" waffles—including multi-grain waffles, organic brands made with flax, hemp, and soy, and fiber-enhanced waffles—seem to be the latest breakfast rage. Bring along a dictionary to decipher the fancy grains. Packaged waffle mixes come in countless new varieties as well. Powdered mixes can easily be enriched with pasteurized instant nonfat dry milk. You will need to experiment to find the right amount to add. When purchasing frozen waffles or packaged waffle mixes look for those fortified with calcium and folic acid. Add fresh, dried, or frozen berries to waffle or pancake batters for a burst of flavor and vitamin C.

▶ *Complete Meal Ideas:* Serve these waffles with:
Fresh fruit or juice of your choice that contains vitamin C
Reduced-fat 2% milk or low-fat yogurt

APPROXIMATE NUTRITIONAL INFORMATION: Serving size: 3 whole wheat pecan waffles; Calories: 372 cals; Protein: 11g; Carbohydrates: 34 g; Fat: 22 g; Fiber: 3.3 g; Sodium: 467 mg; Calcium: 246 mg; Diabetic Exchange: Bread/Starch 2, Fat 4.5, Meat (Medium Fat) 1

french toast banana sandwich

⌒

What's in this for baby and me? Protein, calcium, and folic acid .

THIS QUICK AND easy French toast sandwich is an excellent source of **protein**, **calcium**, and **folic acid**, and a good source of vitamin C, B vitamins, iron, and fiber. It is delicious topped with syrup, honey, cinnamon and sugar, or sliced fresh fruit. This recipe specifies Calcium Rich Roman Meal bread because two slices have as much calcium as one glass of milk! To entice young children to take a bite, try cutting the French toast into cookie cutter shapes, and adding lots of syrup, or letting them sprinkle a confectioners' sugar–cinnamon mix on the toast. This recipe also makes great regular French toast.

makes 4 to 5 slices of toast

2 large eggs

½ cup reduced-fat 2% milk

½ tablespoon unsalted butter or canola oil
    cooking spray, for cooking the French toast

4 to 5 slices of calcium-enriched bread (such as Calcium Rich Roman Meal)

2 bananas, sliced

Maple syrup, jam, or your favorite topping

1. In a bowl, mix the eggs and milk.
2. Melt the butter in a large nonstick skillet over medium-high heat. Place a slice of bread in the egg mixture and turn to coat both sides, then add the slice to the skillet and cook for 2 minutes on each side or until thoroughly cooked and golden brown on both sides. Repeat with the remaining bread.
3. As you cook the toast, add some of the sliced bananas to the skillet and cook them, about 2 minutes on each side.
4. Place a slice of the French toast on each plate, top with some of the banana slices, cover with another piece of toast, and serve with your favorite topping.

▶ *Storage Notes:* Cover any leftovers with plastic wrap and refrigerate. To reheat, place the French toast on a plate and microwave for a few seconds.

▶ *Diabetic Tip:* Omit the banana and top the French toast with low-sugar jam (such as Polaner All Fruit; 2 teaspoons are FREE) or 2 teaspoons (also FREE) Quick Diabetic-Friendly Strawberry-Raspberry Syrup (page 38).

▶ *Complete Meal Ideas:* Serve these French toast sandwiches with:
    Fresh fruit (if not using bananas) or juice of your choice that contains vitamin C
    Reduced-fat 2% milk or low-fat yogurt

APPROXIMATE NUTRITIONAL INFORMATION: Serving size: 2 slices of French toast made from calcium-enriched bread and 1 banana; Calories: 332 cals; Protein: 11 g; Carbohydrates: 53 g; Fat: 10 g; Fiber: 3. g; Sodium: 376 mg; Iron: 2 mg; Calcium: 246 mg; Folic Acid: 87 mcg; Diabetic Exchange: Bread/Starch 3, Fat 2, Fruit .5

healthy bagel toppings

Hard cheese (such as cheddar, Swiss, and Monterey Jack)

Ricotta cheese (whole milk or part-skim)

Neufchâtel cheese

Peanut butter or other nut butters

Hard-boiled or fully cooked eggs

Salmon spread

Egg salad (recipe, page 96)

Tuna salad (recipe, page 101)

Chicken salad (recipe, page 98)

Hummus or bean dips (recipes, pages 148 and 151)

Marmite (see page 31)

yogurt-vanilla pancakes

~

What's in this for baby and me? Protein, calcium, and folic acid.

THESE CRÊPE-LIKE pancakes are an excellent source of **protein**, **calcium**, and **folic acid**, and a good source of iron and B vitamins. They are delicious served with maple syrup, jams, fresh fruit (especially berries), molasses, a sprinkle of confectioners' sugar and cinnamon, or your favorite pancake topping. They can be made in advance and reheated in a microwave oven; or the batter can be refrigerated for up to two days. Let your kids sprinkle the confectioners' sugar mixture on their pancakes and roll them up—a fun way to eat a pancake and at the same time develop their small motor skills. Notes for a **Calcium Boost** follow the recipe.

makes about 12 six-inch pancakes

One 8-ounce container fat-free plain yogurt

1 cup reduced-fat 2% milk

2 large eggs

2 tablespoons canola oil, plus 1 teaspoon
    canola oil or canola oil cooking spray for
    greasing the skillet

1 teaspoon pure vanilla extract

1 tablespoon sugar

⅛ teaspoon salt

¼ teaspoon baking soda

1 cup all-purpose flour

1. Combine the yogurt, milk, eggs, oil, and vanilla extract in a large bowl and whisk together. Add the remaining ingredients and whisk until smooth.
2. Heat the 1 teaspoon canola oil in a large nonstick skillet over medium to medium-high heat until hot, about 3 minutes. Add a little less than ⅓ cup batter to the skillet and immediately swirl the batter to form it into a thin pancake about 6 inches in diameter. Cook the pancake until the surface bubbles and then sets and the underside is golden brown, about 1 minute. Flip the pancake with a wide spatula and cook for one more minute. Serve warm. **Storage Tip:** Cover leftover pancakes with plastic wrap and refrigerate. Reheat in a microwave oven before serving.

▶ *Calcium Boost:* In a measuring cup, combine ⅓ cup pasteurized instant nonfat dry milk with the milk. Mix until the milk powder has dissolved, then follow the directions in Step 2. Pancakes made with powdered milk tend to be slightly denser.

▶ *Diabetic Tip:* Use a low-sugar jam (such as Polaner All Fruit; 2 teaspoons are FREE), or top your pancake with 2 teaspoons (also FREE) Quick Diabetic-Friendly Strawberry Raspberry Syrup (page 38).

▶ *Complete Meal Ideas:* Serve these pancakes with:
Fresh fruit or juice of your choice that contains vitamin C
Reduced-fat 2% milk or low-fat yogurt

APPROXIMATE NUTRITIONAL INFORMATION: Serving size: 4 plain yogurt-vanilla pancakes; Calories: 387 cals; Protein: 16 g; Carbohydrates: 47 g; Fat: 15 g; Fiber: 1 g; Sodium: 368 mg; Calcium: 285 mg; Folic Acid: 94 mcg; Diabetic Exchange: Bread/Starch 3, Fat 3, Meat (Medium Fat) .5

preventing mild hypoglycemia

Hypoglycemia in people who do not have diabetes is far less common than once believed. However, it can occur under certain conditions, such as early pregnancy, prolonged fasting, and long periods of strenuous exercise. A person with hypoglycemia may feel weak, drowsy, shaky, confused, hungry, and dizzy. Paleness, headache, irritability, sweating, rapid heart beat, and a cold, clammy feeling are also signs of low blood sugar.[13]

Hypoglycemia can be a complication of diabetes. Pregnant diabetics or women diagnosed with gestational diabetes should discuss this condition with their doctor and dietitian to develop a coping plan should it occur. Generally, including a source of protein in your breakfast, eating small frequent meals that also include a source of protein, avoiding long periods without eating, and avoiding concentrated sweets, such as sugar, candy, honey, jam, jelly, syrup, and soft drinks may help prevent mild hypoglycemia.

diabetic-friendly
strawberry-raspberry syrup

⌒

What's in this for baby and me? Vitamin C.

THIS QUICK, easy-to-make, syrup is incredible served with any type of store-bought or homemade pancakes, waffles, French toast, or oatmeal. High in **vitamin C**, it is also a wonderful accompaniment to yogurt, frozen yogurt, or ice cream, and it is great on top of the Reduced-Fat Ricotta Cheesecake (page 266). You can use 1 pound of strawberries (about 4 cups) instead of mixing strawberries and raspberries. Frozen berries work too. You might consider adding a little more sugar to please young eaters who like sweet things. This sauce will keep for one week refrigerated.

makes about 2½ cups

½ cup frozen apple juice concentrate

½ cup sugar

2 cups fresh strawberries, washed, hulled, and
  quartered (see Cooking Tip below for
  frozen berries)

2 cups fresh raspberries, rinsed quickly

½ teaspoon pure vanilla extract (optional)

1. Combine the apple juice concentrate and sugar in a large nonstick skillet, stir, and bring to a boil. Reduce the heat and simmer for 5 minutes.
2. Add the berries, stir, and return to a boil. Reduce the heat and simmer, uncovered, for 10 minutes, or until the consistency of a thin syrup. Remove from heat, stir in the vanilla extract, and serve warm or at room temperature. Cover and refrigerate any leftovers.

▶ *Cooking Tip:* Four cups frozen unsweetened berries can be substituted for the fresh berries. Defrost (at room temperature or in a microwave) and drain them, then proceed with the recipe. (Frozen berries may take slightly longer to reach the thin syrup consistency.) Also, you can increase the amount of sugar and eliminate the apple juice concentrate; however, added sugar is not diabetic-friendly.

APPROXIMATE NUTRITIONAL INFORMATION: Serving size: 2 tablespoons strawberry-raspberry syrup; Calories: 81 cals; Carbohydrates: 20 g; Fat: .3 g; Fiber: 2.3 g; Sodium: 4 mg; Vitamin C: 23 mg; Diabetic Exchange: Fruit 1.5, a reduced serving size of 2 teaspoons are FREE

make coffee work for you

~

The amount of caffeine considered safe during pregnancy continues to be a controversial issue. Abstaining from caffeine altogether is the best approach, but some women just need their coffee. At least try limiting yourself to only one cup of any caffeinated beverage per day. To meet your daily calcium requirements and satisfy your coffee craving at the same time, try increasing the amount of milk (soy beverages included) you add to your coffee. In other words, turn your coffee into a calcium-rich café au lait. The following list of caffeine levels in beverages and food comes from the U.S. Food and Drug Administration and the National Soft Drink Association:[17]

	MILLIGRAMS OF CAFFEINE	
ITEM	AVERAGE MG	RANGE OF MG
Coffee (5-oz cup)		
Brewed, drip method	115	60–180
Brewed, percolator	80	40–170
Instant	65	30–120
Decaffeinated, brewed	3	2–5
Decaffeinated, instant	2	1–5
Espresso (single)	100*	
Cappuccino (single)	100*	
Tea (5-oz cup)		
Brewed, major U.S. brands	40	20–90
Brewed, imported brands	60	25–110
Instant	30	25–50
Iced (12-oz glass)	70	67–76
Some soft drinks (6-oz serving)	18	15–30
Cocoa beverage (5-oz cup)	4	2–20
Chocolate milk beverage (8-oz cup)	5	2–7
Milk chocolate (1 oz)	6	1–15
Dark chocolate, semi-sweet (1 oz)	20	5–35
Baker's chocolate (1 oz)	26	26
Chocolate-flavored syrup (1 oz)	4	4

* The values for espresso and cappuccino are taken from the Women's Nutrition Patient Education Resource Manual.

whole wheat popovers

What's in this for baby and me? Protein.

THESE POPOVERS ARE an easy-to-make breakfast or anytime treat, and they are well worth their forty-minute baking time. High in **protein**, and a good source of calcium, iron, folic acid, B vitamins, and fiber, they are best eaten straight from the oven with your favorite jam or marmalade. These popovers can be frozen and reheated for later enjoyment. Notes for a **Calcium Boost** follow the recipe.

makes 6 large popovers

½ cup whole wheat flour	2 teaspoons canola oil
½ cup all-purpose flour	½ teaspoon salt
1 cup reduced fat 2% milk	Canola oil cooking spray for greasing the
2 large eggs plus 1 large egg white	popover pan

1. Preheat the oven to 450°F. Have ready a six-cup nonstick popover pan.
2. In a large mixing bowl, mix the whole wheat and all-purpose flours. Add the remaining batter ingredients and beat with an electric mixer on high speed for 30 seconds. Scrape down the sides of the bowl and beat 15 seconds more. (Note: Don't be concerned if you see tiny lumps of flour. Mash any bigger lumps against the side of the bowl with the back of a spatula.)
3. Preheat the popover pan in the oven for 2 minutes, then remove it and spray with cooking oil. Divide the batter evenly among the popover cups.
4. Bake for 20 minutes, then reduce the heat to 350°F and bake for 20 more minutes, or until golden brown and puffed. Remove the popovers from the oven and serve immediately.

▶ *Cooking Tip:* To freeze, cool completely, then place the popovers in a zip-lock bag and freeze. To reheat, place the popovers on a piece of foil in a preheated 350°F oven for about 10 minutes. Do not microwave.

▶ *Calcium Boost:* In a measuring cup, combine the milk with ⅓ cup pasteurized instant nonfat dry milk. Mix until the milk powder has dissolved, then follow the directions in Step 2. *Note:* Calcium-fortified popovers tend to be considerably heavier than those made according to the basic recipe.

▶ *Variation:* A total of 1 cup all-purpose flour can be used instead of whole wheat flour. Popovers made only with all-purpose flour tend to rise more and are lighter.

▶ **Complete Meal Ideas:** Serve these popovers with:
    Fresh fruit or juice of your choice that contains vitamin C
    Reduced fat 2% milk or low-fat yogurt

APPROXIMATE NUTRITIONAL INFORMATION: Serving size: 2 whole wheat popover; Calories: 265 cals; Protein: 13 g; Carbohydrates: 35 g; Fat: 8 g; Fiber: 3 g; Sodium: 488 g; Diabetic Exchange: Bread/Starch 2.5, Fat 1.5, Meat (Medium Fat) 1

the incredible edible egg

Eggs are an excellent source of protein and vitamin B_{12}, especially for pregnant vegetarians. Following is the nutritional breakdown of one large hard-boiled egg compared to the average recommended daily allowances for pregnant women.

ONE LARGE EGG	RDA/DRI FOR PREGNANT WOMEN*
6.2 g protein	60 g protein
25 mg calcium	1200 mg calcium
.55 mcg vitamin B_{12}	2.6 mg vitamin B_{12}
.25 mg riboflavin	1.4 mg riboflavin

*For a more complete list of the Recommended Daily Allowances (RDAs) and Allowance Intakes (AIs) for pregnant women, see Extra Daily Nutrient Allowances for Pregnancy, page 6.

ricotta cheese pancakes with quick blueberry sauce

What's in this for baby and me? Protein, calcium, and vitamin C.

DON'T BE SURPRISED if these pancakes become a staple on your weekend breakfast menu. No one can turn down a bite of these **protein-** and **calcium-packed** ricotta cheese pancakes topped with **high–vitamin C** blueberry sauce. The key to making these delicate pancakes is to use as little flour as possible. This makes the pancakes harder to flip, but the slightly creamy consistency of the finished pancakes is worth the effort. Little ones seem to love the super-quick blueberry sauce—use a bib to avoid stains. The sauce is also an excellent topping for ice cream or yogurt.

makes nine 2½-inch pancakes

1 cup part-skim ricotta cheese

1 large egg

2 tablespoons sugar

1 teaspoon pure vanilla extract

6 tablespoons all-purpose flour

1 tablespoon orange marmalade or apricot jam

½ tablespoon unsalted butter or canola oil

cooking spray, for cooking the pancakes

Quick Blueberry Sauce (recipe follows)

1. Mix the ricotta cheese, egg, sugar, and vanilla extract in a bowl until smooth. Add the flour and orange marmalade and mix until well blended.
2. Melt the butter in a large nonstick skillet over medium-high heat. Add 1 heaping soupspoonful of the pancake batter for each pancake and flatten slightly with the back of the spoon; do not crowd the pancakes in the pan. Cook for 1½ to 2 minutes, or until the bottoms are golden brown. With a wide spatula, very carefully flip each pancake (using a blunt knife to push the pancake onto the spatula) and continue cooking until golden brown on the second side, about 1½ to 2 minutes longer.
3. Top the pancakes with the blueberry sauce and serve immediately.

not all milks moo

If you are experiencing lactose intolerance, try switching to a soy beverage. There are several varieties on the shelves today that cater to different tastes, convictions, and digestive sensitivities (lactose-free soy beverages range from 70% to 100% lactose free). Also, many soy beverages have added vitamins and nutrients that turn them into a liquid powerhouse.

quick blueberry sauce

yield: 1 cup

1 pint (about 2 cups) fresh blueberries, washed, or 8 ounces frozen unsweetened blueberries (half a 16-ounce bag)
⅓ cup sugar, or to taste

Combine the blueberries and sugar in a saucepan and bring to a boil, stirring occasionally, over high heat. Continue to cook until the syrup has thickened slightly, about 5 minutes. Serve warm. This sauce will keep refrigerated for up to 3 days.

▶ *Variation:* An equal amount of pasteurized farmer's cheese can be substituted for the ricotta cheese, although the calcium value will decrease.

▶ *Complete Meal Ideas:* Serve these pancakes with:
Fresh fruit or juice of your choice
Reduced-fat 2% milk or low-fat yogurt

APPROXIMATE NUTRITIONAL INFORMATION: Serving size: 3 cheese pancakes; Calories: 260 cals; Protein: 13 g; Carbohydrates: 29 g; Fat: 10 g; Fiber: .7 g; Sodium: 128 mg; Calcium: 237 mg; Diabetic Exchange: Bread/Starch 2, Fat 2

APPROXIMATE NUTRITIONAL INFORMATION: Serving size: 5 tablespoons blueberry sauce; Calories: 135 cals; Protein: .6 g; Carbohydrates: 35 g; Fat: .4 g; Fiber: 3 g; Sodium: 6 mg; Vitamin C: 12 mg; Diabetic Exchange: Fruit 2.5

cheese omelet with breakfast chili

What's in this for baby and me? Protein and vitamin C.

Eggs are an excellent source of **protein**, especially for vegetarians or women who have an aversion to meat during pregnancy. This omelet is also a good source of calcium, folic acid, and vitamin A. By altering the amounts of yolks and whites in your omelet, you can increase or decrease your iron and cholesterol intake. If your dietary needs call for lots of iron, use the 2 whole eggs in your omelet, because the iron is in the yolk. If you need to watch your cholesterol, use 1 whole egg and 1 egg white.

An excellent source of **vitamin C** and a good source of protein, calcium, iron, folic acid, and fiber, the breakfast chili is a nutritional powerhouse. The recipe makes a lot, but leftovers are delicious for lunch or dinner over rice, topped with grated cheese, or as a snack with baked tortilla chips and melted cheese. The black beans and tofu are excellent sources of protein, and the beans also contain a hefty supply of iron. Served with corn bread, or any type of whole grain bread, and a salad, the omelet makes a delicious meal at any time of day.

Cheese Omelet

serves 1

2 large eggs
½ teaspoon unsalted butter

2 tablespoons grated cheddar cheese (or any cheese of your choice)
Breakfast Chili (recipe follows)

1. Whisk the eggs and pepper in a bowl; set aside. Melt the butter in a small nonstick skillet over medium-high heat. Add the eggs and allow to cook for about 20 seconds, then, while tilting the skillet, use a spatula to push the cooked egg toward the center of the pan, allowing the raw egg to hit the skillet. Distribute the cheese on top of the eggs, reduce heat to low, and cook for 1 to 2 minutes or until the eggs are cooked through.
2. Flip the omelet in half, cook 10 seconds longer or until there is no visible liquid egg, then transfer to a serving plate. Place some of the breakfast chili on the side and serve immediately.

Breakfast Chili

makes about 4 cups

2 teaspoons canola oil or olive oil

1½ teaspoons chili powder

½ teaspoon ground cumin (optional)

One 14.5-ounce can diced tomatoes (do not drain)

1 cup canned black beans, rinsed and drained

4 ounces extra firm tofu, cut into ½-inch cubes and blotted dry with paper towels

¼ cup chopped fresh cilantro

Heat the oil in a large nonstick skillet over medium-high heat. Add the chili powder and cumin and cook for 30 seconds, then add the tomatoes, beans, and tofu, reduce heat to low, and cook for 5 minutes. Mix in the cilantro, and set aside.

▶ *Cooking Tip:* Any leftover black beans or tofu can be tossed into a salad.

▶ *Health Tip 1:* Be sure to cook your eggs thoroughly (both whites and yolks) during pregnancy (see Eggs and *Salmonella Enteritidis*, page 54).

▶ *Health Tip 2:* If your doctor has restricted your fat intake, use canola oil cooking spray instead of unsalted butter and use a reduced-fat cheese or omit the cheese.

▶ *Complete Meal Ideas:* Serve this omelet with:
Fresh fruit or juice of your choice that contains vitamin C
Reduced-fat 2% milk or low-fat yogurt
2 slices toast (preferably whole wheat)

APPROXIMATE NUTRITIONAL INFORMATION: Serving size: 1 cheese omelet made with 2 large eggs; Calories: 224 cals; Protein: 16 g; Carbohydrates: 1 g ; Fat: 17 g; Fiber: 0 g; Sodium: 214 mg; Diabetic Exchange: Meat/Protein 2, Fat 1

APPROXIMATE NUTRITIONAL INFORMATION: Serving size: ¾ cup breakfast chili; Calories: 128 cals; Protein: 8 g; Carbohydrates: 15 g; Fat: 4 g; Fiber: 5 g; Sodium: 341 mg; Calcium: 95 mg; Vitamin C: 16 mg; Folic Acid: 65 mcg; Diabetic Exchange: Bread/Starch 1, Meat (Medium Fat) 1

swallow your iron supplement with orange juice

Vitamin C aids iron absorption. You can increase the amount of iron your body absorbs by consuming a source of vitamin C with iron-rich foods or with your iron supplement. Try not to take your iron supplement with calcium-fortified juices as calcium can interfere with iron absorption.

brunch casserole
with spinach and red bell peppers

~

What's in this for baby and me? Protein, calcium, vitamins A and C, and folic acid.

A DELICIOUS, NUTRIENT-DENSE entrée for a brunch or a light lunch, this easy-to-make casserole is the ideal dish for family gatherings. The cheese, eggs, and milk are all excellent sources of **protein** and **calcium**, and the spinach and red peppers are high in **vitamins A** and **C** and **folic acid**. This casserole also gets a good rating for iron, B vitamins, and fiber. One of the best features of this dish is that it can be assembled the night before baking. It requires at least one hour, or up to twelve hours, of refrigeration before baking to make sure that the bread absorbs the liquid.

Vary the ingredients to suit your family's tastes. To avoid a soggy mess, be sure that any fresh vegetables that have a high water content, such as mushrooms, bell peppers, or squash, are sautéed before adding. Almost any type of bread can be used; however, stale slices of French or Italian bread work best. Also, any type of good melting cheese, such as Havarti, Gruyère, Monterey Jack, Fontina, or Colby, can be substituted for the sharp cheddar. Leftovers can be reheated in a microwave and enjoyed on a moment's notice. For a decadent splurge, half-and-half can be substituted for the whole milk.

serves 6

1 tablespoon unsalted butter, softened

1 supermarket French or Italian baguette, cut into enough ½-inch slices to make two layers in an 8 x 8 x 2-inch baking dish, spread out on a baking sheet or tray, and left out to dry

One 10-ounce package chopped frozen spinach, thawed and squeezed dry

6 ounces (about 1¾ cups) grated sharp cheddar cheese

½ cup jarred roasted red peppers, drained and chopped

2 scallions, trimmed and thinly sliced (optional)

2 tablespoons chopped fresh dill (optional)

6 large eggs

1¾ cups whole milk

1½ teaspoons salt

Freshly ground pepper, to taste

1. Grease an 8 x 8 x 2-inch Pyrex baking dish with most of the butter. Spread any leftover butter on as many bread slices as possible; set aside.
2. Arrange half of the bread slices in a single layer in the baking dish. Scatter half of the spinach, cheese, red peppers, and optional scallions and dill over the slices. Arrange a second layer of bread on top of the first and cover with the remaining spinach, red peppers, scallions, and dill. Sprinkle half of the remaining cheese on top. Cover the remaining cheese and set aside.

3. Whisk the eggs, milk, salt, and pepper in a bowl. Pour evenly over the casserole and cover with plastic wrap, pressing it directly against the surface. Press gently to make sure that the bread absorbs the liquid. Then place a weight (such as a bag of rice or a couple of cans) on top of the plastic wrap to keep the bread submerged. Refrigerate for at least 1 hour, or overnight.

4. Remove the casserole from the refrigerator and preheat the oven to 350°F.

5. Just before baking, remove the plastic wrap from the casserole and sprinkle the remaining cheese over the top. Bake for 40 minutes, or until puffed and the middle has set. (*Note:* The internal temperature of this casserole should reach 160°F on an instant-read thermometer inserted into the center of the dish.) Remove the casserole from the oven and let cool for 10 minutes before serving.

▶ *Calcium Boost:* In a measuring cup, combine ⅓ cup pasteurized instant nonfat dry milk with the whole milk. Mix until the milk powder has dissolved, then follow the directions in Step 2.

▶ *Health Tip:* If your doctor has restricted your fat intake use margarine instead of unsalted butter, reduced-fat cheddar cheese, and reduced-fat 2% milk.

▶ *Complete Meal Ideas:* Serve this casserole with:
Fresh fruit or juice of your choice that contains vitamin C
Reduced-fat 2% milk or low-fat yogurt
2 slices toast (preferably whole wheat)

APPROXIMATE NUTRITIONAL INFORMATION: Serving size: One-sixth of this brunch casserole; Calories: 453 cals; Protein: 21 g; Carbohydrates: 34 g; Fat: 26 g; Fiber: 3 g; Sodium: 1195 mg; Calcium: 414 mg; Diabetic Exchange: Bread/Starch 2, Fat 2, Meat (Medium Fat) 2

banana muffins with
walnuts and wheat germ

~

What's in this for baby and me? Protein, folic acid, and fiber.

NOTHING BEATS A great banana muffin—any time of day. These muffins are an excellent source of **protein**, **folic acid**, and **fiber**, and a good source of iron, vitamin C, and B vitamins. Refrigerate a week's supply of the muffins, or freeze them for a healthy and delicious breakfast or snack. For an extra protein fix, cut a muffin in half and spread it with 1 tablespoon peanut butter or other nut butter. The mini muffins are designed to be diabetic-friendly.

makes 12 regular muffins or 40 mini muffins

Canola oil cooking spray for greasing the muffin pan, (or use muffin cup liners)

¾ cup whole wheat flour

¾ cup all-purpose flour

⅓ cup toasted wheat germ (optional)

2 teaspoons baking soda

¼ teaspoon salt

½ cup chopped walnuts or pecans

½ cup packed light brown sugar

⅓ cup canola oil

1 large egg

¼ cup reduced-fat 2% milk

1½ cups coarsely mashed ripe bananas (3 to 4
large bananas) (see Cooking Tip)

1. Preheat the oven to 350°F. Spray the muffin cups with cooking spray or line them with muffin liners.
2. In a large bowl, whisk together the flours, wheat germ, if using, baking soda, salt, and walnuts until well combined.
3. In a small bowl, combine the brown sugar, canola oil, egg, and milk and whisk until well blended. Add the bananas and mix well, then add to the flour mixture and mix until well blended.
4. Divide the batter evenly among the muffin cups. Bake until a tester inserted into the center comes out clean: 25 to 30 minutes for regular muffins, 10 to 12 minutes for mini muffins. Transfer the muffins to a rack and cool slightly before eating.

▶ *Cooking Tip:* Ripe bananas can be frozen unpeeled (the skin will turn completely brown when frozen) or peeled and mashed. If freezing peeled bananas, place the measured pulp in a zip-lock freezer bag and mark it with a label. If freezing whole unpeeled bananas, place them in a zip-lock freezer bag. Defrost the pulp or whole bananas at room temperature or in a microwave oven. To facilitate peeling defrosted whole bananas, start at the bottom of the banana rather than at the top stem. Mash the bananas with the back of a fork or a potato masher.

▶ *Variation:* Substitute ¾ cup all-purpose flour for the whole wheat flour.

▶ *Storage Tip:* To freeze the muffins, cool them completely, then place them in a zip-lock bag and freeze. The muffins can be reheated or defrosted in a microwave oven for a few seconds, or in a conventional oven.

▶ *Diabetic Tip:* Omit the nuts and use mini muffin pans for baking. Eat only 1 regular muffin or 2 mini muffins.

▶ *Complete Meal Idea:* Serve these muffins with:
Fresh fruit or juice of your choice that contains vitamin C
Reduced-fat 2% milk or low-fat yogurt (or combine the fruit and
yogurt in a smoothie—see Super Fruit Smoothies, page 57)
Peanut butter

APPROXIMATE NUTRITIONAL INFORMATION: Serving size: 2 regular-size banana muffins; Calories: 432 cals; Protein: 10 g; Carbohydrates: 58 g; Fat: 20 g; Fiber: 5 g; Sodium: 539 mg; Folic Acid: 79 mcg; Diabetic Exchange (values per 1 muffin): Bread/Starch 2, Fat 2

bran muffins with dried cranberries, walnuts, and candied ginger

What's in this for baby and me? Folic acid and fiber.

QUICK, EASY, AND super tasty, these bran muffins are high in **folic acid** and **fiber**, and they are a good source of protein, vitamin C, and B vitamins. The cranberries, ginger, and walnuts are all optional. Feel free to substitute your favorite ingredients—raisins, diced dried apricots or pears, and dried cherries all work well. The batter will keep in the refrigerator for up to two days, and the muffins can be frozen for up to one month. For a protein fix, cut a muffin in half and spread it with 1 tablespoon peanut butter or other nut butter. The mini muffins are designed to be diabetic friendly.

makes 15 regular muffins or about 52 mini muffins

Cooking spray for greasing the muffin pan (or use muffin cup liners)

3½ cups All Bran cereal

1 cup boiling water

¼ cup canola oil

¾ cup sugar

1 cup nonfat buttermilk

1 large egg

1¼ cups all-purpose flour

1¼ teaspoons baking soda

¼ teaspoon salt

½ teaspoon ground ginger (optional)

½ cup dried cranberries or chopped dried apricots (optional)

½ cup chopped walnuts (optional)

⅓ cup chopped candied ginger (optional)

1. Preheat the oven to 400°F. Spray the muffin cups with cooking spray or line with muffin liners.
2. Place the cereal in a small bowl and pour the boiling water over it—do not stir. Set aside.
3. Combine the canola oil and sugar in a large bowl and whisk together. Add the buttermilk and egg and whisk again. Add the flour, baking soda, salt, and powdered ginger, if using, and whisk just until well combined. Add the All Bran mixture and mix with a spoon, then add the remaining cranberries, walnuts, and/or candied ginger, if using, and mix just until combined. (The batter will be quite thick.) Let the batter sit at room temperature for 10 minutes.
4. Gently stir the batter, then divide evenly among the muffin cups. Bake until a tester inserted in the center of a muffin comes out clean: about 20 minutes for regular muffins, about 12 minutes for mini muffins. Transfer the muffins to a rack and cool slightly before eating.

▶ **Storage Tip:** To refrigerate or freeze, cool completely, then place the muffins in a zip-lock bag and refrigerate or freeze. The muffins can be reheated or defrosted in a microwave oven for a few seconds or in a conventional oven.

▶ **Diabetic Tip:** Omit the dried cranberries, walnuts, and candied ginger. Use mini muffin pans for baking.

▶ **Complete Meal Idea:** Serve these muffins with:
Fresh fruit or juice of your choice
Reduced-fat 2% milk or low-fat yogurt (combine the fruit and yogurt into a smoothie—see Super Fruit Smoothies, page 57)
Peanut butter

APPROXIMATE NUTRITIONAL INFORMATION: Serving size: 1 regular bran muffin; Calories: 194 cals; Protein: 5 g; Carbohydrates: 33 g; Fat: 7 g; Fiber: 5 g; Sodium: 203 mg; Diabetic Exchange: Bread/Starch 2, Fat 1.5

choosing the right breakfast cereal

▶ **Look for cereals fortified with 100 percent folic acid and 100 percent iron. (See Cereals that Contain 100 Percent of the Daily Value of Folic Acid, page 301.)**

▶ **Look for cereals containing the following words first on their ingredient lists: whole wheat, whole grain, whole oat flour, or rolled oats. This ensures that the product has not been subject to fiber-robbing refining processes.**

▶ **Look for cereals containing at least 2 grams of fiber per serving. Whole grain products contain fiber, but refined grain cereals do not.**

▶ **Look for cereals low in sugar. A maximum of 5 grams of sugar (about 1 teaspoon) per serving is advised. Cereals containing dried fruit such as raisins are likely to have a higher sugar content, but the nutritional benefits are generally worth the extra sugar.**

▶ **Look for cereals with no more than 2 grams of fat per serving.**

▶ **Vegans and non-meat eaters should look for cereals fortified with 100 percent B_{12}. (See Cereals that Contain 100 Percent of the Daily Value of Vitamin B_{12}, page 302.)**

winter fruit salad

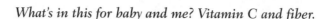

What's in this for baby and me? Vitamin C and fiber.

Unless you live in a tropical climate, or can afford to pay top dollar, summer's sweet fresh fruit becomes a distant memory by late October. Apples, grapes, pears, oranges, and bananas make a wonderful off-season fruit salad. Any type of fruit—fresh or canned (choose fruits packed in light syrup)—can be used, and if imported berries are on sale in your grocery store in the middle of winter, grab them. This salad is an excellent source of **vitamin C** and **fiber** (especially if the apples and pears are left unpeeled), and the optional yogurt provides calcium. A container of fruit salad kept in a cooler is a fantastic snack and an excellent source of hydration for women on bed rest. (*Note*: because of the high water content of the oranges and grapes, this salad does not lend itself to being whipped into a smoothie.)

makes about 4 cups

FRUIT SALAD

2 oranges, peeled and sliced into segments (See Cooking Tip below)

1 apple, washed and diced

1 pear, washed and diced

1 cup red or white seedless grapes, washed

1 ripe banana, sliced

1 kiwi, peeled and sliced

OPTIONAL TOPPINGS

Low-fat plain or fruit yogurt

Honey or molasses

Wheat germ or granola (see Fruit-Filled Granola, page 284)

1. Combine all of the fruit salad ingredients in a large bowl and mix gently. Cover and refrigerate if not serving immediately.
2. To serve, place some fruit salad in a bowl and add one or more toppings, if desired.

▶ **Cooking Tip:** To prepare orange segments: Using a sharp knife, slice off the top and bottom of the orange to expose the flesh. Stand the orange on the counter. Then, working from top to the bottom, and using your first slice as your guide to the thickness of the orange peel, slice the peel off the orange in wide strips. Working over a bowl to catch the juices, hold the orange in one hand and slice out the orange segments from beneath the membranes, holding your knife as close to the membranes as possible; let the segments drop into the bowl. Then squeeze as much juice as possible from the membranes into the bowl.

▶ *Time Saving Tip:* Make fruit salad from a salad bar. Or use canned mandarin orange segments instead of fresh orange slices.

APPROXIMATE NUTRITIONAL INFORMATION: Serving size: 1 cup winter fruit salad; Calories: 144 cals; Protein: 2 g; Carbohydrates: 36 g; Fat: .9 g; Fiber: 5 g; Sodium: 1 mg; Vitamin C: 64 mg; Diabetic Exchange: Fruit 2.5

eggs and salmonella enteritidis

While salmonella can be contracted a number of different ways, contaminated raw eggs are of particular concern for pregnant women. (See page 257 for more information on other causes of salmonellosis.) Unbroken fresh eggs in their shells that appear perfectly normal may contain bacteria called *Salmonella enteritidis* (SE) which can cause food-borne illness. SE silently infects the ovaries of healthy-appearing hens and contaminates the eggs before the shells are formed. Researchers say that, if present, the SE bacteria are usually in the yolk or "yellow," but they can't rule out the bacteria being in egg whites.[14]

People with health problems, the very young, seniors, and pregnant women (the risk is to the unborn child) are particularly vulnerable to SE infections. The symptoms include fever, abdominal cramps, and diarrhea.[15] Proper refrigeration, cooking, and handling of raw eggs should prevent most contamination problems. People can and should enjoy eggs and egg dishes, provided they follow these safe handling guidelines:[16]

▶ Don't eat raw eggs–including raw eggs contained in milk shakes, Caesar salad dressing, Hollandaise sauce, homemade mayonnaise, ice cream, or eggnog. Also, avoid tasting any batters (such as cake and cookie batters) that contain raw egg.

▶ Choose Grade A or AA eggs with clean, uncracked shells. Don't wash eggs.

▶ Buy only refrigerated eggs and keep them refrigerated in their original egg carton in the coldest part of the refrigerator, and not in the door.

▶ Don't keep eggs out of the refrigerator for more than two hours. Bacteria grow rapidly at room temperature.

▶ Use raw eggs within three to five weeks of purchase. Use any leftover yolks or whites within four days. Hard-cooked eggs can be kept in the refrigerator for one week.

▶ Handle eggs safely. Wash hands, utensils, equipment, and work areas with warm soapy water before and after contact with raw eggs and dishes containing raw eggs.

▶ Keep raw eggs separate from other foods that will be cooked.

▶ Cook eggs thoroughly until the yolk and whites are firm. Scrambled eggs should not be runny and there should be no visible liquid egg. Casseroles and other egg-based dishes should be cooked to 160°F on an instant-read thermometer.

▶ Eat eggs promptly after cooking. Refrigerate any leftovers, and consume within three to four days.

Commercially manufactured ice cream and eggnog made with pasteurized eggs have not been linked to SE infections. Dry meringue shells and cookies are safe to eat. It is advisable to avoid meringue-topped pies, chiffon and fruit pies made with raw whipped egg whites, and any custard-based desserts in which the eggs might not have reached a safe internal temperature of 160°F.

summer fruit salad

What's in this for baby and me? Vitamins C and A and fiber.

DURING SUMMER THIS fruit salad, **high in vitamins C** and **A,** and **fiber** (with a good dose of folic acid), is perfect for breakfast or brunch, a snack, or dessert. Use any fresh fruits in any proportions you wish. This recipe calls for raspberries, strawberries, blueberries, cantaloupe, kiwi, and bananas, but you could use peaches, nectarines, apricots, watermelon, honeydew melon, or any other ripe summer fruit. For a tropical twist, with an even more serious supply of vitamins A and C, try combining mangoes, papaya, kiwi, and pineapple with fresh passion fruit juice instead of orange juice. The possibilities are endless!

This fruit salad is best served right after it's made—the berries tend to get a bit soggy if allowed to sit for too long. If there is any leftover salad, throw it in the blender, add some yogurt and pasteurized instant nonfat-dry milk, and whip it into a fruit smoothie (see Super Fruit Smoothies, page 57). For extra calcium, serve the salad topped with low-fat yogurt. A container of fruit salad kept in a cooler is a fantastic snack and an excellent source of hydration for women on bed rest. Talking about the shapes and colors of the fruits in this salad might be a way to get your little one to try a bite.

makes about 4 cups

1 cup fresh raspberries, rinsed quickly

1½ cups fresh strawberries, washed, hulled, and quartered

1 cup fresh blueberries, washed

1½ cups cantaloupe balls or cubes (from about half a melon)

1 kiwi, peeled and sliced

1 banana, sliced

¼ cup orange juice

Combine all of the ingredients in a large bowl and mix gently. Cover and refrigerate if not serving immediately.

▶ *Timesaving Tip:* Make fruit salad from a salad bar.

APPROXIMATE NUTRITIONAL INFORMATION: Serving size: 1 cup summer fruit salad; Calories: 118 cals; Protein: 2 g; Carbohydrates: 29 g; Fat: .9 g; Fiber: 6 g; Sodium: 10 mg; Vitamin C: 97 mg; Vitamin A: 2,113 IU; Diabetic Exchange: Fruit 2

get juiced up

~

Today juices come in seemingly endless varieties, with a spectrum of benefits from which to choose. Some are fortified with calcium and antioxidants, others have low acid and extra pulp, while still others are juice combinations that offer a blast of vitamins and calories. To control your calorie intake, it is advisable to limit your juice consumption to 8 ounces per day. Following is a list of fruit juices (8-ounce servings) and their primary vitamin and calorie values based on the recommended daily allowances (RDA) for a 2,000-calorie diet.

JUICE	VITAMIN	CALORIES
Orange	C = 207%	111 cals
Grapefruit	C = 156%	96 cals
Carrot	A = 539%, C = 35%	98 cals
Mango	C = 130%	130 cals
Tangerine	C = 128%	106 cals
Pineapple	C = 45%	140 cals
Cranberry	C = 149%	144 cals
Tomato	C = 74%, A = 27%	41 cals
V-8 juice	C = 100%, A = 40%	50 cals

super fruit smoothies

What's in this for baby and me? Protein, calcium, and vitamins.

SMOOTHIES ARE IN! Grocery store shelves are lined with enticing prepared smoothies, usually in the dairy section next to the yogurt, and frozen smoothie mixes can be found in freezer sections near the concentrated fruit juices. Be sure to avoid smoothies made with raw eggs (see Eggs and *Salmonella Enteritidis*, page 54). A cool **high-protein**, **high-calcium**, **high-vitamin** power-packed fruit smoothie is great any time of day—and great for kids, too, especially those who don't drink milk regularly!

The following recipe for the Fresh or Frozen Banana Smoothie can be modified to suit your taste. The variations that follow offer some ideas, but feel free to change anything *except* the amounts of yogurt and dry milk. Using these amounts of yogurt and dry milk is equivalent to drinking about 2 cups of milk. Different yogurts can be used, soy instead of regular, and flavored instead of plain.

On the fruit scene, frozen bananas are ideal because they cool the smoothie without using any ice. All of the variations call for half a large fresh or frozen banana combined with approximately ½ cup of another fresh, frozen, or canned fruit. Or, skip the frozen banana and use 1 cup of any type of frozen fruit, such as peaches, strawberries, raspberries, or blueberries. If you use canned fruit, look for fruits packed in their own juices or in light syrup, rather than fruits packed in heavy syrup.

Sweeten your smoothies with apple juice concentrate or plain sugar. The vanilla extract is optional and can be replaced with any other flavoring. If you do not have a blender, you can use a food processor, although the smoothie will not be as thick and whipped. If you use a food processor, mix all of the ingredients *except* the ice cubes, then pour the smoothie over ice. Smoothies are best served ice cold and sipped with a straw.

All of the smoothies make about 2 cups

fresh or frozen basic banana smoothie

¾ cup low-fat plain yogurt

⅓ cup pasteurized instant nonfat dry milk

1 large ripe banana, frozen if desired

1 teaspoon apple juice concentrate or sugar, or to taste

A drop of pure vanilla extract (optional)

1–2 ice cubes

Place all of the ingredients in a blender and process until smooth. Serve immediately.

▶ **Cooking Tip:** Use a paring knife to peel the frozen banana. If the peel is too hard, hold it under running hot water for about 30 seconds.

▶ **Timesaving Tip:** Mix 8 ounces fat-free frozen smoothie mix with ¾ cup low-fat plain yogurt, ⅓ cup pasteurized instant nonfat dry milk, and ice. Add more smoothie mix to taste.

▶ **Calorie Boost:** For a richer, more caloric smoothie, substitute ¾ cup frozen yogurt, ice cream, or soy ice cream for the low-fat plain yogurt; or add Carnation Instant Breakfast powder according to the package directions.

▶ **Diabetic Tip:** Halve the recipe to yield 1 cup smoothie and omit the apple juice concentrate or sugar.

APPROXIMATE NUTRITIONAL INFORMATION: Serving size: 1 banana smoothie (about 2 cups); Calories: 385 cals; Protein: 25 g; Carbohydrates: 65 g; Fat: 4 g; Fiber: 3 g; Sodium: 344 mg; Diabetic Exchange (values per 1 cup smoothie): Skim Milk 2, Fruit .5

FUN VARIATIONS

fresh or frozen strawberry-banana smoothie

¾ cup low-fat plain yogurt

⅓ cup pasteurized instant nonfat dry milk

6 large strawberries (about 1/2 cup), washed
  and hulled

½ large ripe banana, frozen if desired

1 teaspoon apple juice concentrate or sugar,
  or to taste

A drop of pure vanilla extract (optional)

1–2 ice cubes

APPROXIMATE NUTRITIONAL INFORMATION: Serving size: 1 strawberry-banana smoothie (about 2 cups); Calories: 352 cals; Protein: 25 g; Carbohydrates: 57 g; Fat: 4 g; Fiber: 3 g; Sodium: 344 mg; Calcium: 853 mg; Vitamin C: 50 mg; Diabetic Exchange (values per 1 cup smoothie): Skim Milk 2, Fruit .5

fresh or frozen raspberry-banana smoothie

¾ cup low-fat plain yogurt

⅓ cup pasteurized instant nonfat dry milk

½ cup fresh raspberries, rinsed quickly

½ large ripe banana, frozen if desired

1 teaspoon apple juice concentrate or sugar,
  or to taste

A drop of pure vanilla extract (optional)

1–2 ice cubes

APPROXIMATE NUTRITIONAL INFORMATION: Serving size: 1 raspberry-banana smoothie (about 2 cups); Calories: 360 cals; Protein: 25 g; Carbohydrates: 59 g; Fat: 4 g; Fiber: 6 g; Sodium: 343 mg; Calcium: 856 mg; Vitamin C: 25 mg; Diabetic Exchange: (values per 1 cup smoothie) Skim Milk 2, Fruit .5

fresh, frozen, or canned peach-banana smoothie

¾ cup low-fat plain yogurt

⅓ cup pasteurized instant nonfat dry milk

½ small ripe peach, washed and quartered, or
   ½ cup frozen (unthawed) or canned
   peaches

½ large ripe banana, frozen if desired

1 teaspoon apple juice concentrate or sugar,
   or to taste

A drop of pure vanilla extract (optional)

1–2 ice cubes

APPROXIMATE NUTRITIONAL INFORMATION: Serving size: 1 peach-banana smoothie (about 2 cups); Calories: 351 cals; Protein: 25 g; Carbohydrates: 56 g; Fat: 3 g; Fiber: 2 g; Sodium: 343 mg; Calcium: 845 mg; Vitamin C: 13 mg; Diabetic Exchange (values per 1 cup smoothie): Skim Milk 2, Fruit .5

fresh or canned pineapple-banana smoothie

¾ cup low-fat plain yogurt

⅓ cup pasteurized instant nonfat dry milk

½ cup diced fresh pineapple or ½ cup canned
   pineapple in its own juice

½ large ripe banana, frozen if desired

1 teaspoon apple juice concentrate or sugar,
   or to taste

A drop of pure vanilla extract (optional)

1–2 ice cubes

APPROXIMATE NUTRITIONAL INFORMATION: Serving size: 1 pineapple-banana smoothie (about 2 cups); Calories: 400 cals; Protein: 25 g; Carbohydrates: 69 g; Fat: 3 g; Fiber: 2 g; Sodium: 353 mg; Calcium: 843 mg; Vitamin C: 22 mg; Diabetic Exchange (values per 1 cup smoothie): Skim Milk 2, Fruit .5

soups and sandwiches
to savor

⌒

SOUPS

O N A COLD day, there is nothing more homey than walking into a kitchen where soup is simmering on the stove, perfuming the air with each waft of steam. And on a hot day, a bowl of chilled soup is a refreshing treat. Vitamins, minerals, calcium, protein, and fiber—soups have them all, and being pregnant you need them all!

Homemade soups are undoubtedly the best. They are generally healthier than their store-bought cousins, which are usually high in sodium and monosodium glutamate (MSG). However, the recent boom in gourmet, organic, low-fat, and low-sodium canned or long-life boxed soups has created healthier and tastier options for consumers. The vegetable soups in this chapter call for some of the most nutritious vegetables for pregnant women, and the bean soups are as hearty as they are wholesome.

The forgiving, flexible, and versatile nature of soups should put any novice cook at ease in the kitchen. Generally, soups require no special skills and are almost infallible if you follow a few simple steps. Starting and stopping the cooking process usually doesn't affect the outcome of soups, especially the longer-cooking ones. And most important, with some ingredient substitutions, recipes can and should be custom designed to suit your family's tastes.

Soups are a welcome treat any time of day—to accompany a sandwich, as a snack, or for lunch or dinner with friends. Women on bed rest can get a lot of mileage out of soups kept in a thermos at bedside, and women on the go can get a quick and longer-lasting boost from a cup of soup than from coffee. Your young eaters will also benefit from soups, and if they are introduced early in a child's meal plan, they are sure to become a requested item. With a little time, energy, and advance planning, soups can become a great part of your life. So, get out your stockpot and ladle and start a family tradition of eating soups!

SANDWICHES

THE KEY TO making a great sandwich is using the best ingredients you can find. Choosing nutritious, full-bodied bread is essential. Enriched hearty whole grain breads and calcium-fortified whole wheat breads have the best nutritional value. Sourdough breads, whole wheat French bread, whole wheat pita bread, herb breads, and breads laced with black olives, rosemary, and endless other flavors make delectable sandwiches, even though they are not quite as nutritious as enriched whole wheat breads. Rolled and wrapped sandwiches are the latest craze, and green spinach-flavored wraps are a good source of iron.

When choosing sandwich meats, try to avoid those containing nitrites, nitrates, and large amounts of fats, such as bologna and salami. Ham, well-done roast beef, and sliced turkey are good options (see Listeriosis Warning, page 107, for safe cold cuts). Pasteurized cheese is a welcome addition to almost any sandwich. Lettuce, tomatoes, sliced avocado, roasted red bell peppers, and other vegetables add vitamins and roughage to your diet. Dips and spreads make nutritious and tasty additions to sandwiches and can be used in place of light mayonnaise.

It's hard to resist the temptation of a bag of chips with a sandwich, and we all know that sometimes you just have to give in. If that is the case, buy small, lunch-box size bags of chips for portion control. Also, opt for baked tortilla chips or pretzels. Small containers of soups or cold salads (homemade or store-bought) such as potato or macaroni salad, coleslaw, or carrot salad are the perfect accompaniment to any sandwich.

There are a few important points to keep in mind to ensure that your bagged lunch remains as healthy and safe as possible. Harmful bacteria multiply rapidly in the danger zone, temperatures between 40° and 140°F. Any perishable items in your lunch box, including cold cuts, hard-boiled eggs, salads made with mayonnaise, and packaged combos containing luncheon meats and cheese, should be kept cold with an ice pack and refrigerated upon arrival if possible. Food should never be left out at room temperature for more than two hours, one hour if the temperature is over 90°F. Following are a few tips to keep your lunch free of food-borne pathogens.[19]

- Insulated soft-sided lunch boxes or bags are best for keeping foods cold. Use an ice pack or frozen-juice box with any perishable foods.
- Prepare cooked food (such as tuna or egg salad, or mayonnaise-based potato or pasta salads) ahead of time to allow them to be thoroughly chilled before packing. Keep them refrigerated until ready to go. Sandwiches can be prepared the night before and refrigerated.
- Use an insulated container to keep hot foods hot. Fill the container with boiling water, let stand a few minutes, drain, then add the hot food.
- When using a microwave to reheat leftovers, cover food to promote even heating and heat to 165°F. Cook frozen convenience meals according to package directions.
- Don't pack too much food. This will avoid the need to store leftovers.
- Discard all used food packaging and paper bags.

soups and sandwiches to savor

~

SOUPS

Creamy Asparagus-Artichoke Soup

Cheesy Cauliflower-Potato Soup

Great Green Broccoli-Spinach Soup

Butternut Squash–Carrot Soup with Ginger

Greek-Style Chicken, Lemon, and Egg Soup

Black Bean Soup with Cilantro▼

Lentil Soup with Brown Rice and Spinach▼

Turkish-Style Red Lentil Soup▼

Mediterranean Pasta, Bean, and Vegetable Soup

Green Split Pea Soup▼

Beef, Barley, and Vegetable Soup

Gazpacho▼

Basic Chicken Stock

Basic Vegetable Stock▼

SANDWICHES

Pr-egg-o Salad Sandwich

Chicken Salad with Dried Apricots and Almonds

Grilled Cheese Sandwich

Tuna Salad Sandwich

Wraps and Rolls

▼ Vegan recipe

RECIPE NOTES

Soups

"SOUPS AND SANDWICHES to Savor" offers a healthy collection of vegetable soups that are easy to prepare for a weekday meal, yet elegant enough to serve at a dinner party. Ideally, fresh vegetables should be used to prepare these soups, but frozen vegetables—broccoli florets, spinach, corn, or peas—work fine in most soups. Canned tomatoes and beans are indispensable, and prepackaged washed, peeled, and cut vegetables, such as baby carrots, broccoli and cauliflower florets, or butternut squash save time and energy. Vegetables from a salad bar—sliced or shredded carrots, celery, and peas—are ideal for purchasing in small portions, or if you just don't feel like chopping.

Some of the vegetable soups here are pureed, but pureeing is optional. It is easier and more efficiently accomplished with a blender than a food processor. If you don't already own one, a blender is a worthwhile investment. It is ideal for making smoothies, milk shakes, crushes, and other cool drinks, and after your baby arrives you can use it to puree baby foods. If you do not plan to puree a soup, be sure to cut the vegetables and other ingredients into bite-size pieces before cooking them.

To increase the calcium content of creamy vegetable soups without increasing the fat, use any kind of milk (including buttermilk) mixed with pasteurized instant nonfat dry milk (about ⅓ cup). If you are lactose intolerant, buttermilk is easier to digest than milk or half-and-half. All soups may be thinned with additional stock, water, or milk.

Any soup can be adapted for a vegetarian diet by using vegetable stock and omitting the meat products. Healthy garnishes—such as grated cheddar or Parmesan cheese, plain yogurt, nuts, sesame or pumpkin seeds, wheat germ, tofu, or croutons—are an easy way to add a splash of protein, calcium, or grain to your diet and a new dimension to your soup. If you have been advised to watch your salt intake, use low-sodium canned stock, limit the number of bouillon cubes, and go easy on the salt.

Some notes about the soup recipes in this chapter:

- The recipes can be cut in half for a smaller yield.
- For convenience, soups can be frozen in meal-size portions in plastic containers or freezer bags. Be sure to label and date all frozen foods.
- Vegetable soups should be frozen *after* they are pureed and *before* adding dairy products such as buttermilk or half-and-half.
- Margarine can be substituted for unsalted butter.

- Choose fat-free, low-sodium canned stocks whenever possible.
- Bouillon cubes (meat, poultry, or vegetable) dissolved in water can be substituted for the amount of stock or water called for in the recipes. They are cheaper than canned stock and take up less storage space in kitchen cupboards. Some brands are MSG free.
- Use ultra-pasteurized half-and-half.
- Check to make sure that all dairy products are fresh before adding them to soup. To prevent curdling, scald any questionable liquid products, such as milk or half-and-half, before adding them to the soup.
- All herbs and spices are optional. Young children may object to green things in their soup or they may prefer a blander flavor.
- Thin soups to the desired consistency very gradually, adding about 2 tablespoons of liquid at a time. It is always easier to thin a soup than to thicken one. To thicken a soup, add a quick-dissolving thickener, such as Wondra or Pillsbury Shake and Blend, according to the package directions.
- A flame tamer buffers the heat for longer-cooking soups.
- As a general rule, soups cooked in a slow cooker require less water than those cooked on the stove as there is almost no evaporation. Vegetables take a surprisingly long time to cook in a slow cooker, so they should be thinly sliced and placed on the bottom of the pot. Meat should follow the vegetables. Because it is impossible to predict their liquid absorption, avoid adding uncooked pasta, rice, or any other raw grain to soups cooked in a slow cooker unless you follow specific directions in a recipe. Also, while sautéing onions, garlic, and other vegetables and seasonings before adding them to the cooker may seem like more work, it greatly improves the flavor of the finished soup.

SANDWICHES

SANDWICHES CAN BE as exciting or as boring as you make them. For a delicious lunch or snack, make sandwiches with pasteurized cheeses, fresh lettuce, fresh herbs, spreads, and lean, high-quality deli meats or leftovers from the night before (such as grilled chicken, steak, lamb, or meat loaf). Use the tastiest, heartiest, healthiest bread you can find. Remember to keep your lunch refrigerated, especially during the hot summer months.

Filling Suggestions

Sliced turkey, ham, roast beef (well-done), chicken, or your favorite deli meats or tofu provide protein. Purchase home-style or all-natural meats, because they contain little or no preservatives. To prevent listeriosis, be sure to thoroughly heat all lunch meats before eating them (see Listeriosis Warning, page 107). Try to avoid the following sandwich meats because of their high fat, nitrite, or nitrate content: salami, bacon, Spam, corned beef, and bologna. Pasteurized cheese is a tasty addition to any sandwich. Choose low-fat varieties (less than 2 grams of fat per ounce) if you need to restrict your fat intake.

Salad Suggestions

Egg, chicken, salmon, tuna, crab, shrimp, or lobster salads (homemade or store-bought) make delicious sandwiches and add some protein to your diet. All mayonnaise-based salads require refrigeration.

Spread Suggestions

As an alternative to high-quality light mayonnaise, try pasteurized cheese spreads such as Boursin or other flavored cheese spreads, pasteurized goat cheese (*chevre*), Neufchâtel, or flavored cream cheeses, plain ricotta cheese or Ricotta Cheese and Red Pepper Dip (page 146), guacamole (store-bought or Homemade Guacamole, page 145), hummus (store-bought or Healthy Hummus, page 148), pesto (store-bought or Basil Pesto, page 121), or any other prepared spread, to give your sandwich a special flavor.

Vegetable Suggestions

Salad—romaine, loose-leaf, Boston, Bibb, mesclun, and watercress—tomatoes, cucumbers, green peppers, and shredded carrots are all great sources of fiber and vitamins. Leftover grilled, roasted, or stir-fried vegetables are a fabulous addition to any sandwich, particularly wraps. (Keep in mind that romaine lettuce has the highest folic acid content of all the greens listed above.)

Bread Suggestions

Choose whole grain, bran, or calcium-enriched bread whenever possible. Flat breads or tortillas are perfect for wrap sandwiches. Try to stay away from white bread that has little nutritional value unless it is fortified with calcium, iron, or other nutrients.

pantry items for
soups and sandwiches to savor

SOUP PANTRY

Fresh Produce

Asparagus

Baby spinach (5- and 6-ounce packages)

Broccoli and broccoli florets

Butternut squash

Carrots (peeled baby carrots or regular carrots)

Cauliflower

Celery

Cucumbers

Fresh herbs: cilantro, dill, and parsley

Garlic

Ginger

Lemons

Mushrooms (preferably cremini)

Onions: regular and Vidalia or other sweet onions

Potatoes (any kind)

Scallions

Swiss chard

Tomatoes

Zucchini

Dairy and Soy Products

Cheese: grated Fontina, Monterey Jack, Parmesan, and/or sharp cheddar

Extra firm tofu

Grade A large eggs

Half-and-half (preferably ultra-pasteurized)

Low-fat or fat-free plain yogurt

Nonfat buttermilk

Unsalted butter

Whole milk

Canned, Bottled, and Jarred Staples

Artichoke hearts packed in water or brine (13.75-ounce can)

Balsamic vinegar or any other vinegar

Black beans (19-ounce can)

Canola oil

Fat free low-sodium stock (any kind)

Great Northern white beans (15.5-ounce can)

Olive oil

Peeled and diced tomatoes (14.5-ounce can)

Roasted red peppers

V-8 juice (low-sodium preferred) or tomato juice

Dry Staples

Brown rice and any other rice except instant

Croutons

Dried apricots

Green lentils

Green split peas

Pasteurized instant nonfat dry milk

Pearl barley

Red lentils

Saltine crackers

Small pasta (such as ditalini or alphabet pasta)

Herbs and Spices

Bay leaves

Bouillon cubes (any flavor)

Chili powder

Dried marjoram
Dried mint
Dried oregano
Dried tarragon
Dried thyme
Garlic powder (not garlic salt)
Ground cumin
Ground ginger
Paprika or red pepper
Pesto (store-bought or homemade)

Frozen Staples
Artichoke hearts
Spinach (6-, 8-, or 10-ounce package)

Meats and Poultry
Beef shank, bone-in (1 pound)
Chicken tenders (½ pound)
Whole chicken (3½ pounds)

From the Salad Bar
Broccoli florets
Cauliflower florets
Diced onions
Sliced mushrooms

SANDWICH PANTRY
Fresh Produce
Avocados
Bananas
Celery
Cucumbers
Fresh herbs: cilantro, dill, and parsley
Lemons
Lettuce
Red bell peppers
Scallions
Tomatoes

Dairy
2% Milk Singles (cheese slices)
Cheese for sandwiches
Grade A large eggs
Grated Parmesan cheese

Canned, Bottled, and Jarred Staples
Caesar salad dressing (preferably reduced-fat)
Canola oil
Chunk white tuna in spring water
Hoisin sauce
Light mayonnaise
Mustard (any kind)
Peanut butter (preferably reduced-fat)
Roasted red peppers
Salsa
Thai-style peanut sauce

Dry Staples
Dried apricots
Sliced almonds
Bread for sandwiches
Burrito-size tortillas (10-inch)
Calcium-enriched bread (such as Calcium Enriched Roman Meal)

Miscellaneous Staples
Chicken tenders or leftover cooked chicken
Hummus (store-bought or homemade)
Tabbouleh (store-bought or homemade)
Lunch meats

From the Salad Bar
Sliced cucumbers
Sliced red bell peppers
Sliced tomatoes
Washed lettuce

creamy asparagus-artichoke soup

What's in this for baby and me? Vitamin C and folic acid.

IF YOUR CHILDREN are fond of green vegetables, don't be surprised if they acquire a taste for this simple-to-make soup. High in **vitamin C** and **folic acid**, and a good source of protein, vitamin A, and fiber, the soup is elegant enough to be served at a dinner party, yet simple enough for lunch or a snack. If tarragon does not appeal to you, omit it or substitute your favorite herb. For a bit of texture and protein, add cooked shrimp, crabmeat, or cheese. Asparagus tips, diced tomatoes, or croutons are nice garnishes. Serve this soup hot or chilled.

serves 6 (makes about 7 cups)

3 tablespoons unsalted butter	(see Cooking Tip below to use the aspara-
1 medium onion, chopped	gus tips as garnish)
1 medium potato, peeled and diced	One 13.75-ounce can artichoke hearts, drained
4 cups fat-free low-sodium stock	1½ teaspoons dried tarragon (optional)
½ teaspoon salt, or to taste	½ cup half-and-half or whole milk (optional)
1 pound green asparagus, washed, tough ends	Freshly ground pepper, to taste
trimmed, and stalks cut into 1-inch pieces	Squeeze of fresh lemon juice (optional)

1. Melt the butter in a 6-quart saucepan over medium-high heat. Add the onion and sauté for 3 minutes. Add the potato, stock, and salt and bring to a boil. Add the asparagus, artichoke hearts, and tarragon, if using, and return to a boil, then reduce the heat and simmer, uncovered, for 10 to 15 minutes, or until the potatoes are tender. Remove from the heat.
2. Allow the soup to cool slightly, then puree it. Return the pureed soup to the rinsed-out saucepan, add the half-and-half, if using, and bring just to a boil over medium-high heat. Adjust the seasoning, add the lemon juice, if desired, and serve immediately, or let cool to room temperature, refrigerate, and serve chilled.

▶ *Timesaving Tip:* Use 1 pound frozen asparagus instead of the fresh. Rinse the frozen asparagus under hot water to dissolve large chunks of ice, then proceed with the recipe.

▶ *Cooking Tip:* To add some texture, reserve the asparagus tips rather than cooking them in the soup. Then microwave, steam, or boil the tips (do not overcook), and add them to the finished soup.

▶ *Storage Tip:* This soup keeps refrigerated for about 5 days. It can be frozen, *before* the half-and-half or whole milk is added, for up to 1 month.

▶ *Health Tip:* If your doctor has restricted your fat intake, substitute margarine for the butter and additional fat-free stock or water for the half-and-half.

▶ *Complete Meal Ideas:* Serve this soup with:
> 3 ounces protein (you might want to try the Tomato and Mozzarella Salad with Fresh Basil, page 132)
> Whole wheat bread
> Reduced-fat 2% milk or low-fat yogurt
> Fresh fruit

APPROXIMATE NUTRITIONAL INFORMATION: Serving size: 1 cup asparagus-artichoke soup; Calories: 152 cals; Protein: 6 g; Carbohydrates: 15 g; Fat: 9 g; Fiber: 4 g; Sodium: 284 mg; Vitamin C: 19 mg; Folic Acid: 86 mcg; Diabetic Exchange: Bread/Starch 1, Fat 2

cheesy cauliflower-potato soup

What's in this for baby and me? Protein, calcium, and vitamin C.

THIS SOUP IS rich in **protein**, **calcium**, and **vitamin C**, and it is a good source of vitamin A, folic acid, and fiber. For a chunkier soup, puree all but 2 cups of the soup. Garnish with chopped fresh cilantro or parsley for a lovely finishing touch.

serves 6 (makes about 7 cups)

3 tablespoons unsalted butter

1 medium onion, chopped

4 cups cauliflower florets (about 1 pound),
   washed and cut into small florets

1 medium-large potato, peeled and diced

½ teaspoon salt, or to taste

4 cups fat-free low-sodium stock

1 ½ cups whole milk

1 cup grated sharp cheddar cheese, Fontina,
   or Monterey Jack

Freshly ground pepper, to taste

¼ cup chopped fresh parsley or cilantro

1   Melt the butter in a 6-quart saucepan over medium-high heat. Add the onion and sauté for 3 minutes. Add the cauliflower florets, potato, salt, and stock and bring to a boil, then reduce the heat and simmer for 15 to 20 minutes, or until the potatoes and cauliflower are tender. Remove from the heat.

2   Allow the soup to cool slightly, then puree it. Return the pureed soup to the rinsed-out saucepan. Add the milk and bring just to a boil over medium-high heat. Add the cheese, reduce the heat to low, and stir until the cheese is melted—do not let the soup boil after adding the cheese.

3   Adjust the seasoning, garnish with the parsley, and serve.

▶ **Storage Tip:** This soup keeps refrigerated for about 5 days. Do not freeze.

▶ **Complete Meal Ideas:** Serve this soup with:
   Green salad (you might want to try the Spinach Salad with Mandarin Oranges and Toasted Almonds, page 138, or a tossed salad with French-Style Tarragon Vinaigrette, page 141)
   Whole wheat bread
   Reduced-fat 2% milk or low-fat yogurt
   Fresh fruit

APPROXIMATE NUTRITIONAL INFORMATION: Serving size: 1 cup cheesy cauliflower-potato soup; Calories: 221 cal.; Protein: 10 g; Carbohydrates: 15 g; Fat: 14 g; Fiber: 3 g; Sodium: 395 mg; Vitamin C: 42 mg; Calcium: 219 mg; Diabetic Exchange: Bread/Starch 1, Fat 3, Whole Milk 1.5

food aversions and cravings

What? All of a sudden you've lost your taste for vegetables? Fruits? Fish? Chicken? But you used to love a good steak with a baked potato smothered in sour cream: Fear not. Food aversions are just as common as food cravings during pregnancy. And, like cravings, they can last for an hour, a day, weeks, or even months. Also, don't be surprised if your food aversion on Monday becomes your craving on Friday, or the other way around.

The taste for certain foods varies from person to person and can change without warning at any time during pregnancy. This is usually not a problem, but some food aversions may require effort to replace lost nutrients. For example, if you have an aversion to fruit, increase your intake of vegetables—and vice versa. If chicken or beef turn you off, increase your intake of peanut butter, eggs, cheese, dried beans and peas, or tofu. If a food aversion lasts longer than one month, or the appropriate substitutions are not meeting your daily nutrient requirements, discuss the situation with your doctor or a dietitian.

great green broccoli-spinach soup

What's in this for baby and me? Calcium, vitamins A and C, and fiber.

Tasty and healthy, this broccoli-spinach soup is high in **calcium**, **vitamins A** and **C**, and **fiber**, and it is a good source of protein, iron, and folic acid. Garnish with grated cheese or croutons.

serves 6 (makes about 7 cups)

3 tablespoons unsalted butter

1 medium onion, chopped

1 pound (about 8 cups) broccoli florets,
   washed and trimmed (see Timesaving Tip
   below)

1 medium potato, peeled and diced

4 cups fat-free low-sodium stock

1 teaspoon salt, or to taste

One 6-ounce package baby spinach, washed,

or 6–8 ounces frozen chopped spinach,
   thawed, drained, and squeezed

1 cup nonfat buttermilk

⅓ cup pasteurized instant nonfat dry milk
   (optional)

Freshly ground pepper, to taste

Shredded sharp cheddar cheese or your
   favorite cheese, for garnish

1. Melt the butter in a 6-quart saucepan over medium-high heat. Add the onion and sauté for 3 minutes. Add the broccoli, potato, stock, and salt and bring to a boil, then reduce the heat and simmer, covered, for about 15 minutes, or until the potatoes are tender. During the last 5 minutes, stir the spinach into the soup. Remove from the heat

2. Allow the soup to cool slightly, then puree it in batches in a blender or food processor. Return the pureed soup to the rinsed-out saucepan.

3. In a large measuring cup or small bowl, combine the buttermilk and dry milk and whisk until smooth. Add to the pureed soup and bring the soup just to a boil over medium-high heat. Adjust the seasoning, garnish with the cheese, and serve immediately.

▶ *Timesaving Tip:* Pick up broccoli florets from a salad bar or use 1 pound frozen broccoli florets and frozen spinach.

▶ *Storage Tip:* This soup keeps refrigerated for about 5 days. It can be frozen, before the half-and-half is added, for up to one month.

▶ *Complete Meal Ideas:* Serve this soup with:

> 3 ounces protein (you might want to try the Grilled Cheese Sandwich, page 97)
> Whole wheat bread
> Reduced-fat 2% milk or low-fat yogurt
> Fresh fruit that contains vitamin C

APPROXIMATE NUTRITIONAL INFORMATION: Serving size: 1 cup broccoli-spinach soup; Calories: 160 cals; Protein: 9 g; Carbohydrates: 17 g; Fat: 7 g; Fiber: 6 g; Sodium: 563 mg; Calcium: 206 mg; Vitamin A 2,930 IU; Vitamin C: 87 mg; Diabetic Exchange: Bread/Starch .5, Fat 1, Low-Fat Milk 1

butternut squash–carrot soup with ginger

~

What's in this for baby and me? Vitamins A and C.

THIS VELVETY SMOOTH soup is the perfect prelude to dinner, and a delicious companion to a sandwich. Butternut squash and carrots are excellent sources of **vitamins A and C**. Peeled and cut-up fresh butternut squash, found in the refrigerated produce section of many grocery stores, is ideal for this soup. If it is unavailable in your area, see the **Cooking Tip** below for instructions on using a whole squash. For a zippier soup, feel free to replace the fresh and ground ginger with 1½ teaspoons mild curry powder.

serves 6 to 8 (makes about 8½ cups)

2 tablespoons unsalted butter	⅓ cup dried apricots (optional)
1 medium onion, chopped	5 cups fat-free low-sodium stock
2 tablespoons minced fresh ginger	½ teaspoon salt, or to taste
1¼ pounds peeled and cut-up butternut squash	1 teaspoon ground ginger (optional)
	½ cup half-and-half (optional)
3 carrots, peeled and chopped, or 1½ cups sliced peeled baby carrots	¼ cup chopped fresh cilantro, for garnish (optional)

1. Melt the butter in a 6-quart saucepan over medium heat. Add the onions and fresh ginger and sauté for 3 minutes. Add the squash, carrots, apricots, if using, stock, salt, and ground ginger, if using. Bring to a boil, then reduce the heat and simmer for 10 to 15 minutes, or until the squash and carrots are tender.
2. Remove the soup from the heat and allow to cool slightly, then puree in batches. Return the pureed soup to the rinsed-out saucepan, add the half-and-half, and reheat over medium-high heat just until the soup reaches a boil. Garnish with the cilantro, if desired, and serve immediately.

▶ *Cooking Tip:* To use a whole butternut squash for this soup, preheat the oven to 375°F. Line a baking dish large enough to accommodate the squash with foil and grease the foil with 2 tablespoons canola oil. Using a sharp knife, cut a 1½-pound butternut squash lengthwise in half. Scoop out the seeds and then place the two halves cut-side down in the baking dish. Bake for 45 minutes, or until the pulp is tender. Allow the squash to cool slightly, then scoop out the flesh; you should have at least 2½ cups; set aside.

▶ *Storage Tip:* This soup keeps refrigerated for about 5 days. It can be frozen, before the half-and-half is added, for up to one month.

▶ *Complete Meal Ideas:* Serve this soup with:

    3 ounces protein (you might want to try the Pr-egg-o Salad Sandwich, page 96;
        the iron in this sandwich will be enhanced by the vitamin C in the soup)
    Whole wheat bread
    Reduced-fat 2% milk or low-fat yogurt
    Fresh fruit

APPROXIMATE NUTRITIONAL INFORMATION: Serving size: 1 cup butternut squash–carrot soup; Calories: 135 cals; Protein: 3 g; Carbohydrates: 19 g; Fat: 6 g; Fiber: 2 g; Sodium: 230 mg; Vitamin A 14,224 IU; Vitamin C: 21 mg; Diabetic Exchange: Bread/Starch 1, Fat 1

greek-style chicken, lemon, and egg soup

~

What's in this for baby and me? Protein and vitamin A.

THIS RICH, CREAMY-TEXTURED soup is an amazing source of **protein** and **vitamin A** and a good source of vitamin C, iron, and fiber. It is a cinch to make, especially if you have leftover chicken or turkey. Vegetarians can use vegetable stock and substitute additional vegetables for the chicken.

serves 6 (makes about 8 cups)

7 cups fat-free low-sodium stock

4 carrots, peeled and thinly sliced, or 2 cups sliced peeled baby carrots

1 celery stalk, washed and thinly sliced (optional)

½ cup uncooked rice (any kind except instant)

½ pound chicken tenders, sliced into thirds, or 1½ cups diced cooked chicken

3 large eggs

¼ cup freshly squeezed lemon juice (from about 1½ lemons), or to taste

½ teaspoon salt, or to taste

Freshly ground pepper, to taste

¼ cup chopped fresh parsley or dill, for garnish (optional)

1. Place the chicken stock in a 6-quart saucepan and bring to a boil. Add the carrots, celery, if using, rice, and chicken tenders or cooked chicken and bring to a boil. Reduce heat and simmer, uncovered, for 25 minutes, or until the rice is tender. Reduce the heat to low and prepare the egg-lemon mixture.
2. In a medium bowl, beat the eggs with the lemon juice until light and frothy. Gradually whisk in 3 ladlefuls of the soup broth, then add the egg mixture to the soup, stirring constantly. Stir and cook for 5 minutes longer to cook the egg *completely*.
3. Adjust the seasoning, including the lemon, garnish with the parsley, if desired, and serve immediately.

pica: an unusual craving

It has been suggested that pica, the craving for inappropriate substances with little or no nutritional value, may be associated with iron deficiency anemia. The most common non-food substances that pregnant women crave are dirt, clay, laundry starch, and ice. Other less common cravings include chalk, air fresheners, charcoal, and mothballs. Whether pica is the cause or effect of anemia remains unknown, but the condition usually clears when the anemia is treated. Consult your doctor or health-care provider if you experience the desire to consume non-food substances.[25, 26]

▶ **Storage Tip:** This soup keeps refrigerated for about 3 days. Do not freeze.

▶ **Complete Meal Ideas:** Serve this soup with:
> 3 ounces protein (such as hard cheese) if you are not using chicken
> Whole wheat bread
> Green salad (you might want to try a tossed salad with the French-Style Tarragon Vinaigrette, page 141)
> Reduced-fat 2% milk or low-fat yogurt
> Fresh fruit that contains vitamin C

APPROXIMATE NUTRITIONAL INFORMATION: Serving size: 1 cup Greek-style chicken soup; Calories: 189 cals; Protein: 19 g; Carbohydrates: 18 g; Fat: 4 g; Fiber: 2 g; Sodium: 344 mg; Vitamin A: 11,598 IU; Diabetic Exchange: Bread/Starch 1, Fat 1, Meat (Lean) 2

black bean soup with cilantro

What's in this for baby and me? Protein, vitamins A and C, folic acid, and fiber.

THIS SOUP IS a fabulous source of **protein**, **vitamins A** and **C**, **folic acid**, and **fiber**, and a good source of iron. Canned beans are a real time-saver. The spices and garnishes are optional (especially for young eaters), but they add color and a burst of flavor. Pureeing some cups of the soup is optional too, though it gives it a wonderful consistency. In addition to fresh cilantro, other traditional garnishes include grated cheddar cheese and (reduced-fat) sour cream. **Slow Cooker Instructions** follow.

serves 8 (makes about 8 cups)

2 tablespoons canola oil

1 large onion, chopped

4 carrots, peeled and sliced, or 2 cups sliced peeled baby carrots

¼ cup diced jarred roasted red peppers (optional)

3 garlic cloves, crushed (optional)

2 teaspoons ground cumin (optional)

2 teaspoons dried oregano (ground or whole)

or dried basil (optional)

½ teaspoon chili powder (optional)

Two 19-ounce cans black beans, drained

5 cups fat-free low-sodium stock or water, or more as needed

1 cup V-8 juice

Salt and freshly ground pepper, to taste

Chopped fresh cilantro, for garnish (optional)

1. Heat the canola oil in a 6-quart saucepan over medium-high heat until hot. Add the onion and sauté for 3 minutes. Add the carrots, and the optional red peppers, garlic, cumin, oregano, and chili powder and sauté for 3 minutes. Add the beans, stock, and V-8 juice and bring to a boil, then reduce the heat and simmer, uncovered, for 20 minutes, or until the carrots are tender.
2. Allow the soup to cool slightly, then puree 3 cups of it. Return the pureed soup to the saucepan and stir. Add stock or water to thin the soup if desired.
3. Adjust the seasoning, add the cilantro, and serve immediately.

▶ *Cooking Tip:* Stock or water can be substituted for the V-8 juice.

▶ *Storage Tip:* This soup keeps refrigerated for about 1 week, and it can be frozen for up to 1 month.

▶ *Slow Cooker Instructions: Use 3½ cups stock instead of 5 cups. Because this recipe calls for canned black beans, the cooking time is short, even in a slow cooker. When the carrots are soft, the soup is essentially ready, usually after 4 hours on high heat.*

1. Using a large nonstick skillet instead of a saucepan, sauté the onion as directed in Step 1, then add the carrots, and the optional bell peppers, garlic, cumin, oregano, and chili powder, and sauté for 3 minutes.
2. Transfer the contents of the skillet to the slow cooker, then add the black beans, stock, and V-8 juice. Cover and cook on high for 6 hours. Finish the soup as directed in Steps 2 and 3.

▶ *Complete Meal Ideas:* Serve this soup with:
  Corn bread or whole wheat bread (you might also want to try the Cheese and Spinach Quesadillas, page 184)
  Green salad
  Reduced-fat 2% milk or low-fat yogurt
  Fresh fruit that contains vitamin C

APPROXIMATE NUTRITIONAL INFORMATION: Serving size: 1 cup black bean soup; Calories: 211 cals; Protein: 11 g; Carbohydrates: 30 g; Fat: 6 g; Fiber: 10 g; Sodium: 160 mg; Vitamin A: 8,892 IU; Vitamin C: 18 mg; Folic Acid: 163 mcg; Diabetic Exchange: Bread/Starch 1.5, Fat 2

lentil soup with brown rice and spinach

⌒

What's in this for baby and me? Protein, iron, vitamin A, folic acid, and fiber.

The combination of lentils, brown rice, and spinach provides a powerhouse of **protein**, **iron**, **vitamin A**, **folic acid**, and **fiber**. For a lighter soup, omit the rice and increase the lentils to 1⅓ cups. Kids might prefer the soup without the spinach. The balsamic vinegar added to the soup at the last minute gives it a wonderful tang, and the olive oil adds richness. **Slow Cooker Instructions** follow.

serves 8 (makes about 10 cups)

2 tablespoons olive oil

1 medium onion, finely chopped

2 garlic cloves, crushed

4 carrots, peeled and finely diced, or 2 cups sliced peeled baby carrots

½ cup uncooked brown rice (or any rice except instant)

1 tablespoon dried thyme

2 bay leaves (optional)

10 cups fat-free low-sodium stock or water, or more as needed

1 cup green lentils, picked over and rinsed

One 5-ounce bag baby spinach, washed, or 5 ounces (half a 10-ounce package) frozen spinach, thawed and drained

Salt and freshly ground pepper, to taste

Balsamic or red wine vinegar, to taste, for garnish (optional)

Olive oil, to taste, for garnish (optional)

1. Heat the olive oil in a 6-quart saucepan over medium heat. Add the onion and sauté for 3 minutes. Add the garlic, carrots, brown rice, thyme, and optional bay leaves and sauté for 3 minutes. Add the stock and lentils, stir, and bring to a boil. Skim off the foam with a spoon, then reduce the heat and simmer for about 35 minutes, or until the lentils are cooked. After 25 minutes of cooking, remove the bay leaves from the soup (if using), stir in the spinach.
2. If the finished soup is too thick, add more stock or water ¼ cup at a time.
3. Add a couple of drops of vinegar and olive oil, adjust the seasoning, and serve immediately.

▶ *Timesaving Tip:* Add diced vegetables to a packaged lentil soup mix and season with dried herbs and oil and vinegar if desired.

▶ *Storage Tip:* This soup keeps refrigerated for about 5 days, and can be frozen for up to 1 month.

▶ **Health Tip:** If your doctor has restricted your fat intake, omit the olive oil garnish to the finished soup.

▶ **Slow Cooker Instructions:** *Use 9 cups of stock instead of 10. (If you are not omitting the brown rice and increasing the amount of lentils to 1½ cups, use 8 cups of stock.)*

1. Using a large nonstick skillet instead of a saucepan, sauté the onion as directed in Step 1, then add the garlic, carrots, thyme, and optional bay leaves and sauté for 3 minutes more.

2. Transfer the contents of the skillet to the slow cooker, then add the lentils and stock. Cover and cook on high for 6 hours, or until the carrots and lentils are soft. Add the brown rice and spinach and cook 30 minutes longer. (*Note:* Do not leave the slow cooker unattended while cooking the brown rice.) Thin the soup with stock or water if desired, and finish the soup as directed in Step 3.

▶ **Complete Meal Ideas:** Serve this lentil soup with:
    Whole wheat bread
    Reduced-fat 2% milk or low-fat yogurt
    Fresh fruit that contains vitamin C (you might want to try the Orange, Blueberry, and Date Salad with Frozen Yogurt, page 283)

APPROXIMATE NUTRITIONAL INFORMATION: Serving size: 1 cup lentil soup with brown rice and spinach; Calories: 176 cals; Protein: 11 g; Carbohydrates: 25 g; Fat: 4 g; Fiber: 10 g; Sodium: 246 mg; Iron 4 mg; Vitamin A: 1,841 IU; Folic Acid: 110 mcg; Diabetic Exchange: Bread/Starch 1.5, Fat, 1

turkish-style red lentil soup

What's in this for baby and me? Protein, iron, vitamin A, folic acid, and fiber.

THIS QUICK-COOKING earthy soup is delicious any time of year. The lentils are an excellent source of **protein**, **iron**, **vitamin A**, **folic acid**, and **fiber**, and a good source of vitamin C. The sautéed mint and paprika garnish is optional, but it adds a distinctive flavor to the soup. If you are short on time, simply add the mint and paprika directly to the soup during the last twenty minutes of cooking time. Or, garnish the soup instead with chopped fresh cilantro or parsley and a swirl of low-fat plain yogurt. This soup can be pureed for a finer consistency. **Slow Cooker Instructions** follow.

serves 6 to 8 (makes about 7 cups)

2 tablespoons unsalted butter

1 medium onion, chopped

2 garlic cloves, crushed

3 carrots, peeled and sliced, or 1½ cups sliced peeled baby carrots

1½ cups red lentils, picked over and rinsed

7 cups fat-free low-sodium stock or water, or more as needed

Salt and freshly ground pepper, to taste

Garnish (optional)

    1½ tablespoons unsalted butter

    1 teaspoon dried mint

    Dash of paprika or red pepper

1. Melt the butter in a 6-quart saucepan over medium-high heat. Add the onion and sauté for 3 minutes. Add the garlic, carrots, lentils, and stock and bring to a boil. Reduce the heat and simmer, uncovered, for 30 minutes, or until the carrots are soft and the lentils are mushy.
2. Thin the finished soup with additional stock or water if desired. Adjust the seasoning and keep warm while you prepare the garnish.
3. To prepare the garnish, melt the butter in a small saucepan over medium-high heat. Add the mint and paprika and cook for 10 to 20 seconds, or just until fragrant. Add the garnish to individual soup bowls (or add it to the soup in the saucepan). (*Note:* You can also add the mint and paprika directly to the soup during the last 20 minutes of cooking.)

▶ *Cooking Tip:* The bright orange lentils will lose some of their color during cooking and the finished soup will be a golden yellow color.

▶ *Storage Tip:* This soup keeps refrigerated for about 1 week, and it can be frozen for up to 1 month.

▶ *Variation:* Add your favorite diced vegetables or dried herbs and spices to this soup when you add the carrots in Step 1. Substitute a dash of mild curry powder for the chili powder.

▶ *Slow Cooker Instructions:* *Use 6½ cups stock instead of 7.*
1. Melt the butter in a large nonstick skillet over medium-high heat. Add the onions and sauté for 3 minutes, then add the garlic and carrots and sauté for 2 minutes.
2. Transfer the contents of the skillet to the slow cooker. Add the lentils and stock, cover, and cook on high for 4 hours, or until the carrots are tender. Follow Step #3 to finish the soup, or omit the butter and add the mint and paprika directly to the soup during the last 20 minutes of cooking.

▶ *Complete Meal Ideas:* Serve this soup with:
Whole wheat bread
Vegetable that contains vitamin C (you might want to try the Tomato and Mozzarella Salad with Fresh Basil, page 132)
Reduced-fat 2% milk or low-fat yogurt
Fresh fruit that contains vitamin C

APPROXIMATE NUTRITIONAL INFORMATION: Serving size: 1 cup red lentil soup; Calories: 236 cals; Protein: 15 g; Carbohydrates: 34 g; Fat: 5 g; Fiber: 6 g; Sodium: 280 mg; Vitamin A: 8,756 IU; Iron: 4 mg; Folic Acid: 106 mcg; Diabetic Exchange: Bread/Starch 2, Fat .5, Meat (Lean) 1

mediterranean pasta, bean, and vegetable soup

~

What's in this for baby and me? Iron, vitamins A and C, and fiber.

THIS THICK AND hearty soup is sure to become a family favorite—kids love it with alphabet pasta (add about 1½ cups) or any other small pasta. This soup is loaded with **iron, vitamins A** and **C**, and **fiber**. It is also a good source of protein, folic acid, and B vitamins. Don't be put off by the long ingredient list—many of the ingredients are optional. For a real treat, or an elegant first course, garnish this soup with pesto (homemade, page 121, or store-bought) and grated Parmesan cheese. This soup is even better on the second day, and it freezes well. A pureed or strained version (without the pesto and cheese) makes a super meal for young eaters. **Slow Cooker Instructions** follow.

serves 6 (makes about 8 cups)

3 tablespoons olive oil or canola oil

1 medium onion, finely diced

2 garlic cloves, crushed (optional)

5 carrots, peeled, cut lengthwise in half, and sliced, or 2 cups sliced peeled baby carrots

2 teaspoons dried thyme, oregano, basil, or herbes de Provence

1 teaspoon salt, or to taste

5 cups fat-free low-sodium stock (6 cups if omitting the V-8 juice, or more if needed)

1½ cups V-8 or tomato juice (see Vegetable Variation below)

One 14.5-ounce can diced tomatoes (do not drain) or 2 cups diced fresh tomatoes

One 15.5-ounce can Great Northern white beans (or any other small canned beans), drained

1 medium zucchini, washed, quartered lengthwise, and sliced

¾ cup ditalini pasta, or other small pasta

1 small bunch (about 10 ounces) Swiss chard, spinach, beet greens, or arugula, washed, stems removed, and thinly sliced (optional) (see Timesaving Tip below about using frozen greens)

Freshly ground pepper, to taste

Pesto, for the table (optional)

Grated Parmesan cheese or your favorite cheese, for the table (optional)

1. Heat the olive oil in a 6-quart saucepan over medium-high heat. Add the onion and sauté for 2 minutes. Add the garlic, if using, carrots, and thyme and sauté for 3 minutes. Add the salt, stock, and V-8 juice, if using, and bring to a boil. Reduce the heat and simmer, uncovered, for 10 minutes.

2. Add the tomatoes, beans, zucchini, and pasta, reduce the heat, and simmer for 15 to 20 minutes, or until the pasta is cooked. Add the greens during the last 10 minutes of cooking.

3. Adjust the seasoning, and thin the soup with stock or water if desired. Serve immediately and pass the pesto and cheese at the table, if desired.

▶ **Timesaving Tip:** Use one 10-ounce package frozen spinach or other greens in place of fresh. Microwave or defrost and drain well, then add to the soup during the last 5 minutes of cooking.

▶ **Vegetable Variation:** Add any favorite vegetables that require a longer cooking time (such as potatoes, winter squash, or leeks) with the carrots in Step 1; add any quick-cooking vegetables (such as broccoli or cauliflower florets, summer squash, corn, peas, and green beans or wax beans) with the zucchini in Step 3. Add any greens (fresh or frozen) during the last 5 minutes of cooking time. For a less "tomato-y" soup, omit the V-8 juice and use 7 cups stock.

▶ **Protein Variation:** Add sautéed tofu (see Instructions for Sautéing Tofu, page 189), diced cooked chicken or turkey, or any other cooked meat during the last 10 minutes of Step 2.

▶ **Storage Tip:** This soup keeps refrigerated for about 1 week, and it can be frozen for up to 1 month.

▶ **Slow Cooker Instructions:** *Reduce the stock by ½ cup. Use only ½ cup pasta.*
   1. Using a nonstick skillet instead of a saucepan, sauté onion as directed in Step 1, then add the garlic, if using, carrots, and thyme and sauté for 3 more minutes.
   2. Transfer the contents of the skillet to the slow cooker, and add the salt, stock, V-8 juice, and diced tomatoes. Cover and cook on high for 6 hours. During the last 30 minutes of cooking, add the beans, pasta, and Swiss chard. (*Note*: Do not leave the slow cooker unattended while cooking the pasta.) Finish the soup as directed in Step 3.

▶ **Complete Meal Ideas:** Serve this soup with:
   3 ounces protein (you might want to try the Grilled Cheese Sandwich, page 97, or the Hummus-Tabbouleh Roll, page 105)
   Whole wheat bread
   Reduced-fat 2% milk or low-fat yogurt
   Fresh fruit that contains vitamin C

APPROXIMATE NUTRITIONAL INFORMATION: Serving size: 1 cup pasta, bean, and vegetable soup; Calories: 210 cals; Protein: 9 g; Carbohydrates: 31 g; Fat: 6 g; Fiber: 8 g; Sodium: 667 mg; Vitamin A: 10,877 IU; Vitamin C: 32 mg; Iron: 5 mg; Diabetic Exchange: Bread/Starch 2, Fat 1

green split pea soup

What's in this for baby and me? Protein, vitamin A, folic acid, and fiber.

SPLIT PEA SOUP is an excellent source of **protein**, **vitamin A**, **folic acid**, and **fiber**, and a good source of iron. If you insist that green split pea soup needs a ham bone for flavor, this lighter recipe might convince you otherwise. Croutons make a nice garnish (see Homemade Croutons, page 140). **Slow Cooker Instructions** follow.

serves 6 (makes about 7 cups)

3 tablespoons unsalted butter

1 medium onion, finely chopped

2 garlic cloves, crushed

4 carrots, peeled and sliced, or 2 cups sliced
    peeled baby carrots

2 celery stalks, washed and sliced (optional)

1 teaspoon dried thyme (optional)

1 teaspoon dried marjoram (optional)

2 bay leaves (optional)

8 cups fat free low-sodium stock or water, or
    more as needed

1½ cups (10 ounces) green split peas (see
    Cooking Tip below)

Salt and freshly ground pepper, to taste

1. Heat the butter in a 6-quart saucepan over medium heat. Add the onion and sauté for 3 minutes. Add the garlic, carrots, and optional celery, thyme, marjoram, and bay leaves and sauté for 3 minutes longer.
2. Add the stock and peas, stir, and bring to a boil. Skim off the foam with a spoon, then reduce the heat and simmer for about 2 hours, or until the peas are tender.
3. If the soup is too thick, add more stock or water, 2 tablespoons at a time. Adjust the seasoning, remove the bay leaves and serve immediately.

▶ *Cooking Tip:* Pick over and rinse the peas, then soak them for 8 to 12 hours in 5 cups water. Or, for faster results, place the peas in a 3-quart saucepan, add water to cover by at least 2 inches, and bring to a boil. Cook for 2 minutes, then remove from the heat and let stand, covered, at room temperature, for at least 1 hour or up to 6 hours. Drain, rinse again, and proceed with the recipe.

▶ *Timesaving Tip:* Use packaged instant split pea soup. Add your favorite cooked, diced vegetables or seasonings suggested here.

▶ *Storage Tip:* This soup keeps refrigerated for about 5 days, and it can be frozen for up to 1 month.

▶ *Slow Cooker Instructions: It is essential to soak the peas before adding them to the slow cooker. The amount of time it takes for the peas to cook will vary;, it may take up to 10 hours. Use 6 cups stock instead of 8.*

1. Follow the instructions in the **Cooking Tip** above to soften the peas before cooking.
2. Using a large nonstick skillet instead of a saucepan, follow the instructions in Step 1.
3. Transfer the contents of the skillet to the slow cooker. Add the drained soaked peas and the stock, cover, and cook on high for 8 hours, or possibly up to 10 hours, until the peas are soft. Finish the soup as directed in Step 3.

▶ *Complete Meal Ideas:* Serve this soup with:
Whole wheat bread (you might want to try the Veggie Cheese Wrap, page 103)
Reduced-fat 2% milk or low-fat yogurt
Fresh fruit that contains vitamin C

APPROXIMATE NUTRITIONAL INFORMATION: Serving size: 1 cup green split pea soup; Calories: 203 cals; Protein: 11 g; Carbohydrates: 26 g; Fat: 7 g; Fiber: 10 g; Sodium: 306 mg; Vitamin A: 11,721 IU; Folic Acid: 100 mcg; Diabetic Exchange: Bread/Starch 1.5, Meat (Medium Fat) 1

buying canned soups

The canned soup market is booming, and manufacturers are producing healthier products. Choose canned, jarred, or boxed soups low in sodium and fat and high in protein (containing 8 to 10 g). High-protein soups usually contain poultry, meat, or beans. Read labels carefully and opt for all-natural soups whenever possible. For a calcium boost, add powdered milk to milk-based soups (canned or homemade), such as cream of mushroom, asparagus, or cream of tomato. Also, as an alternative to canned soups, look for packaged protein- and iron-rich instant bean, lentil, and mixed bean soups.

beef, barley, and vegetable soup

What's in this for baby and me? Protein and vitamins A and C.

THE SOUP IS an excellent source of **protein** and **vitamins A** and **C**, as well as a good source of iron, B vitamins, and fiber. Any vegetables, from potatoes and turnips to broccoli and spinach, can be added in place of the beef to make this a hearty vegetarian soup. Grated Parmesan cheese is a lovely garnish. This soup is even better the second day. **Slow Cooker Instructions** follow.

serves 6 to 8 (makes about 8 cups)

2 tablespoons canola oil or olive oil

1 medium onion, finely diced

4 carrots, peeled and sliced, or 2 cups sliced
   peeled baby carrots

½ cup uncooked pearl barley, rinsed under hot
   water

1 pound beef shank, bone-in

One 14.5-ounce can peeled and diced tomatoes (do not drain) or 1½ cups peeled and

diced fresh tomatoes

8 cups fat-free low-sodium stock, or more as
   needed

1 zucchini, washed, halved lengthwise, and
   sliced

Salt and freshly ground pepper, to taste

¼ cup chopped fresh parsley, for garnish
   (optional)

1. Heat the canola oil in a 6-quart saucepan over medium-high heat. Add the onion and sauté for 3 minutes. Add the carrots and barley and sauté for 3 minutes. Add the beef, tomatoes, and stock and bring to a boil. Reduce the heat and simmer, uncovered, for 20 minutes.
2. Add the zucchini and simmer for about 25 minutes longer, or until the barley and meat are tender.
3. Remove the shank from the soup, and when it is cool enough to handle, remove the meat from the bone. Cut the meat into small pieces and return it to the soup.
4. Add more canned stock or water to thin the soup, if desired, and adjust the seasoning and heat through before serving. Garnish with the parsley, if desired, and serve immediately.

▶ **Storage Tip:** This soup keeps refrigerated for about 3 days, and it can be frozen for up to 1 month.

▶ **Slow Cooker Instructions:** *Use 6 cups stock instead of 8. Drain the diced tomatoes.*
1. Using a large nonstick skillet instead of a saucepan, sauté the onion as directed in Step 1. Add the carrots and barley and sauté for 3 minutes.

2. Transfer the contents of the skillet to the slow cooker, then add the beef shank, *drained* diced tomatoes, zucchini, and stock. Cover and cook on high for 6 hours.

3. Finish the soup as directed in steps 3 and 4.

▶ *Complete Meal Ideas:* Serve this soup with:

3 ounces protein (such as hard cheese) if you are not using the beef shank (you might want to try the Roasted Red Pepper and Cheese Dip, page 146, with your bread)

Whole wheat bread

Reduced-fat 2% milk or low-fat yogurt

Fresh fruit that contains vitamin C

APPROXIMATE NUTRITIONAL INFORMATION: Serving size: 1½ cups beef, barley, and vegetable soup: Calories: 240 cals; Protein: 18 g; Carbohydrates: 17 g; Fat: 11 g; Fiber: 4 g; Sodium: 312 mg; Vitamin A: 9,994 IU; Vitamin C: 18 mg; Diabetic Exchange: Bread/starch 1, Fat .5, Meat (Medium Fat) 2

gazpacho

What's in this for baby and me? Vitamins A and C.

GAZPACHO IS A fantastic source of **vitamins A** and **C**, and a good source of folic acid and fiber. A quick and easy soup that involves no cooking, it is the ideal first course for a summer meal, or a refreshing snack any time of day. Saltine crackers, a staple snack food for most pregnant women, are used in this soup instead of traditional bread. Puree to a chunky or smooth consistency, then add diced cucumber, tomatoes, radishes, or avocado for additional texture if desired. Serve well chilled.

serves 2 (makes about 2 cups)

4 saltine crackers

1 pound (about 3) vine-ripened tomatoes, quartered

¾ cup peeled and sliced seedless cucumber

¼ cup jarred roasted red peppers

A dash of garlic powder (optional)

¼ cup water, fat-free low-sodium stock, or V-8 juice

Leaves from 4 sprigs of fresh cilantro (optional)

Salt and freshly ground pepper, to taste

A few drops of olive oil

A few drops of balsamic vinegar

1. Combine all of the ingredients except the olive oil and balsamic vinegar in a blender or food processor and pulse until desired consistency.
2. Transfer to a bowl, cover, and refrigerate until well chilled, at least 1 hour. Stir in the olive oil and balsamic vinegar, adjust the seasoning, and serve.

▶ *Storage Tip:* This soup keeps refrigerated for up to 3 days. Do not freeze.

▶ *Health Tip:* If your doctor has restricted your fat intake, omit the olive oil.

▶ *Complete Meal Ideas:* Serve this gazpacho with:
> 3 ounces protein (you might want to try the Tuna Salad, page 101, or the Grilled Cheese Sandwich, page 97)
> Whole wheat bread
> Reduced-fat 2% milk or low-fat yogurt
> Fresh fruit

APPROXIMATE NUTRITIONAL INFORMATION: Serving size: 1 cup gazpacho; Calories: 103 cals; Protein: 3 g; Carbohydrates: 17 g; Fat: 4 g; Fiber: 3 g; Sodium: 100 mg; Vitamin A: 2,133 IU; Vitamin C: 74 mg; Diabetic Exchange: Bread/Starch 1, Fat 1

drink plenty of water

~

Fluid intake is vital throughout pregnancy. A pregnant woman needs to drink 1 quart (4 cups) to 1½ quarts (6 cups) of water every day *in addition* to milk. Fruit juices are high in calories (for a list of the calorie content of juices, see Get Juiced Up, page 56), so one or two servings per day is fine, but do not drink fruit juice in place of water.

Why Is Water So Important?

To aid with digestion

To ensure proper hydration

To avoid constipation

To reduce the risk of urinary tract infections

To eliminate toxins and keep your system clean

To regulate your body temperature

To reduce swelling

To prevent dry skin

basic chicken stock

~

What's in this for baby and me? Vitamin A.

THERE IS NOTHING quite like the soul-warming aroma of chicken stock simmering on the stove. The key to this low-fat stock is to allow time to chill it before using it. Chilling congeals the fat on the surface of the stock, which makes it easy to remove. Use this recipe as a blueprint—add or omit any vegetables, herbs, or spices to suit your taste. The cooked chicken from this recipe can be used for Greek-Style Chicken, Lemon, and Egg Soup (page 76), Chicken Salad with Diced Apricots and Almonds (page 98). **Slow Cooker Instructions** follow.

makes 7 to 8 cups

One 3¼- to 3½-pound chicken or 3¼ pound
   chicken parts, rinsed and any large chunks
   of fat removed
1 medium onion, quartered
1 large carrot, scrubbed and quartered
1 celery stalk, washed and quartered
   (optional)

5 fresh parsley sprigs (optional)
2 bay leaves (optional)
2 teaspoons salt, or to taste
10 to 12 cups water, or enough to completely
   cover all ingredients
Freshly ground pepper, to taste

1. In a large stockpot, combine all of the ingredients and bring to a boil. Reduce the heat and simmer, uncovered, for 1½ hours. If the water level drops below the height of the stock ingredients before the stock has simmered for 1 hour, add ½ cup of water at a time, or just enough to keep the ingredients covered.
2. Transfer the chicken to a plate; set aside. Strain the stock into a heatproof bowl. Allow the stock to cool to room temperature, then refrigerate until chilled.
3. When the chicken is cool enough to handle, remove the meat from the bones. (This is more easily done while the chicken is still warm.) Cover and refrigerate for another use.
4. Once the stock has chilled, remove it from the refrigerator and, using a large spoon, scrape off as much fat from the surface as possible. Refrigerate until needed.

▶ *Storage Tip:* This stock keeps for about 3 days refrigerated, and it can be frozen for up to 3 months. If you do not plan to use the frozen stock all at once, freeze it in smaller containers so you can defrost only what you need.

▶ *Slow Cooker Instructions: Use a 3- to 3¼-pound whole chicken and 8 cups of water instead of 10 to 12 cups.*

1. Coarsely chop the onion, carrot, and celery stalk. Arrange the onions, carrots, and celery in the bottom of a slow cooker. Add the chicken or 3¼ pounds chicken parts and the remaining ingredients. Cover and cook on high for 8 hours, or until the chicken is tender and falling off the bone.
2. Finish the stock as directed in Steps 2 through 4.

APPROXIMATE NUTRITIONAL INFORMATION: *Serving size: 1 cup basic chicken stock; Calories: 30 cals; Protein: 4 g; Carbohydrates: 3 g; Fat: 0 g; Fiber: 0 g; Sodium: 885 mg; Diabetic Exchange: 1 cup FREE

*Ten cups of fat free low-sodium chicken broth were used to calculate the nutritional information instead of a whole cooked chicken.

basic vegetable stock

What's in this for baby and me? Vitamins A and C.

THIS VEGETABLE STOCK, which is high in **vitamins A** and **C**, is so good, you can eat it as a soup, with your favorite additions. Before you begin the stock, think about what you would like the dominant flavor to be. Herbs—such as rosemary, sage, cilantro, and even lemongrass—can be used to flavor your stock. For a fabulous Asian-style vegetarian soup, add miso to the finished stock, along with vegetables, sautéed tofu (see Instructions for Sautéing Tofu, page 189), soba noodles, and fresh herbs.

makes about 6 cups

3 tablespoons olive oil or canola oil

1 medium onion, quartered

2 carrots, scrubbed and coarsely chopped

2 large garlic cloves, crushed

6–8 ounces mushrooms (preferably cremini), washed and cut into thick slices

1 cup boiling water

12 cups water

2 bay leaves (optional)

½ teaspoon each dried oregano and dried thyme (or 1 teaspoon of either herb)

One 14.5-ounce can peeled and diced tomatoes (do not drain) or 1½ cups peeled and diced fresh tomatoes, with their juice (optional)

1 teaspoon salt, or to taste

1. Preheat the oven to 425°F.
2. Place the olive oil in a large baking dish, add the onion, carrots, garlic, and mushrooms, and stir to lightly coat the vegetables with the oil. Roast for 30 to 40 minutes, or until the vegetables are nicely browned.
3. Transfer the roasted vegetables to a 6-quart saucepan. Add the boiling water to the baking dish and scrape up as much of the roasted bits in the bottom of the pan as possible, then add the liquid to the saucepan.
4. Add the remaining ingredients and bring to a boil, then reduce the heat and simmer gently for 1 hour, or until the stock is slightly reduced and the flavors have had a chance to develop.
5. Strain the stock into a heatproof bowl; use the back of a ladle or spoon to press against the solids to extract as much liquid as possible. Allow the stock to cool to room temperature, and refrigerate until ready to use.

▶ *Storage Tip:* This stock keeps for about 3 days refrigerated, and it can be frozen for up to 3 months. If you do not plan to use the frozen stock all at once, freeze it in smaller containers so you can defrost only what you need.

APPROXIMATE NUTRITIONAL INFORMATION: Serving size: 1 cup basic vegetable stock; Calories: 99 cals; Protein: 2 g; Carbohydrates: 8 g; Fat: 7 g; Fiber: 2 g; Sodium: 617 mg; Vitamin A: 5,799 IU; Vitamin C: 14 mg; Diabetic Exchange: Fat 1, Vegetable 1

pr-egg-o salad sandwich

What's in this for baby and me? Protein, iron, folic acid, and fiber.

A SIMPLE EGG salad sandwich is a wonderfully easy way to get **protein**, **iron**, **folic acid**, and **fiber** into your diet, especially if you're a vegetarian. This sandwich is also a good source of B vitamins and calcium. Serve this egg salad in a sandwich, or as a salad on top of a bed of lettuce. Doctor it up with your favorite seasonings, herbs, or vegetables, or keep it simple. This recipe can easily be doubled.

makes 1 sandwich (makes about ½ cup salad)

2 hard-boiled large eggs, chopped
2 tablespoons diced celery (optional)
1 tablespoon light mayonnaise, or to taste
Salt and freshly ground pepper, to taste

2 slices hearty whole wheat bread or calcium-enriched bread (such as Calcium Enriched Roman Meal)

1. Gently mix the eggs, celery, if using, mayonnaise, and salt and pepper in a small bowl.
2. Spread the egg salad on one of the slices of bread, top with the remaining bread, and cut in half. (Refrigerate any leftovers.)

▶ *Variation:* For an herbal touch, add 1 tablespoon sliced scallions or chives and 1 tablespoon chopped fresh parsley, dill, tarragon, or chervil to the egg salad. Or, for a more full-flavored taste, add a dash of paprika, curry powder, mustard, or Tabasco, or a few capers or olives. For a colorful salad, add diced fresh red bell peppers or jarred red peppers.

▶ *Complete Meal Ideas:* Serve this sandwich with:
A raw or cooked vegetable, vegetable soup, or green salad (you might want to try the Creamy Asparagus-Artichoke Soup, page 68, or the Great Green Broccoli-Spinach Soup, page 72.)
Reduced-fat 2% milk or low-fat yogurt
Fresh fruit that contains vitamin C

APPROXIMATE NUTRITIONAL INFORMATION: Serving size: 1 egg salad sandwich (½ cup) on 2 slices whole wheat bread; Calories: 446 cals; Protein: 20 g; Carbohydrates: 47 g; Fat: 21 g; Fiber: 6 g; Sodium: 822 mg; Iron: 4 mg; Folic Acid: 80 mcg; Diabetic Exchange: Bread/Starch 3, Fat 2, Meat (Medium Fat) 2

grilled cheese sandwich

What's in this for baby and me? Protein, calcium, and fiber.

No NEED TO reinvent the wheel—but spreading the mayonnaise on the *outside* of the bread prevents sticking while using a minimal amount of fat. The cheese and calcium-enriched bread are great sources of **protein**, **calcium**, and **fiber**. To entice young children to try a bite, cut the sandwich into their favorite shapes with cookie cutters.

makes 1 sandwich

1 teaspoon light mayonnaise

2 slices of hearty whole grain bread or
   enriched bread (such as Calcium Enriched
   Roman Meal)

2 ounces sliced favorite high-calcium cheese

(such as 2 to 3 slices 2% Milk Singles
reduced-fat pasteurized process cheese
with added calcium)

Mustard, to taste (optional)

1. Place a small nonstick skillet over medium-high heat. Thinly spread half of the mayonnaise on one side of a bread slice, then place the slice *mayonnaise-side down* in the skillet. Arrange the cheese slices on top of the bread. Spread mustard, if using, on one side of the second bread slice and the rest of the mayonnaise on the *other side*, and place the bread *mayonnaise-side up on top of the cheese.*
2. Cook the first side until nicely browned and the cheese is beginning to melt (check by lifting up the sandwich). Flip the sandwich and cook the other side until nicely browned and the cheese is entirely melted. Cut in half and serve.

▶ *Complete Meal Ideas:* Serve this sandwich with:
   A raw or cooked vegetable, a vegetable soup, or a green salad (you might want to try the Mediterranean Pasta, Bean, and Vegetable Soup, page 84, or the Gazpacho, page 90.)
   Reduced-fat 2% milk or low-fat yogurt
   Fresh fruit

APPROXIMATE NUTRITIONAL INFORMATION: Serving size: 1 grilled cheese sandwich on whole grain bread; Calories: 354 cals; Protein: 17 g; Carbohydrates: 48 g; Fat: 13 g; Fiber: 6 g; Sodium: 1,220 mg; Calcium 346 mg; Diabetic Exchange: Bread/Starch 3, Fat 2, Meat (Medium Fat) 1

chicken salad
with dried apricots
and almonds

What's in this for baby and me? Protein and vitamin C.

HIGH IN **protein** and **vitamin C** and a good source of vitamin A and fiber, this chicken salad is terrific on toasted whole grain bread or on a bed of mixed greens. The almonds are optional, but, especially when toasted, they add depth of flavor. This salad is not designed for children, but a serving of the plain cooked chicken and diced apricots could be set aside to make a perfect meal for a young eater. This recipe can be halved.

makes 4 to 6 sandwiches (makes about 3 cups salad)

2 teaspoons canola oil (if using the chicken tenders)

1 pound chicken tenders or boneless, skinless chicken breasts, cut into 1-inch cubes, or about 2½ cups finely diced cooked chicken or turkey

Salt and freshly ground pepper, to taste

⅓ cup chopped dried apricots

2 tablespoons chopped fresh herbs, such as cilantro or dill (optional)

½ red bell pepper, finely diced, or ¼ cup chopped jarred roasted red peppers

½ cup sliced almonds, toasted

½ cup light mayonnaise, or to taste

1. If using chicken tenders, heat the canola oil in a large nonstick skillet over medium-high heat. Add the chicken, season with salt and pepper, and sauté for 7 minutes, or until completely cooked; transfer to a bowl to cool. Dice the cooked chicken, or tear the meat into bits with your fingers, and return to the bowl.
2. Combine the diced chicken and the remaining ingredients in a bowl and mix well. Adjust the seasoning. Refrigerate if not serving immediately. (Any leftovers should be covered and refrigerated.)

▶ *Timesaving Tip:* Buy a rotisserie chicken and cut or tear the meat into small pieces.

▶ *Variation:* Feel free to add your favorite spices, herbs, and other ingredients to the salad. Some nice additions are diced celery, toasted pine nuts, and curry powder.

▶ *Complete Meal Ideas:* Serve this salad with:

Green salad (you might want to try a tossed salad with the Sun-Dried Tomato and Basil Dressing, page 142, or romaine lettuce with the Caesar Salad Dressing, page 143)

Whole wheat roll or bread

Reduced-fat 2% milk or low-fat yogurt

Fresh fruit

APPROXIMATE NUTRITIONAL INFORMATION: Serving size: ¾ cup chicken salad (not including bread): Calories: 307 cals; Protein: 25 g; Carbohydrates: 13 g; Fat: 17 g; Fiber: 3 g; Sodium: 199 mg; Vitamin C: 15 mg; Diabetic Exchange: Bread/Starch 1, Fat 1, Meat (Medium Fat) 3

the perfect brown-bag lunch

Quick and easy peanut butter (or other nut butter) sandwiches made with whole wheat bread remain one of America's healthiest and most beloved sandwiches.

THE PERFECT BROWN BAG LUNCH

Peanut butter or other protein-rich sandwich

Vegetable sticks or V-8 juice

A couple of healthy oatmeal cookies

A piece of fresh fruit

8 ounces of low-fat yogurt or a glass of reduced-fat 2% milk

APPROXIMATE NUTRITIONAL INFORMATION: 1 peanut butter and jelly sandwich on whole wheat bread made with 3 tablespoons peanut butter and 2 teaspoons jam; Calories: 445 cals; Protein: 17 g; Carbohydrates: 41 g; Fat: 27 g; Sodium: 491 mg; Fiber: 6 g; Diabetic Exchange: Bread/Starch 2, Meat (High Fat) 1.5, Fat 2

tuna salad sandwich

What's in this for baby and me? Protein and fiber.

LIGHT, FRESH, AND high in **protein** and **fiber**, this deli-style salad would also be perfect served on its own on a bed of lettuce.

makes 2 sandwiches

One 6–6½-ounce can chunk white tuna in spring water, drained, rinsed, and drained again

2 tablespoons thinly sliced scallions (green part only)

2 tablespoons finely diced celery (optional)

3 tablespoons light mayonnaise, or to taste

1 tablespoon freshly squeezed lemon juice, or to taste

Salt and freshly ground pepper, to taste

4 slices hearty whole grain bread or calcium-enriched bread (such as Calcium Enriched Roman Meal)

1. Combine all of the ingredients except the bread in a bowl and mix until well blended. Cover and refrigerate any leftovers.
2. To make each sandwich, spread the salad on one of the slices of bread, top with the remaining bread, and cut in half.

▶ *Variation:* Add chopped fresh dill, parsley, or your favorite fresh herb, a few small capers (drained), or finely diced green peppers to the salad.

▶ *Complete Meal Ideas:* Serve this sandwich with:
   A raw or cooked vegetable, vegetable soup, or tossed salad (you might want to try Romaine Lettuce with the Olive Oil–Lemon Dressing, page 144, or raw vegetables with the Spinach Dip, page 147, or the Artichoke-Spinach Dip, page 148)
   Reduced-fat 2% milk or low-fat yogurt
   Fresh fruit

APPROXIMATE NUTRITIONAL INFORMATION: Serving size: 1 tuna salad sandwich on whole wheat bread; Calories: 415 cals; Protein: 29 g; Carbohydrates: 47 g; Fat: 15 g; Fiber: 6 g; Sodium: 1,141 mg; Diabetic Exchange: Bread/Starch 3, Fat 1, Meat (Medium Fat) 4

indigestion and heartburn

Indigestion and heartburn are very common complaints during pregnancy, especially during the first and third trimesters. During the first trimester, heartburn is caused by increased hormone levels and smooth muscle relaxation, which allow acids to reflux (come back up) more easily. During the third trimester, decreased stomach capacity limits the space for food and stomach juices, resulting in indigestion and heartburn.

TIPS FOR COPING

▶ Avoid greasy, fatty, spicy, or fried foods.

▶ Avoid gas-forming foods such as cabbage and beans.

▶ Avoid all caffeinated beverages and chocolate.

▶ Avoid all citrus fruits and juices.

▶ Sit down when you eat and try to relax.

▶ Eat slowly and chew thoroughly.

▶ Don't eat and drink at the same time. Wait thirty to sixty minutes after eating to drink a beverage.

▶ Don't lie down after eating. Take a walk instead.

▶ Try not to eat three hours prior to bedtime.

▶ Eat more frequent smaller meals instead of three large ones.

▶ Sip a cup of plain hot water after meals.

▶ If indigestion keeps you awake at night, try to sleep propped up with pillows.

▶ Wear loose-fitting clothing, especially around the abdomen and waist.

▶ Avoid bending over at the waist. Bend at the knees.

▶ Never take any medication for heartburn without consulting your doctor or nurse.

▶ Avoid preparations containing sodium or sodium bicarbonate.

wraps and rolls

veggie cheese wrap

What's in this for baby and me? Protein, calcium, vitamins A and C, folic acid, and fiber.

A DELICIOUS WAY to get your **protein**, **calcium**, **vitamins A** and **C**, **folic acid**, and **fiber**, not to mention a good dose of B vitamins. Create your own masterpiece and watch others drool over your lunch! Any leftover roasted or stir-fried vegetables are wonderful in this veggie-cheese wrap. Using a spinach wrap or an organic sprouted-wheat burrito-size tortilla (available in whole foods stores) adds a nice dose of iron. **Complete Meal Ideas** for all of the following wraps and rolls include reduced-fat 2% milk or low-fat yogurt and fresh fruit.

makes 1 wrap

4 slices of provolone, Swiss, or any cheese
   that melts easily

1 burrito-size (10-inch) tortilla

3 tomato slices

2 strips jarred roasted red peppers (optional)

A couple of avocado slices

A handful of lettuce leaves

1 tablespoon salsa, or to taste

Arrange the cheese over the tortilla and microwave for a few seconds to melt the cheese. Top with the remaining ingredients, roll up, and slice in half.

APPROXIMATE NUTRITIONAL INFORMATION: Serving size: 1 veggie cheese wrap; Calories: 416 cals; Protein: 20 g; Carbohydrates: 36 g; Fat: 22 g; Fiber: 15 g; Sodium: 884 mg; Calcium: 476 mg; Vitamin A: 1,950 IU; Vitamin C: 22 mg; Folic Acid: 91 mcg; Diabetic Exchange: Bread/Starch 2, Fat 2, Meat (High Fat) 2

chicken caesar wrap

What's in this for baby and me? Protein, vitamins A and C, and fiber.

THIS CHICKEN WRAP is loaded with **protein**, **vitamins A** and **C**, and **fiber**, and it is a good source of calcium and folic acid. Use your favorite store-bought Caesar salad dressing or the Caesar Salad Dressing on page 143.

makes 1 wrap

½ cup diced cooked chicken, or 4 ounces
   (about 4 slices) sliced turkey breast
A handful of sliced romaine leaves
3 tomato slices

1 burrito-size (10-inch) tortilla
2 tablespoons grated Parmesan cheese, or to
   taste
1 tablespoon Caesar salad dressing

Distribute the chicken, lettuce, and tomato slices evenly over the tortilla. Top with the Parmesan cheese and salad dressing. Roll up and slice in half.

APPROXIMATE NUTRITIONAL INFORMATION: Serving size: 1 chicken Caesar wrap; Calories: 377 cals; Protein: 31 g; Carbohydrates: 29 g; Fat: 15 g; Fiber: 11 g; Sodium: 757 g; Vitamin A: 1,190 IU; Vitamin C: 18 mg; Diabetic Exchange: Bread/Starch 2, Fat 1, Meat (Medium Fat) 3

asian-style turkey wrap

What's in this for baby and me? Protein, vitamins A and C, and fiber.

A SMALL AMOUNT of hoisin and Thai peanut sauce is the secret of this yummy Asian-style turkey wrap, which is high in **protein**, **vitamins A** and **C**, and **fiber**, and a good source of folic acid. Fresh cilantro adds the perfect punch.

makes 1 wrap

1 teaspoon hoisin sauce
1 teaspoon Thai peanut sauce
1 burrito-size (10-inch) tortilla
4 ounces (about 4 slices) sliced turkey breast

2–3 strips of jarred roasted red peppers
   (optional)
A handful of lettuce leaves
A couple sprigs of fresh cilantro (optional)

Mix the hoisin and peanut sauces in a small dish. Spread evenly over the tortilla. Top with the turkey slices and the remaining ingredients, roll up, and slice in half.

hummus-tabbouleh roll

What's in this for baby and me? Protein, vitamins A and C, folic acid, and fiber.

ROLLS DON'T GET much better or healthier than this. This hummus-tabbouleh roll is an excellent source of **protein**, **vitamins A** and **C**, **folic acid**, and **fiber**, and a good source of iron. If you have the time and energy to make homemade hummus and tabbouleh, see the recipes on page 148 for Healthy Hummus and on page 126 for Best-Ever Tabbouleh Salad. If not, don't feel guilty—store-bought varieties work just as well.

makes one roll

⅓ cup hummus (any flavor)

1 burrito-size (10-inch) tortilla or large whole
   wheat pita round

⅓ cup tabbouleh salad

3 tomato slices

A few cucumber slices

A handful of lettuce leaves

A squeeze of fresh lemon juice

Spread the hummus on the tortilla or cut open one edge of the pita bread and spread the hummus inside. Top with the remaining ingredients, roll up, and slice in half.

rachel hudson's peanut butter and banana roll

What's in this for baby and me? Protein and fiber.

A QUICK, SIMPLE, satisfying roll, created by an eleven-year-old.

makes 1 roll

3 tablespoons peanut butter
1 burrito-size (10-inch) tortilla

½ banana, sliced

Spread the peanut butter on the tortilla. Add the banana slices, roll up, and slice in half.

APPROXIMATE NUTRITIONAL INFORMATION: Serving size: 1 peanut butter and banana roll; Calories: 459 cals; Protein: 17 g; Carbohydrates: 48 g; Fat: 25 g; Fiber: 14 g; Sodium: 575 mg; Diabetic Exchange: Bread/Starch 2, Fat 3, Fruit 1, Meat (High Fat) 1.5

listeriosis warning

LISTERIOSIS IS A food-borne illness that is caused by a bacterium called *Listeria monocytogenes,* found in soil and water. The bacteria are very resistant to common food preservation agents such as heat, nitrites, nitrates, and acids, and they can continue to multiply in refrigerated foods. *Listeria* is often present in the intestines of seemingly healthy animals. The bacteria can contaminate milk and meat products from infected animals and can also contaminate vegetables fertilized with tainted manure. It is important to note that "contaminated food may not look, smell, or taste different from uncontaminated food" (U.S. Food and Drug Administration (FDA), July 1997).[20]

Healthy people are generally resistant to listeriosis, but pregnant women are about twenty times more likely than other healthy adults to get listeriosis. About one-third of listeriosis cases happen during pregnancy. Infected pregnant women may experience only a mild, flu-like illness (including fever or a stiff neck); however, infections during pregnancy can lead to premature delivery, infection of the newborn, or even stillbirth.[21] Because the symptoms of listeriosis can take a few days or even weeks to appear and can be mild, you may not even know you have it. That is why it is important to take appropriate food safety precautions during pregnancy. Following is a list of guidelines to prevent listeriosis infection provided by the USDA's Food Safety and Inspection Service and the U.S. Food and Drug Administration:[22, 23, 24]

- ▶ Do not eat hot dogs, luncheon meats, or deli meats unless they are reheated until steaming hot.
- ▶ Do not eat soft cheeses such as unpasteurized feta or unpasteurized fresh mozzarella, Brie, Camembert, blue-veined cheeses, and Mexican-style cheeses such as *queso fresco* (also called *queso blanco*) and *asadero.* Pasteurized hard cheeses, semi-soft cheeses (such as part-skim low-moisture mozzarella and feta), processed cheese slices and spreads, cream cheese, and cottage cheese can be consumed safely.
- ▶ Do not eat refrigerated pâté or meat spreads. Canned or shelf-stable pâté and meat spreads can be eaten.
- ▶ Do not eat refrigerated smoked seafood unless it is an ingredient in a cooked dish such as a casserole. Examples of refrigerated smoked seafood include salmon, trout, whitefish, cod, tuna, and mackerel, which are most often labeled as "nova-style," "lox," "kippered," "smoked," or "jerky." Canned fish such as salmon and tuna or shelf-stable smoked seafood may be eaten safely.
- ▶ Do not drink raw (unpasteurized) milk or eat foods that contain unpasteurized milk.
- ▶ Use all perishable items that are precooked or ready-to-eat as soon as possible. Observe all expiration dates.
- ▶ Wash the insides of refrigerators regularly, and be sure to thoroughly clean liquid spills, such as spills from hot dog and luncheon meat packages.
- ▶ Use a refrigerator thermometer to make sure that your refrigerator always stays at 40°F or below.
- ▶ Wash all fruits and vegetables with water.
- ▶ After handling raw foods, wash your hands with warm soapy water, and wash the utensils, cutting boards, and dishes you used with hot soapy water before using them again.
- ▶ Cook foods to well-done temperatures (see Well-Done Temperature Guide, page 303).

salads and dips
for munching and crunching

~

SALADS

IF YOU LOVE salads, you're in luck. All types of salads, from simple greens and raw or cooked vegetables to grain- or pasta-based salads, provide vitamins and nutrients beneficial to pregnant women—and their families. The roughage from greens, vegetables, and grains is essential for good digestion as well as for controlling constipation.

Like soups, salads require no special skills to make and they allow loads of room for creativity. Salads can be eaten as a snack between meals or as a side dish, or, with a little imagination, they can become a well-balanced entrée for lunch or dinner. There are numerous ways to transform a simple salad into a healthy main course by adding a bit of protein and a grain. Following are some ideas to help you jazz up your own salads and boost their nutritional value.

Tips for Making Healthier Salads

▶ *Protein Suggestions*

Cooked (preferably baked, grilled, or broiled) poultry or meat (cooked well-done), cooked or canned fish (such as tuna or salmon), cooked shellfish, hard-boiled eggs, pasteurized hard cheese, part-skim cottage cheese, beans (such as kidney beans, soybeans, chickpeas, or lima beans), tofu, or nuts and seeds (such as pumpkin or sesame seeds).

▶ *Grain Suggestions*

Enriched whole wheat bread, tortillas, wheat germ, rice, enriched pasta, kasha, quinoa, tabbouleh, bulgar, wheat berries, or croutons.

▶ **Dairy Suggestions**

Low-fat or nonfat plain yogurt, grated or cubed pasteurized hard cheese, part-skim cottage or ricotta cheese, or any safe-for-pregnancy cheese of your choice. (See Listeriosis Warning, page 107, for more information on safe cheeses.)

▶ **Power Greens**

Romaine, Boston, Bibb, loose-leaf, spinach, arugula, beet greens, escarole, Belgian endive, sorrel, dandelion, mustard greens, or sliced cabbage.

Most grocery stores, restaurants, and even fast food chains offer salad bars or prepared salads (avoid those with preservatives), an easy way to pick up lunch, dinner, or a side dish without having to expend energy on washing greens and chopping vegetables. It's up to you to make healthy choices. Here are a few tips for navigating the salad bar.

Healthy Choices at the Salad Bar

- Scan the salad bar to check for cleanliness and a well-maintained general appearance.
- Avoid composed salads made with mayonnaise unless they are in well-chilled containers.
- Choose romaine, Boston, Bibb, loose-leaf, or iceberg lettuce (in that order).
- Try to include a grain (such as pasta, rice, tabbouleh, couscous, or croutons) and a protein (chickpeas, beans, grated or cubed pasteurized hard cheese or hard-boiled eggs) in your salad.
- Choose a low-fat or reduced-fat salad dressing that has been kept well chilled, especially if it is mayonnaise-based (such as ranch). Or, make your own oil and vinegar dressing.
- Top your salad with sesame seeds, pumpkin seeds, or nuts (unless you are on a low-sodium diet).
- Avoid bacon bits, whether real or artificial.
- Compose a plain fruit salad for dessert, breakfast, or snack.
- Avoid tofu unless it is stored in clean water and kept well chilled.

There is no substitute for homemade salad dressings, and once you've been spoiled by the real thing, the store-bought varieties pale in comparison. But convenience counts, and store-bought salad dressings are definitely convenient. The dizzying variety of prepared salad dressings on the market today can make choosing one a daunting task. When selecting a dressing, first let your taste buds guide you, then look for those low in fat, sodium, and preservatives. Read labels carefully. The most important thing to remember, no matter what dressing you choose, is to use salad dressings in *moderation*—don't drown your salad.

DIPS

ACCOMPANIED BY NUTRITIOUS whole grain crackers or breads, vegetables, or low-fat chips (preferably baked, not fried), dips make a great snack for pregnant women, especially those on bed rest or on the go. Dips are the perfect cocktail food for entertaining, and they work wonders as a hunger buffer when dinner is running late. Almost all of the dips in this section can be made in advance, with the exception of guacamole, which tends to lose its fresh green color quickly. Most keep for at least three days under refrigeration.

The desire to dip starts at a young age, with french fries dipped in ketchup (some kids eat more ketchup than french fries!). Try going one step healthier by introducing kids to peeled baby carrots with reduced-fat sour-cream ranch dip, guacamole with chips, or their favorite crackers with hummus. You'd be surprised at what you can get away with by making food a little playful.

Grocery stores, gourmet food stores, and restaurants offer countless choices of dips, but many store-bought varieties contain high levels of sodium, MSG, and fat. It is important to strike a balance between the nutritional benefits of the vegetables, whole grain crackers, or breads that accompany the dip and the dip itself. As with store-bought salad dressings, *moderation* is the key. Feel free to jazz up store-bought dips or to experiment with dips by adding your favorite herbs, grated or diced vegetables, spices, and plain low-fat yogurt or pasteurized instant nonfat dry milk powder for extra calcium. Make dips and smart dippers part of your family's meal plan.

salads and dips for munching and crunching

~

SALADS

Asian-Style Pasta and Vegetable Salad▼

Best-Ever Tabbouleh Salad▼

Quinoa Salad▼

Pasta Salad with Basil Pesto

Noodles with Spinach, Red Peppers, and Sesame Dressing▼

Couscous Salad with Chickpeas and Vegetables▼

Kids' Favorite Three-Bean Salad▼

Vegetables with Lemon, Olive Oil, and Fresh Herbs▼

Pink Potato Salad

Tomato and Mozzarella Salad with Fresh Basil

Roasted Beets with Goat Cheese, Walnuts, and Baby Greens

Asparagus, Hearts of Palm, and Tomato Salad▼

Spinach Salad with Mandarin Oranges and Toasted Almonds▼

Four Delicious Homemade Salad Dressings

DIPS

Homemade Guacamole▼

Roasted Red Pepper and Cheese Dip

Healthy Hummus▼

Spinach Dip

Artichoke-Spinach Dip

Black Bean Dip▼

▼ Vegan recipe

RECIPE NOTES

SALADS AND DIPS are quick, easy, and nutritious foods for the whole family. They are the perfect way to get additional vitamins and fiber into your diet. While green salads are not ideal for young eaters, many of the other salads in this chapter, particularly the pasta and grain and bean salads, work well for preschoolers and older kids. Getting your kids involved in making some of the simple salads and dips might entice them to try a bite and maybe even eat a vegetable or two at the same time.

Some notes about the recipes in this chapter:

- Always use the freshest greens and vegetables you can find.
- Be sure to wash all greens and vegetables thoroughly (see Tips for Washing and Storing Greens, page 315).
- Be sure to keep any salad or salad dressings that contain mayonnaise refrigerated at all times.
- Choose enriched pastas and breads. Read labels for folic acid and iron content.
- Feel free to use any kind of olive oil, from extra-light to heavy, full-bodied Greek olive oils.
- Substitute your favorite oil for canola oil in any recipe.
- When making any type of vinaigrette, for best results, combine all of the ingredients except the oil with the vinegar, stir to dissolve, then add the oil, whisking to emulsify.
- Use artichoke hearts packed in water or brine, not oil.
- Rinse all canned beans and other canned vegetables to remove some of the salt.
- Use *only* pasteurized cheeses, particularly in the case of mozzarella, feta, or goat cheese.
- Use reduced-fat sour cream or yogurt, or a mixture of both, for dips and salads.
- If you are a vegetarian, you can substitute tofu-based sour cream or tofu-based mayonnaise.

pantry items for salads and dips
for munching and crunching

SALAD PANTRY

Fresh Produce

Avocados

Baby greens

Baby spinach

Broccoli florets

Carrots

Cauliflower florets

Cherry or grape tomatoes

Fresh herbs: basil, cilantro, dill, mint, and parsley

Garlic

Ginger

Green asparagus

Green Beans

Lemons

Limes

Oranges

Potatoes

Red beets

Red bell peppers

Romaine lettuce

Scallions

Tomatoes

Watercress

Zucchini

Dairy and Soy Products

Grade A large eggs

Parmesan cheese (grated)

Pasteurized feta cheese

Pasteurized goat cheese

Pasteurized part-skim low-moisture mozzarella cheese

Canned, Bottled, and Jarred Staples

Anchovy paste

Artichoke hearts packed in water or brine

Balsamic vinegar

Canola oil

Chickpeas

Deli-style dill pickles

Dijon mustard

Fat-free low-sodium stock (any kind)

Hearts of palm

Light mayonnaise

Mandarin oranges in light syrup

Olive oil

Olives (any kind)

Orange juice

Red kidney beans

Red or white wine vinegar

Reduced-fat smooth peanut butter

Rice vinegar (plain or seasoned)

Sesame oil (preferably toasted)

Soy sauce (regular or light)

Sun-dried tomatoes packed in oil

Worcestershire sauce

Dry Staples

Quinoa (such as Ancient Harvest brand)

Couscous

Shaped pasta (such as fusilli) and thin pasta (such as linguine or capellini)

Pine nuts

Sliced or slivered almonds

Tabbouleh mix

Udon noodles (brown rice or buck-
 wheat)
Walnuts

Condiments, Herbs, and Spices
Basil pesto
Dried basil
Dried oregano
Dried tarragon
Ground cumin
Italian seasoning

From the Salad Bar
Artichoke hearts
Baby spinach
Broccoli florets
Cauliflower florets
Cooked red beets
Deli-style pickles
Hard-boiled eggs
Lettuce
Shredded or grated carrots
Sliced olives
Sliced red bell peppers
Sliced romaine lettuce
Sliced scallions

DIP PANTRY

Fresh Produce
Baby spinach
Fresh herbs: cilantro and parsley
Garlic

Hass avocados
Lemons
Limes
Red onions
Scallions
Tomatoes

Dairy and Soy Products
Parmesan cheese (grated)
Part-skim ricotta cheese
Pasteurized feta cheese
Reduced-fat sour cream

Canned, Bottled, and Jarred Staples
Anchovy paste or fillets
Artichoke hearts packed in water or
 brine (14-ounce can)
Black beans (15.5-ounce can)
Canola oil
Chickpeas (15-ounce can)
Light mayonnaise
Olive oil
Pimentos
Roasted red bell peppers
Tahini

Condiments
Ground cumin
Tabasco sauce

Frozen Staples
Chopped spinach (10-ounce package)

choosing the right greens

All greens are not created equal. Here are four common greens listed in order of nutrients found in a 1 cup serving.

ROMAINE

8 cals
1,456 IU Vitamin A
13 mg Vitamin C
76 mcg Folic Acid

BOSTON, BIBB,
or BUTTERHEAD

7 cals
534 IU Vitamin A
4 mg Vitamin C
40 mcg Folic Acid

LOOSE-LEAF

10 cals
1,064 IU Vitamin A
10 mg Vitamin C
28 mcg Folic Acid

ICEBERG

7 cals
182 IU Vitamin A
2 mg Vitamin C
30 mcg Folic Acid

asian-style pasta and vegetable salad

What's in this for baby and me? Vitamins A and C.

LOADED WITH **vitamins A** and **C**, and a good source of protein, folic acid, and fiber, this tasty, colorful dish is sure to please the whole family. Sautéed tofu (see Instructions for Sautéing Tofu, page 189), or any source of protein (such as cooked scallops, shrimp, salmon, or chicken), can be added to turn this salad into a main course. If you are short on time, pick up the shredded carrots and broccoli florets at a salad bar, or substitute fresh baby spinach leaves for the broccoli. Consider omitting the scallions, ginger, red bell peppers, and cilantro for young eaters.

serves 8 (makes about 8 cups)

1 pound thin pasta (such as linguine or
    capellini)
1 tablespoon canola oil
2 teaspoons sesame oil (optional)
½ cup sliced scallions
2 tablespoons grated fresh ginger
¾ cup reduced-fat low-sodium stock
¼ cup reduced-fat smooth peanut butter
¼ cup soy sauce

1 tablespoon seasoned rice vinegar or freshly
    squeezed lime juice
1 teaspoon brown sugar
1 cup shredded carrots
½ cup finely diced red bell pepper
1½ cups broccoli florets, cooked until crisp-
    tender
¼ cup chopped fresh cilantro

1. Cook the pasta according to the package directions; drain and rinse quickly under cool water. Drain again, place in a large bowl and set aside.
2. Heat the canola oil and sesame oil, if using, in a medium skillet over medium heat until hot. Add the scallions and ginger and sauté for 1 minute. Add the stock and peanut butter and stir until smooth, then add the soy sauce, rice vinegar, and brown sugar, and bring to a boil. Reduce the heat and simmer for 2 minutes.
3. Add the sauce to the pasta, along with the remaining ingredients. Stir and toss until well combined. Adjust the seasoning and serve cold or at room temperature.

▶ *Storage Tip:* This salad keeps for 3 days refrigerated.

▶ *Health Tip:* If your doctor has restricted your salt intake, use low-sodium soy sauce. If your fat intake has been restricted, go easy on the peanut butter and reduce the amount of canola oil to 1 teaspoon.

▶ *Diabetic Tip:* Reduce the portion size to ½ cup.

▶ *Complete Meal Ideas:* Serve this salad with:

    3 ounces protein (you might want to try the Chicken with Homemade Barbecue
        Sauce, page 236, or the Sautéed Tofu and Portobello Mushrooms on a Bed of
        Greens, page 188)
    Green salad
    Reduced-fat 2% milk or low-fat yogurt
    Fresh fruit

APPROXIMATE NUTRITIONAL INFORMATION: Serving size: 1 cup Asian-style pasta and vegetable salad; Calories: 184 cals; Protein: 8 g; Carbohydrates: 25 g; Fat: 7 g; Fiber: 3 g; Sodium: 532 mg; Vitamin A: 7,366 IU; Vitamin C: 43 mg; Diabetic Exchange (values per ½ cup serving): Bread/Starch 1.5, Fat 1, Vegetable 1

quinoa salad

~

What's in this for baby and me? Vitamins A and C and iron.

IF YOU'VE NEVER tried quinoa, this salad is sure to make a quinoa-convert out of you. Quinoa (pronounced *keen-wa*) is an easy-to-cook grain that has an earthy taste and pop-in-your-mouth texture (see important washing instruction below). This salad is a great source of **vitamins A** and **C** and **iron**, and a good source of protein and fiber. Use this recipe as a guideline—add your family's favorite vegetables, and for extra protein, try adding sautéed tofu (see Instructions for Sautéing Tofu, page 189). It is advisable to purchase boxed quinoa (such as Ancient Harvest Quinoa) rather than buy it in bulk because boxed grains tend to be larger, cleaner, sweeter, and more fluffy when cooked.

serves 4 to 6 (makes about 5 cups)

1 cup quinoa, thoroughly rinsed under hot water (see Cooking Tip below)

⅓ cup finely diced red bell pepper (optional)

½ cup shredded or grated carrots

½ cup sliced black olives (optional)

¼ cup thinly sliced scallions (optional)

¼ cup chopped fresh cilantro or 2 tablespoons

finely chopped fresh mint

1 tablespoon grated orange zest

3 tablespoons freshly squeezed orange juice

2 tablespoons seasoned rice vinegar

2 tablespoons canola oil

Salt, to taste

1. Prepare the quinoa according to the package directions. (If you do not have package directions, combine the thoroughly rinsed quinoa with 2 cups water in a saucepan and bring it to a boil. Reduce the heat and simmer, covered, for 15 to 20 minutes, or until the grains look transparent and the spiral-like germ has separated. Remove from heat and let stand for 5 minutes, then fluff with a fork and transfer to a large bowl.
2. Add the remaining ingredients to the quinoa and mix gently until well incorporated. Adjust the seasoning and serve chilled or at room temperature.

▶ *Cooking Tip:* It is absolutely essential to rinse quinoa before cooking it to remove the bitter natural outer coating on each grain. Most of this coating is removed before sale; however, there may be a small residue left on the grain. Rinse the quinoa in a fine-mesh strainer under cold running water for about 1 minute, or place it in the saucepan you plan to cook it in, add water, and swish the grains with your hands for about 1 minute; drain.

▶ *Storage Tip:* This salad keeps for 2 days refrigerated.

▶ *Complete Meal Ideas:* Serve this salad with:

> Salad or vegetable soup (you might want to try the Black Bean Soup with Cilantro, page 78, or the Tomato, Mozzarella, and Fresh Basil Salad, page 132)
>
> Reduced-fat 2% milk or low-fat yogurt
>
> Fresh fruit that contains vitamin C

APPROXIMATE NUTRITIONAL INFORMATION: Serving size: 1 cup quinoa salad; Calories: 260 cals; Protein: 6 g; Carbohydrates: 35 g; Fat: 11 g; Fiber: 4 g; Sodium: 162 mg; Vitamin A: 4,029 IU; Vitamin C: 22 mg; Diabetic Exchange: Bread/Starch 2, Fat 2

pasta salad with basil pesto

~

What's in this for baby and me? Protein, calcium, and folic acid.

Rᴵᴄʜ ɪɴ **protein**, **calcium**, and **folic acid**, and a good source of vitamin C, iron, B vitamins, and fiber, this pasta salad makes the perfect lunch or dinner for a pregnant woman and her family. The recipe makes a fantastic pesto sauce, but if pesto does not appeal to you, try the Sun-Dried Tomato Dressing on page 142, or use your favorite home-made or store-bought dressing.

serves 6 (makes about 8 cups)

4½ to 5 cups cooked fusilli or your favorite
    shaped pasta, rinsed briefly under cold
    water. (Note: 2½ cups dry fusilli yields
    about 4½ cups cooked pasta)
1 vine-ripened tomato, cut into small wedges,
    or about 1 cup cherry or grape tomatoes
One 13.75-ounce can artichoke hearts, drained
    and cut into small wedges (optional)
8 ounces pasteurized mozzarella cheese (see
    Health Tip below), cubed (about 1½ cups)
½ cup olives (any kind) (optional)
½ cup Basil Pesto (recipe follows) or store-
    bought pesto, or to taste
Salt and freshly ground pepper, to taste

Combine all of the ingredients in a large bowl and toss gently until well combined. Adjust the seasoning and serve.

▶ *Variation:* Substitute your favorite cheese for the mozzarella, and use any vegetables or greens in place of the artichokes, such as steamed or sautéed broccoli or zucchini, or fresh spinach or arugula.

▶ *Storage Tip:* This salad keeps for 3 days refrigerated. The pesto will lose its bright green color, but the taste will remain unaffected. Bring just to room temperature before serving.

▶ *Health Tip:* Do *not* use unpasteurized fresh mozzarella cheese stored in water (see Listeriosis Warning, page 107).

▶ *Complete Meal Ideas:* Serve this pasta salad with:
    Green salad or green vegetable (you might want to try the Vegetables with
        Lemon, Olive Oil, and Fresh Herbs, page 128, or romaine lettuce with the
        Caesar Salad Dressing, page 143)
    Reduced-fat 2% milk or low-fat yogurt
    Fresh fruit that contains vitamin C

APPROXIMATE NUTRITIONAL INFORMATION: Serving size: 1 cup pasta salad with basil pesto; Calories: 241 cals; Protein: 13 g; Carbohydrates: 32 g; Fat: 7 g; Fiber: 3 g; Sodium: 336 mg; Calcium: 219 mg; Folic Acid: 103 mcg; Diabetic Exchange: Bread/Starch 2, Fat .5, Meat (Medium Fat) 1

basil pesto

WATER IS SUBSTITUTED for some of the oil in this recipe, resulting in a superb, reduced-fat pesto that is scrumptious on hot linguine, fish, or poultry, as well as pasta salads. For a wonderful fresh basil punch, use pesto in sandwiches instead of mayonnaise. To preserve the bright green color of freshly made pesto, make sure that the plastic wrap is directly against the surface of the pesto.

makes about 1 cup

2 cups tightly packed fresh basil leaves (about 2 ounces)

¼ cup plus 1 tablespoon olive oil or canola oil

3 tablespoons grated Parmesan cheese

⅓ cup pine nuts, toasted

1 large garlic clove, crushed

Salt and freshly ground pepper, to taste

2 tablespoons water

In a food processor pulse all of the ingredients until smooth, scraping down the sides of the bowl as necessary. Do not overmix, or the pesto will be gummy. Adjust the seasoning. Transfer to a bowl and cover the pesto with plastic wrap directly against the surface. Refrigerate until needed.

▶ **Storage Tip:** This pesto keeps for 5 days refrigerated, and it can be frozen for up to 1 month. Unless you plan to use it all at once, freeze it in portion-size servings in small or snack-size zip-lock bags.

APPROXIMATE NUTRITIONAL INFORMATION: Serving size: 2 tablespoons basil pesto; Calories: 24 cals; Protein: 1 g; Carbohydrates: .6 g; Fat: 2 g; Fiber: .2 g; Sodium: 54 mg; Diabetic Exchange: FREE

noodles with spinach, red bell peppers, and sesame dressing

⌒

What's in this for baby and me? Vitamins A and C, and folic acid.

THIS NOODLE SALAD is an excellent source of **vitamins A** and **C** and **folic acid**, and a good source of protein, iron, B vitamins, and fiber. Feel free to add your favorite ingredients, including grated carrots, broccoli florets, or zucchini slices cooked until crisp-tender. This salad can be made a day ahead, but, in that case, the spinach should be added just before serving. If serving to children, omit the red pepper and possibly the garlic. If not, add a drop or two of hot oil for a good punch.

serves 4 (makes about 4½ cups)

8 ounces linguine or udon noodles

2 tablespoons toasted sesame oil

2 tablespoons soy sauce, or to taste

1 tablespoon seasoned rice vinegar, or to taste

½ cup thinly sliced red bell pepper

1½ cups tightly packed baby spinach leaves or 1 bunch watercress leaves, trimmed (use top leafy part only), washed, and dried

1 very small garlic clove, crushed (optional)

1. Cook the noodles according to the package directions. Drain and rinse quickly under cold water. Drain again, then place in a large bowl.
2. Add the sesame oil, soy sauce, and rice vinegar to the noodles and toss to coat. Add the remaining ingredients and toss gently until well combined. Adjust the seasoning and serve.

▶ *Storage Tip:* This salad keeps for 3 days refrigerated, although the spinach will wilt.

▶ *Complete Meal Ideas:* Serve these noodles with:
   3 ounces protein (you might want to try the Asian-Style Turkey Wrap, page 104, or the Old Bay Tofu Cakes with Cocktail Sauce, page 186.)
   Reduced-fat 2% milk or low-fat yogurt
   Fresh fruit that contains vitamin C

APPROXIMATE NUTRITIONAL INFORMATION: Serving size: 1 cup noodles with sesame dressing; Calories: 253 cals; Protein: 8 g; Carbohydrates: 39 g; Fat: 7 g; Fiber: 3 g; Sodium: 438 mg; Vitamin A: 1,880 IU; Vitamin C: 30 mg; Diabetic Exchange: Bread/Starch 2.5, Fat 1.5, Vegetable 1

choosing store-bought dips
and smart dippers

⁓

Let your taste buds guide you, but opt for dips low in fat. Unfortunately, most prepared dips have little nutritional value, so be sure to eat them with healthful foods. Read labels to ensure smart choices; some packaged dips are MSG-free. You can also reduce the fat by mixing a prepared dip with low-fat or nonfat plain yogurt or reduced-fat sour cream. Kids love dipping just about anything in anything, so don't forget to offer them some!

SMART DIPPERS

Grains: Whole wheat crackers, whole wheat pita bread or pita chips, flat breads, fat-free bagel chips, Melba toast, matzo, tortillas, or homemade croutons (see Homemade Croutons, page 140).

Vegetables: Ready-cut carrots and celery sticks; peeled baby carrots; cherry tomatoes; radishes; broccoli and cauliflower florets; sliced bell peppers, fennel, jicama, or kohlrabi; or quick-cooked (blanched or steamed) asparagus, green beans, or snow peas; or any other vegetables you like.

couscous salad with chickpeas and vegetables

~

What's in this for baby and me? Protein, iron, vitamin C, folic acid, and fiber.

COUSCOUS SALAD MAKES an easy and delicious side dish for just about any main course. When combined with vegetables and herbs as in this salad, it is an excellent source of **protein**, **iron**, **vitamin C**, **folic acid**, and **fiber**, and a good source of vitamin A and B vitamins. Don't let the long list of ingredients intimidate you—use your favorite vegetables and herbs in place of the ones called for. A source of protein such as cooked chicken or shrimp, sautéed tofu (see Instructions for Sautéing Tofu, page 189), or cheese is always a welcome addition. Any small-grained pasta, such as orzo, acini di pepe, or quinoa (see instructions for cooking quinoa on page 118), can be used in place of the couscous.

serves 4 (makes about 4 cups)

3 cups cooked couscous (about ¾ cup uncooked couscous)

2 tablespoons wine vinegar

1 small garlic clove, crushed (optional)

½ teaspoon Dijon mustard (optional)

3 tablespoons olive oil or canola oil

1 vine-ripened tomato, cut into wedges, or 12 cherry or grape tomatoes, halved

½ cup diced red bell pepper (optional)

⅔ cup (one 7¾-ounce can) chickpeas

⅔ cup canned or jarred artichoke hearts, quartered (optional)

½ cup olives (any kind) (optional)

⅓ cup pine nuts, toasted (optional)

¼ cup chopped fresh parsley (optional)

¼ cup finely sliced scallions (optional)

Fresh lemon juice, to taste

Salt and freshly ground pepper, to taste

1. Cook the couscous according to the package directions. In general, about ¾ cup of couscous and 1¼ cups of water yield 3 cups cooked couscous. Transfer the couscous to a large bowl and allow to cool. Then fluff with a fork or your hands to separate the grains.
2. In a small bowl, mix the vinegar and optional garlic and mustard until well blended. Add the olive oil, mix well, and set aside.
3. Add the remaining ingredients except the lemon juice and salt and pepper to the couscous, then add the dressing and mix gently until all of the ingredients are well combined. Add lemon juice to taste, adjust the seasoning, and serve.

▶ *Timesaving Tip:* Pick up your favorite cleaned and ready-cut vegetables, such as grated carrots, peppers, zucchini, broccoli florets, cucumbers, tomatoes, or chickpeas, from a salad bar and add them to the couscous salad.

▶ *Storage Tip:* This salad keeps for 3 days refrigerated.

▶ *Health Tip:* If your doctor has restricted your salt or fat intake, use less olive oil and omit the olives, pine nuts, and salt.

▶ *Diabetic Tip:* Reduce the portion size to ½ cup.

▶ *Complete Meal Ideas:* Serve this couscous salad with:
> 3 ounces protein (you might want to try the Healthy Hummus, page 148, or the
> > Marinated Grilled or Broiled Lamb Chops, page 244)
> Reduced-fat 2% milk or low-fat yogurt
> Fresh fruit that contains vitamin C

APPROXIMATE NUTRITIONAL INFORMATION: Serving size: 1 cup couscous salad with chickpeas and vegetables; Calories: 397 cals; Protein: 12 g; Carbohydrates: 47 g; Fat: 19 g; Fiber: 9 g; Sodium: 364 mg; Vitamin C: 36 mg; Folic Acid: 115 mcg; Iron: 4 mg; Diabetic Exchange (values per ½ cup serving): Bread/Starch 1.5, Fat 2, Vegetable .5

best-ever tabbouleh salad

~

What's in this for baby and me? Vitamins A and C.

TABBOULEH IS A super-healthy Middle Eastern dish made from bulgur wheat (which is steamed, dried, and crushed) and vegetables. This salad is an excellent source of **vitamins A** and **C**, and a good source of protein, iron, folic acid, and fiber. Packaged tabbouleh mixes are convenient and tasty, and a good starting point for adding other ingredients, such as brown rice, wheat berries, grated carrots, or cucumbers. Tabbouleh is an excellent side dish for just about any main course, particularly grilled dishes. It makes a great salad on its own, on a bed of greens, and a nice sandwich in a pita pocket (see Hummus-Tabbouleh Roll, page 105). If you have mint growing in your garden, add some.

serves 4 to 6 (makes about 4 cups)

One 6-ounce package tabbouleh (Middle Eastern wheat salad mix)

2 tablespoons freshly squeezed lemon juice, or to taste

3 tablespoons olive oil or canola oil

2 vine-ripened tomatoes, cut into small dice

⅔ cup finely diced red bell pepper (½ red bell pepper) (optional)

½ cup chickpeas or your favorite canned beans, rinsed (optional)

½ cup pine nuts, toasted (optional)

Salt and freshly ground pepper, to taste

1. Place the contents of the tabbouleh package in a medium bowl and add boiling water (not cold water) in the amount stated on the package. Stir, then cover with plastic wrap and let sit for 20 minutes.
2. Add the remaining ingredients and mix thoroughly. Adjust the seasoning and serve.

▶ **Storage Tip:** This salad keeps for 2 days refrigerated.

▶ **Diabetic Tip:** Reduce the portion size to ½ cup.

▶ **Complete Meal Ideas:** Serve this salad with:
   3 ounces protein (you might want to try the Healthy Hummus, page 148, or the Marinated Grilled or Broiled Lamb Chops, page 244)
   Whole wheat pita bread and cheese, or cheese toasts
   Reduced-fat 2% milk or low-fat yogurt
   Fresh fruit that contains vitamin C

APPROXIMATE NUTRITIONAL INFORMATION: Serving size: 1 cup tabbouleh salad; Calories: 259 cals; Protein: 6 g; Carbohydrates: 16 g; Fat: 21 g; Fiber: 4 g; Sodium: 220 mg; Vitamin A: 1,424 IU; Vitamin C: 52 mg; Diabetic Exchange (values per ½ cup serving): Bread/Starch .5, Fat 2, Vegetable .5

kids' favorite three-bean salad

What's in this for baby and me? Vitamin C, folic acid, and fiber.

DON'T TELL YOUR kids that their favorite three-bean salad is packed with **vitamin C**, **folic acid**, and **fiber** and is a good source of protein, vitamin A, and iron as well—they might reject it simply because it's too healthy! Allowing finicky eaters to help make this salad might be a way to entice them to try the beans. Chickpeas and kidney beans are called for in this recipe because they seem to be the most readily available in small ("salad topper" 7.5-ounce) can sizes. However, feel free to add your family's favorites, from black-eyed peas to cannellini beans.

serves 4 (makes about 4 cups)

8 ounces green beans, washed, ends trimmed,
    cut into ½-inch pieces, and cooked until
    crisp-tender

⅔ cup (one 7.5-ounce can) red kidney beans,
    rinsed and drained

⅔ cup (one 7.5-ounce can) chickpeas, rinsed
    and drained

½ cup cherry or grape tomatoes, sliced in half

¼ cup chopped fresh cilantro (optional)

2 tablespoons olive oil or canola oil

1 tablespoon freshly squeezed lime or lemon
    juice, or to taste

A dash of ground cumin (optional)

Salt and freshly ground pepper, to taste

Combine all of the ingredients in a bowl and mix well. Adjust the seasoning and serve.

▶ **Timesaving Tip:** Omit the olive oil, lime juice, and cumin and use your favorite bottled dressing. Use frozen green beans instead of fresh; cook them according to package directions.

▶ **Storage Tip:** This salad keeps four days refrigerated. The lime juice will cause a slight discoloration of the green beans and cilantro, but this does not affect the taste.

▶ **Complete Meal Ideas:** Serve this with:
    3 ounces protein (you might want to try the Chicken Caesar Wrap, page 104, or
        the Spinach and Cheese Quesadillas, page 184.)
    Reduced-fat 2% milk or low-fat yogurt
    Fresh fruit that contains vitamin C

APPROXIMATE NUTRITIONAL INFORMATION: Serving size: 1 cup three-bean salad; Calories: 180 cals; Protein: 7 g; Carbohydrates: 22 g; Fat: 8 g; Fiber: 8 g; Sodium: 334 mg; Vitamin C: 18 mg; Folic Acid: 100 mcg; Diabetic Exchange: Bread/Starch 1.5, Fat 1

vegetables with lemon, olive oil, and fresh herbs

~

What's in this for baby and me? Vitamins A and C, folic acid, and fiber.

THIS VEGETABLE SIDE dish, which can be served warm or at room temperature, goes well with any main course. Cauliflower, broccoli, green beans, or zucchini, all good to excellent sources of **vitamins**, **folic acid**, and **fiber** (depending on the vegetable), lend themselves to this simple preparation. You can serve one vegetable or a mixture. Be sure to drain the vegetables well and blot them dry with paper towels before adding the dressing. The fresh herbs really add to this dish, so don't leave them out.

serves 4 (makes about 4 cups)

12–16 ounces fresh vegetables, washed (see below)

2 tablespoons olive oil

2 tablespoons freshly squeezed lemon juice,
or to taste

Salt and freshly ground pepper, to taste

2 tablespoons chopped fresh parsley, cilantro, or your favorite fresh herb

▶ *Cauliflower or Broccoli* (12 to 16 ounces equals about 5 cups broccoli florets and about 6 cups cauliflower florets)

Boil, steam, or microwave the florets until crisp-tender. Drain well and blot dry with paper towels. Put in a bowl, add the olive oil, and toss gently. Add the remaining ingredients and toss again. Adjust the seasoning and serve.

APPROXIMATE NUTRITIONAL INFORMATION: Serving size: 1 cup cauliflower florets; Calories: 116 cals; Protein: 6 g; Carbohydrates: 11 g; Fat: 8 g; Fiber: 6 g; Sodium: 197 mg; Vitamin A: 2,807 IU; Vitamin C: 152 mg; Folic Acid: 101 mcg; Diabetic Exchange: Fat 1.5, Vegetable 2

APPROXIMATE NUTRITIONAL INFORMATION: Serving size: 1 cup broccoli florets; Calories: 116 cals; Protein: 6 g; Carbohydrates: 11g; Fat: 7 g; Fiber: 6 g; Sodium: 197 mg; Vitamin A: 2,807 IU; Vitamin C: 152 mg; Diabetic Exchange: Fat 1, Vegetable 2

▶ *Green Beans* (16 ounces equals about 4 cups)

Trim the ends of the beans, then boil, steam, or microwave them until crisp-tender. Drain well and blot dry with paper towels. Put in a bowl, add the olive oil, and toss gently. Add the remaining ingredients and toss again. Adjust the seasoning and serve.

APPROXIMATE NUTRITIONAL INFORMATION: Serving size: 1 cup green beans; Calories: 102 cals; Protein: 2 g; Carbohydrates: 10 g; Fat: 7 g; Fiber: 4 g; Sodium: 150 mg; Diabetic Exchange: Fat 1, Vegetable 2

▶ **Zucchini** (16 ounces equals about 3 small zucchini. *Note:* It is important to use young, small zucchini rather than the large overgrown squash that are abundant at the end of the summer.)

1. Cook the whole zucchini in boiling salted water for about 8 to 10 minutes, or until tender. Check tenderness by piercing the middle of a zucchini with the tip of a knife. (See **Cooking Tip 2** for microwave instructions.)
2. Drain carefully (the zucchini skin tears easily) and cool slightly. When cool enough to handle, trim the ends, then cut the zucchini into ¼-inch slices and place in a serving bowl. Add the olive oil and toss gently, then add the remaining ingredients and toss again. Adjust the seasoning and serve.

APPROXIMATE NUTRITIONAL INFORMATION: Serving size: 1 cup zucchini; Calories: 80 cals; Protein: .8 g; Carbohydrates: 5 g; Fat: 7 g; Fiber: 2 g; Sodium: 150 mg; Diabetic Exchange: Fat 1, Vegetable 1

▶ **Cooking Tip 1:** The lemon will cause a slight discoloration of the broccoli, zucchini skin, green beans, and parsley. This does not affect the taste.

▶ **Cooking Tip 2:** To microwave the zucchini, cut in half, place in a microwaveable container with about 2 tablespoons water, and microwave on high. Cooking time will be around 5 to 7 minutes, depending on your microwave.

▶ **Storage Tip:** This salad keeps for 2 days refrigerated.

▶ **Complete Meal Ideas:** Serve these vegetables with:

  3 ounces protein (you might want to try the Tilapia Mediterranean Style, page
    256, or the Vegetarian Omelet for One, page 190.)
  Reduced-fat 2% milk or low-fat yogurt
  Fresh fruit that contains vitamin C

pink potato salad

What's in this for baby and me? Vitamins A and C.

THE BEETS MAKE this potato salad healthier and prettier than regular potato salad. High in **vitamins A** and **C**, and a good source of folic acid and fiber, it is delicious served on a bed of lettuce alongside a sandwich. The pickles and chopped dill give the salad a wonderful tang and may just satisfy your pickle craving.

serves 4 to 6 (makes about 4 cups)

2 medium red beets, scrubbed (see Timesaving Tip below)

1 large potato, scrubbed

3 large carrots, scrubbed

1–2 hard-boiled eggs, chopped (optional)

1 large deli-style kosher dill pickle, cut into small dice, or to taste

⅓ cup light mayonnaise, or to taste

Salt and freshly ground pepper, to taste

3 tablespoons chopped fresh parsley or dill

1. Place the beets, potato, and carrots in a large saucepan, cover with water, and bring to a boil. Cook until tender (pierce the vegetables with a knife to check for doneness), about 20 to 25 minutes for the potato and the carrots, 30 to 40 minutes for the beets. Drain and cool.

2. Peel the beets, potatoes, and carrots and cut into ¼-inch cubes (see **Cooking Tip 2** for advice on peeling the carrots). Place in a large bowl.

3. Add the remaining ingredients and gently mix. Cover with plastic wrap and refrigerate until well chilled, about 2 hours. Adjust the seasoning and serve.

▶ *Timesaving Tip:* In a pinch, you can substitute canned or jarred beets, or plain cooked beets from a salad bar, for the fresh beets. Drain them well. (*Note:* If using canned or jarred beets, the pink color of the salad will probably not be as intense.) Buy pre-sliced sandwich dill pickles to save a bit of time on the chopping.

▶ *Cooking Tip 1:* You can boil the eggs in the same saucepan as the vegetables. The eggshells will turn a grayish color from the beets, but the eggs will not be affected.

▶ *Cooking Tip 2:* To peel the cooked carrots, using a paring knife, remove the skin from around the carrot, rather than using a top-to-bottom peeling motion.

▶ *Storage Tip:* This salad keeps for 3 days refrigerated. The intensity of the pink color will increase with time.

▶ *Complete Meal Ideas:* Serve this salad with:

> 3 ounces protein (you might want to try the Tuna Salad Sandwich, page 101, or the Spice-Rubbed Pork Chops, page 242)
> Green salad or vegetable
> Reduced-fat 2% milk or low-fat yogurt
> Fresh fruit

APPROXIMATE NUTRITIONAL INFORMATION: Serving size: ¾ cup pink potato salad; Calories: 150 cals; Protein: 3 g; Carbohydrates: 18 g; Fat: 8 g; Fiber: 3 g; Sodium: 671 mg; Vitamin A: 13,149 IU; Vitamin C: 14 mg; Diabetic Exchange: Bread/Starch 1, Fat 1.5, Vegetable .5

tomato and mozzarella salad
with fresh basil

~

What's in this for baby and me? Protein, calcium, and vitamin C.

IF YOU GROW tomatoes in your garden, you probably already know what a joy this salad is during the summer months. High in **protein**, **calcium**, and **vitamin C**, and a good source of vitamin A, this simple-to-prepare salad can't be beat! Because each ingredient speaks for itself, quality and freshness are of utmost importance. Present the salad on a bed of baby greens for added fiber, or use it as a topping on toasted or grilled hearty bread, to make the Italian dish called *bruschetta*.

serves 4 (makes about 4 cups)

2 large vine-ripened tomatoes, cubed, or
 about 1¾ cups halved cherry or grape
 tomatoes
8 ounces pasteurized part-skim low-moisture
 mozzarella cheese (see Health Tip below),
 cut into ½-inch cubes (about 1½ cups)
⅓ cup thinly sliced fresh basil leaves

1 tablespoon red or white wine vinegar, or to
 taste
A couple of drops of balsamic vinegar
 (optional)
2 tablespoons olive oil, or to taste
Salt and freshly ground pepper, to taste

Combine all of the ingredients in a bowl, mix gently, and serve. (Refrigerate any leftovers.)

▶ *Health Tip:* Use only pasteurized mozzarella cheese. Do not use unpasteurized fresh mozzarella cheese stored in water (see Listeriosis Warning, page 107).

▶ *Storage Tip:* This salad is best eaten the day it is made.

▶ *Complete Meal Ideas:* Serve this salad with:
 Whole wheat bread or roll
 Green salad, green vegetable, or green soup (you might want to try the Creamy
  Asparagus-Artichoke Soup, page 68, or the Artichoke-Spinach Dip, page 150,
  with whole wheat bread or crackers)
 Reduced-fat 2% milk or low-fat yogurt
 Fresh fruit

APPROXIMATE NUTRITIONAL INFORMATION: Serving size: 1 cup tomato and mozzarella salad; Calories: 234 cals; Protein: 16 g; Carbohydrates: 5 g; Fat: 17 g; Fiber: .8 g; Sodium: 451 mg; Vitamin C: 12 mg; Calcium: 423 mg; Diabetic Exchange: Fat 1.5, Meat (Medium Fat) 2, Vegetable 1

roasted beets with goat cheese, walnuts, and baby greens

~

What's in this for baby and me? Protein, calcium, vitamin A, and folic acid.

IF YOU LIKE beets, you'll love this salad, which is high in **protein**, **calcium**, **vitamin A**, and **folic acid**, and a good source of vitamin C and fiber. This recipe calls for roasting the beets, but you can boil them, if you prefer. In a pinch, canned or jarred beets also work. Toasting the walnuts is optional, but it does enhance their flavor. You might consider setting aside a few beet pieces for young children. Many kids like the sweet taste!

serves 2 to 3

3 beets, leaves and roots trimmed, scrubbed
1 tablespoon red wine vinegar
½ teaspoon Dijon mustard
2 tablespoons olive oil or canola oil
3 to 4 cups baby greens, washed and dried

2.5 ounces pasteurized goat cheese (see Health Tip below), broken into small chunks
2 tablespoons walnuts (optional)
Salt and freshly ground pepper, to taste

1. Preheat the oven to 425°F. Line a baking dish with foil.
2. Place the beets in the dish and bake for 45 minutes to 1 hour, or until tender. Check for tenderness by inserting the tip of a knife into the middle of a beet. Let cool slightly.
3. When cool enough to handle, remove the skin from the beets. Slice the beets into matchsticks and place them in a bowl (be careful not to stain your clothing with the beet juice).
4. Mix the vinegar with the mustard in a small bowl, then whisk in the olive oil. Set aside.
5. Arrange the baby greens in a serving bowl or on a platter. Place the beets on top of the greens. Drizzle the dressing evenly over the top, then garnish with the goat cheese and walnuts, if using. Sprinkle with salt and pepper and serve immediately.

▶ *Health Tip:* Use only pasteurized goat cheese (see Listeriosis Warning, page 107).
▶ *Complete Meal Ideas:* Serve this salad with:
   Whole wheat bread or roll
   Reduced-fat 2% milk or low-fat yogurt
   Fresh fruit

APPROXIMATE NUTRITIONAL INFORMATION: Serving size: half of the beet salad (without the dressing); Calories: 243 cals; Protein: 15 g; Carbohydrates: 9 g; Fat: 17 g; Fiber: 3 g; Sodium: 174 mg; Vitamin A: 1,500 IU; Diabetic Exchange: Fat 3.5, Vegetable 2

APPROXIMATE NUTRITIONAL INFORMATION: Serving size: 1 tablespoon salad dressing; Calories: 82 cals; Protein: 0 g; Carbohydrates: 0 g; Fat: 9 g; Fiber: 0 g; Sodium: 5 mg; Diabetic Exchange: Fat 2, Meat (Medium Fat) 2, Vegetable 2

asparagus, hearts of palm, and tomato salad

~

What's in this for the baby and me? Vitamins A and C and folic acid.

THIS QUICK, EASY, colorful, and tasty salad is loaded with **vitamins A** and **C** and **folic acid**, and it is also a good source of protein, iron, and fiber. Canned or jarred hearts of palm are found in the canned vegetable or international food section of most grocery stores. This salad is best eaten the day it is made.

serves 4 (makes about 4 cups)

1 pound asparagus, washed, tough ends
   trimmed, and cut into 1½-inch pieces
One 14-ounce can hearts of palm, drained and
   cut into ½-inch slices
1–2 vine-ripened tomatoes, diced
4 cups baby greens, washed and dried

(optional)
2 tablespoons red wine vinegar
½ teaspoon Dijon mustard
¼ cup olive oil or canola oil
Salt and freshly ground pepper, to taste

1. Boil, steam, or microwave the asparagus until crisp-tender. The cooking time will depend on the cooking method, but the average cooking time is about 5 minutes. Drain, place in a bowl, and cool.
2. Add the hearts of palm and tomatoes to the asparagus; set aside. Arrange the baby greens on a serving platter; set aside.
3. In a small bowl, mix the vinegar and mustard. Add the olive oil and mix until well blended. Add most of the dressing to the salad and toss gently. Adjust the seasoning. Drizzle the remaining dressing evenly over the baby greens, place the asparagus salad in the center, and serve immediately.

▶ *Timesaving Tip:* Use presliced "salad cut" hearts of palm if available. Frozen, canned, or jarred asparagus can be substituted for the fresh (follow package directions for preparation)—although the texture and taste will not equal that of the fresh.

▶ *Diabetic Tip:* Reduce the portion size to ½ cup.

> ▶ **Complete Meal Ideas:** Serve this salad with:

    3 ounces protein (you might want to try the Pr-egg-o Salad Sandwich, page 96, or the Flank Steak with Salsa Verde, page 222)

    Whole wheat bread

    Reduced-fat 2% milk or low-fat yogurt

    Fresh fruit that contains vitamin C

APPROXIMATE NUTRITIONAL INFORMATION: Serving size: 1 cup asparagus, hearts of palm, and tomato salad; Calories: 176 cals; Protein: 5 g; Carbohydrates: 10 g; Fat: 14 g; Fiber: 4 g; Sodium: 252 mg; Vitamin A: 1,314 IU; Vitamin C: 26 mg; Diabetic Exchange (values per ½ cup serving): Fat 1.5, Vegetable 1

travel tips

Whether you are traveling near or far, it is important to use common sense and advance planning during pregnancy. Be sure to inform your doctor of your travel plans. While traveling in an airplane is almost always safe during pregnancy, it is not recommended for women who have obstetrical medical conditions that could result in an emergency. Some complications include pregnancy-induced hypertension, poorly controlled diabetes, sickle cell disease, a history of premature labor, placental abnormalities, or weakened cardiovascular systems.[27]

PLANNING AHEAD

▶ Ask your doctor if it is safe for you to travel and if you should carry a copy of your medical records with you.

▶ Ask your doctor about immunizations (some are safe, others are not) and what types of medications to include in your first aid kit, especially those for diarrhea and constipation.

▶ Preferably before you leave, or as soon as you arrive, determine the hospitals, doctors, and pharmacies that would be available should you require medical care.

▶ Check with your airline for travel restrictions during pregnancy, and order special meals (such as vegetarian, low-sodium, diabetic, or kosher) if your diet requires one.

PACKING YOUR BAG

▶ Carry all medications and important items in your carry-on luggage.

▶ Take along favorite foods that may be hard to find.

▶ Carry emergency snacks—crackers, cookies, fruit (fresh or dried), fruit cups, sliced vegetables, juice boxes, peanut butter, energy bars, cereal, and granola bars.

▶ Carry bottled water if the tap water is unsafe or if bottled water is unavailable in stores. Don't forget to include enough water for brushing your teeth.

▶ Pack loose clothing and comfortable shoes. Wear support hose if possible.

▶ Take powdered milk, long-life milk, or calcium supplements if you foresee a problem meeting your calcium needs.

▶ Pack sun block if you are headed to a sunny destination. Avoid prolonged exposure to the sun, which may lead to dizziness, fainting, dehydration, heat stroke, and sunburn (not to mention skin cancer).

GETTING THERE

▶ Wear loose travel clothing and comfortable shoes (preferably slip-ons, so you don't have to bend over), which allow your feet to swell.

▶ During long flights, train trips, or car rides, be sure to stretch your legs at least *every two hours*. This is important during the later stages of pregnancy, when blood clots are more likely.

▶ Be sure to drink plenty of (bottled) water throughout your journey.

▶ Don't hold it in—find a bathroom, or go behind a bush if you have to. The last thing you need is a urinary tract infection.

▶ Don't lift heavy bags. Hire a porter if necessary.

SAFE EATING

▶ Make sure you can identify everything you eat and that it is cooked *well-done*. Do not eat any raw meat (such as beef carpaccio or salmon gravalax) or raw fish (such as sushi or sashimi).

▶ If you are traveling to a less-developed country, eat only fruits or vegetables with a peel—apples, oranges, bananas, pineapples, mangoes, papayas, tangerines, etc.—and wash all fruit before you peel it.

▶ Stay hydrated. If the water is unsafe, drink only bottled water. If safe water is unavailable, drink canned or bottled fruit juice or other beverages. Do not drink sodas, beer, or any other beverages from a tap.

▶ Do not use ice cubes if the drinking water is unsafe.

▶ Brush your teeth with bottled water if the drinking water is unsafe.

▶ Follow the Tips for Eating in Restaurants (page 207) when dining out.

▶ Explain your dietary needs to your waiter. Most restaurants will fix a special dish following your dietary restrictions.

▶ If you think you may have food poisoning (severe vomiting or diarrhea), seek medical help *immediately*. Do not wait until you are dehydrated.

spinach salad with mandarin oranges and toasted almonds

~

What's in this for baby and me? Vitamins A and C and fiber.

AN AMAZING COMBINATION! This spinach salad is packed with **vitamins A** and **C** and **fiber**, and it is a good source of protein and iron. The Asian-style dressing complements the sweet oranges, but feel free to use your favorite vinaigrette or your favorite citrus fruit, such as fresh grapefruit or regular orange segments. For extra protein, you can add some sautéed tofu (see Instructions for Sautéing Tofu, page 189) to the salad. Oh, and toasting the almonds is essential.

serves 2 to 3

dressing

1 teaspoon soy sauce

1 tablespoon seasoned rice vinegar

3 tablespoons canola oil

A few drops of toasted sesame oil

1 very small garlic clove, crushed (optional)

Freshly ground pepper, to taste

spinach salad

2 cups packed baby spinach (one 6-ounce bag), washed and dried (see Timesaving Tip)

⅓ cup sliced or slivered almonds, toasted (see Cooking Tip)

½ cup mandarin oranges in juice (no added sugar), drained

1. To make the salad dressing, combine all of the ingredients in a small bowl and mix well. Set aside.
2. To make the salad, combine the spinach, almonds, and mandarin oranges in a salad bowl. Add the dressing, toss gently, and serve immediately.

▶ *Timesaving Tip:* Use packaged prewashed baby spinach leaves.

▶ *Cooking Tip:* To toast the almonds, place them in a small nonstick skillet over medium heat and stir until golden brown. Or, place the almonds on a baking sheet under a broiler for a minute or two—watch them carefully, because they tend to burn quickly.

▶ *Diabetic Tip:* Omit the almonds and use only one-quarter of the dressing.

▶ **Complete Meal Ideas:** Serve this salad with:

> 3 ounces protein (you might want to try the Sautéed Shrimp with Pasta, page 246, or the Homemade Tofu-Bean Burritos, page 182)
> Whole wheat bread
> Reduced-fat 2% milk or low-fat yogurt
> Fresh fruit that contains vitamin C

APPROXIMATE NUTRITIONAL INFORMATION: Serving size: half of the spinach salad; Calories: 170 cals; Protein: 6 g; Carbohydrates: 15 g; Fat: 11 g; Fiber: 6 g; Sodium: 42 mg; Vitamin A: 2,222 IU; Vitamin C: 20 mg; Diabetic Exchange: Fat 2, Vegetable 3

APPROXIMATE NUTRITIONAL INFORMATION: Serving size: half of the dressing; Calories: 187 cals; Protein: .3 g; Carbohydrates: .4 g; Fat: 20 g; Fiber: 0; Sodium: 154 mg; Diabetic Exchange (values per one-quarter of the salad dressing): Fat 2

homemade croutons

Fat-free homemade croutons are a wonderful snack any time of day. They are perfect "dippers" and a welcome addition to almost any soup. Any type of bread (fresh or stale) can be used to make croutons. French baguettes make light, delicate croutons, while hearty country, sourdough, rosemary, olive, and whole wheat breads make more robust, flavorful croutons.

To make croutons, preheat the oven to 350°F. Cut bread into cubes. Distribute the bread cubes evenly on a baking sheet and bake for 20 minutes. Turn the croutons, and continue baking for 5 to 10 minutes, or until hard and light golden brown. Cool, then store in an airtight container or zip-lock bag.

four delicious salad dressings

~

Having a bunch of washed and chilled lettuce on hand, along with a jar of home-made salad dressing, makes creating a fabulous salad an effortless task. Once you've tried these homemade dressings you will find it hard to go back to the store-bought bottled stuff. The Tarragon Vinaigrette has the longest shelf life of these dressings, about three weeks, so you can make it in a large batch. Shake or mix well before serving and dressing your salad.

french-style tarragon vinaigrette

The red wine vinegar can be replaced with sherry vinegar, rice vinegar, or any other flavored vinegar. Balsamic vinegar adds a rich, sweet flavor to dressings, but it should be used sparingly so as not to overpower the vinaigrette. The garlic can be replaced with minced shallots, the sugar with some honey, and the oil with plain or flavored oil. Feel free to play around with this basic recipe, but make sure not to add too many different flavors, which can begin to cancel out each other.

makes about ⅔ cup

2 teaspoons Dijon mustard, or to taste	¼ teaspoon salt
1 small garlic clove, smashed (optional)	Pinch of sugar
¼ cup red wine vinegar	Freshly ground pepper, to taste
½ teaspoon dried tarragon, basil, or oregano (optional)	¼ cup canola oil
	¼ cup olive oil

Combine the mustard, garlic, if using, vinegar, tarragon, if using, salt, sugar, and pepper in a jar with a lid or in a small bowl and shake or whisk until well blended. Add the canola oil and olive oil and shake or whisk until emulsified.

▶ **Cooking Tip:** This recipe can easily be doubled.

▶ **Storage Tip:** This dressing will keep refrigerated for up to 3 weeks.

APPROXIMATE NUTRITIONAL INFORMATION: Serving size: 1 tablespoon French-style tarragon vinaigrette; Calories: 99 cals; Protein: 0 g; Carbohydrates: 0 g; Fat: 11 g; Fiber: 0 g; Sodium: 64 mg; Diabetic Exchange: Fat 2

sun-dried tomato and basil dressing

THIS DRESSING IS great on boiled or steamed vegetables (especially potatoes), on a firm-leaved green salad (such as sliced romaine leaves or red leaf lettuce), or on a pasta salad with chunks of pasteurized feta or pasteurized goat cheese. It also makes a delicious sandwich spread. For a thicker sauce that is mouthwatering with fish, crab cakes, hamburgers, veggie burgers, or tofu cakes (see Old Bay Tofu Cakes, page 186), add 1 tablespoon light mayonnaise and reduce the water to ¼ cup.

makes about ¾ cup

⅓ cup sun-dried tomatoes packed in oil

2 teaspoons red wine vinegar

2 teaspoons balsamic vinegar

¼ cup canola oil

¼ cup plus 3–4 tablespoons boiling water

½ teaspoon dried oregano or Italian seasoning

Salt and freshly ground pepper, to taste

Combine all of the ingredients in a blender or food processor and process until smooth. The dressing can be thinned with additional hot water, 3 to 4 tablespoons, if desired.

▶ **Health Tip:** If your doctor has restricted your fat intake, use less oil and more water.

APPROXIMATE NUTRITIONAL INFORMATION: Serving size: 1 tablespoon sun-dried tomato and basil dressing; Calories: 48 cals; Protein: 0 g; Carbohydrates: 0 g; Fat: 5 g; Fiber: .2 g; Sodium: 8 mg; Diabetic Exchange: Fat 1

caesar salad dressing

W<small>HO CAN RESIST</small> a really good Caesar salad? This recipe uses a tablespoon of light mayonnaise instead of the traditional eggs. Do *not* use uncooked eggs in your dressing or eat any Caesar salad dressing prepared with uncooked eggs—ask your waiter about uncooked eggs if you are dining out (see Eggs and *Salmonella Enteritidis,* page 54). This dressing is delicious on sliced romaine lettuce with lots of Parmesan cheese, croutons, and some chopped fresh dill, or on any other lettuce with your favorite cheese, croutons, and fresh herbs. The amounts of olive oil and canola oil can be adjusted to suit your taste. Stick with these amounts if you like a rich olive oil taste.

makes about ½ cup

1 tablespoon light mayonnaise

2 tablespoons freshly squeezed lemon juice,
or to taste

1 teaspoon Worcestershire sauce

1 small garlic clove, squeezed through a garlic
press or minced

½ teaspoon anchovy paste (optional)

¼ teaspoon salt

Freshly ground pepper, to taste

⅓ cup olive oil

2 tablespoons canola oil

Combine all of the ingredients except the olive oil and canola oil in a small bowl and whisk until smooth. Gradually add the olive oil and canola oil, whisking until emulsified.

▶ *Cooking Tip:* This salad dressing will separate as it sits. Whisk or shake it to re-emulsify it.

▶ *Storage Tip:* This dressing will keep refrigerated for up to 3 days.

APPROXIMATE NUTRITIONAL INFORMATION: Serving size: 1 tablespoon Caesar salad dressing: Calories: 117 cals; Protein: 0 g; Carbohydrates: 0 g; Fat: 13 g; Fiber: 0 g; Sodium: 96 mg; Diabetic Exchange: Fat 2.5

What's in this for baby and me? Vitamins A and C, folic acid, and fiber.

Rᵢᴄʜ ɪɴ **vitamins A** and **C**, **folic acid**, and **fiber**, and a good source of protein and calcium, this power-packed salad is surprisingly quick and easy to assemble. The order in which you add the ingredients is vital to the success of this salad. Adding the olive oil first coats the leaves so they are not "burned" by the acid of the lemon juice.

serves 2

4 cups washed and sliced romaine lettuce
¼ cup grated Parmesan cheese
1 ripe avocado, peeled, pitted, and sliced

1½ tablespoons olive oil, or to taste
Juice of ½ a fresh lemon, or to taste
Salt and freshly ground pepper, to taste

Place the romaine lettuce, Parmesan cheese, and avocado in a salad bowl. Drizzle the olive oil evenly over the top, then toss gently. Add the lemon juice and salt and pepper and toss gently again. Serve immediately.

▶ *Diabetic Tip:* Reduce the portion size to 1 cup salad.

APPROXIMATE NUTRITIONAL INFORMATION: Serving size: half of this salad; Calories: 304 cals; Protein: 8 g; Carbohydrates: 10 g; Fat: 28 g; Fiber: 6 g; Sodium: 205 mg; Vitamin A: 3,504 IU; Vitamin C: 41 mg; Folic Acid: 211 mcg; Diabetic Exchange (values per 1 cup serving of salad): Fat 3, Vegetable 1

homemade guacamole

What's in this for baby and me? Vitamin C.

HIGH IN **vitamin C** and a good source of folic acid and fiber, homemade guacamole is delicious served as a dip for sliced fresh vegetables and baked tortilla chips, or with fajitas, quesadillas, tacos, or any grilled main course. It is also wonderful spread on sandwiches instead of mayonnaise.

makes 2½ cups

3 ripe avocados, preferably Hass

3 tablespoons very finely chopped red onion or sweet white onion (such as Vidalia)

1 large vine-ripened tomato, cut into small dice

2 tablespoons freshly squeezed lime juice, or to taste

3 tablespoons chopped fresh cilantro (optional)

1 small garlic clove, crushed (optional)

Dash of Tabasco sauce or freshly ground pepper to taste

Salt, to taste

1. Cut the avocados in half and remove the pits. Cut the halves into quarters, then peel them and place in a small bowl. Using the back of a fork, mash the avocados to a chunky consistency. (Do not use a food processor or blender.)
2. Add the remaining ingredients and mix until well combined. Season to taste, cover with the plastic wrap placed flush against the surface of the guacamole, and refrigerate a couple hours before serving.

▶ *Storage Tip:* This dip keeps refrigerated for 1 day. Some discoloration will occur, but the taste will not be affected.

▶ *Diabetic Tip:* Reduce the portion size to 2 tablespoons.

APPROXIMATE NUTRITIONAL INFORMATION: Serving size: ¼ cup guacamole; Calories: 158 cals; Protein: 2 g; Carbohydrates: 8 g; Fat: 15 g; Fiber: 4 g; Sodium: 12 mg; Vitamin C: 13 mg; Diabetic Exchange (values per 2 tablespoon serving): Fat 1.5

roasted red pepper and cheese dip

What's in this for baby and me? Vitamin C.

TASTY AND EASY to prepare, this dip makes a perfect snack or sandwich spread. It is a great source of **vitamin C** and a good source of protein, calcium, and vitamin A. The feta cheese gives the dip a great consistency and the perfect tang. Serve with your favorite raw vegetables or whole wheat crackers for a vitamin and fiber fix.

makes about 1 cup

⅓ cup part-skim ricotta cheese

⅔ cup (about 4 ounces) crumbled pasteurized feta cheese (see Health Tip below)

⅓ cup sliced jarred roasted red peppers

Salt and freshly ground pepper, to taste

Combine all of the ingredients in the bowl of a food processor and pulse, scraping down the sides of the bowl as needed, until smooth and creamy. Do not overmix, or the dip will be runny. (Refrigerate any leftovers.)

▶ *Health Tip:* Use only pasteurized feta cheese (see Listeriosis Warning, page 107)

▶ *Storage Tip:* This dip keeps for 3 days refrigerated.

APPROXIMATE NUTRITIONAL INFORMATION: Serving size: ¼ cup roasted red pepper and cheese dip; Calories: 105 cals; Protein: 6 g; Carbohydrates: 3 g; Fat: 8 g; Fiber: .1 g; Sodium: 388 mg; Vitamin C: 19 mg; Diabetic Exchange: Fat 1, Meat (Medium Fat) 1

spinach dip

~

What's in this for baby and me? Vitamin A.

THIS SPINACH DIP is high in **vitamin A** and a good source of vitamin C, calcium, and folic acid. Fresh vegetables for dipping provide additional vitamins and fiber. This recipe can be cut in half to serve fewer people or doubled to feed a crowd. If your kids like dip, this one could be a winner—but you might want to leave out the anchovy paste.

makes about 2 cups

One 10-ounce package frozen chopped
   spinach, thawed, drained, and squeezed
   dry

¼ cup sliced scallions

¼ cup fresh parsley leaves

1½ teaspoons anchovy paste, or to taste
   (optional)

3 tablespoons freshly squeezed lemon juice,
   or to taste

⅓ cup part-skim ricotta cheese

½ cup reduced-fat sour cream

2 tablespoons light mayonnaise

Salt and freshly ground pepper, to taste

Combine the spinach, scallions, parsley, anchovy paste, if using, and lemon juice in the bowl of a food processor and process until fairly smooth. Add the ricotta cheese, sour cream, and mayonnaise and pulse just until blended. Season and serve; refrigerate leftovers.

▶ *Variation:* Use about 12 ounces of fresh spinach in place of the frozen spinach. Cook the spinach (sauté, steam, microwave, or boil), drain, and squeeze out as much liquid as possible before proceeding with the recipe.

▶ *Storage Tip:* This dip keeps for 2 days refrigerated. The spinach will lose its bright green color from the acid of the lemon juice, but the taste is unaffected.

▶ *Health Tip:* If your doctor has restricted your salt intake, omit the anchovy paste and go easy on the salt. If you need to reduce your fat intake, omit the mayonnaise and use low-fat ricotta cheese and nonfat yogurt or nonfat sour cream instead of reduced-fat sour cream. Yogurt produces a less creamy dip.

APPROXIMATE NUTRITIONAL INFORMATION: Serving size: ¼ cup spinach dip; Calories: 61 cals; Protein: 3 g; Carbohydrates: 4 g; Fat: 4 g; Fiber: 1 g; Sodium: 87 mg; Vitamin A: 2,982 IU; Diabetic Exchange: Fat 1, Vegetable 1

healthy hummus

~

What's in this for baby and me? Protein, folic acid, and fiber.

AN EXCELLENT SOURCE of **protein**, **folic acid**, and **fiber**, and a good source of vitamin C and iron, hummus is a wonderful addition to any pregnant woman's diet, and many kids love it. Serve hummus with toasted whole wheat pita bread, Melba toast, whole wheat crackers, or sliced fresh vegetables. For a delicious vegetarian sandwich, see the Hummus-Tabbouleh Roll on page 105. If your dietary needs call for extra calories, or if you are serving small children who don't need to watch their fat intake, feel free to substitute additional olive oil or canola oil for the water.

makes about 2 cups

One 15-ounce can chickpeas, rinsed and
   drained
1 small garlic clove, crushed (optional)
½ teaspoon ground cumin (optional)
¼ cup freshly squeezed lemon juice, or to
   taste

2 tablespoons canola oil or olive oil
1 tablespoon tahini
A few drops of Tabasco sauce (optional)
2–3 tablespoons water (add more or less to
   desired consistency)
Salt, to taste

Combine all of the ingredients in the bowl of a food processor or blender and process until completely smooth, scraping down the sides of the bowl as needed. Season and serve; refrigerate leftovers.

▶ **Cooking Tip 1:** For a slightly higher yield, use a 19-ounce can of chickpeas and increase the following ingredients: 2 small garlic cloves, 3 tablespoons canola oil or olive oil, 2 tablespoons tahini, and ¼ cup water.

▶ **Cooking Tip 2:** If serving this hummus as an appetizer, garnish it with 2 tablespoons chopped fresh parsley and a dash of cayenne pepper. Or, dribble extra olive oil on top and sprinkle with olives or toasted pine nuts.

▶ **Storage Tip:** This dip keeps for 3 days refrigerated.

▶ **Health Tip:** If your doctor has restricted your fat intake, substitute water for the olive oil.

APPROXIMATE NUTRITIONAL INFORMATION: Serving size: ½ cup homemade hummus; Calories: 261 cals; Protein: 10 g; Carbohydrates: 31 g; Fat: 12 g; Fiber: 8 g; Sodium: 154 mg; Folic Acid: 189 mcg; Diabetic Exchange: Bread/Starch 2, Fat 2.5, Meat (Lean) .5

constipation

Constipation is a common problem for pregnant women. Like indigestion and heart-burn, it usually occurs during the first and third trimesters. During the first trimester, increased hormonal levels tend to cause constipation, while during the third trimester, smooth-muscle relaxation and cramped and compressed abdominal space slow down waste elimination. It is important to include high-fiber foods in your diet and to drink plenty of fluids, including water, milk, and (some) fruit juice.

TIPS FOR COPING

▶ Increase high-fiber foods in your diet, such as whole grain cereals and breads, beans, lentils, peas, raw fruits and vegetables, and dried fruit. A good fiber intake is about 25 to 30 g per day.

▶ Increase fluids—drink at least 8 glasses of water per day, and ideally a total of 12 cups of fluid per day.

▶ With permission from your doctor, get regular exercise, which helps get your intestines moving.

▶ Go for walks after meals.

▶ Try a glass of prune juice or some prunes in the morning.

▶ Iron supplements cause constipation in some women. Try taking your supplement at different times of the day.

▶ Do *not* take any form of laxative, bulk-forming supplemental fiber (such as psyllium and methylcellulose) or mineral oil without the consent of your doctor.

artichoke-spinach dip

What's in this for baby and me? Vitamin C and A and folic acid.

AN EXCELLENT SOURCE of **vitamin C** and **A** and **folic acid** and a fine source of **calcium** and fiber, this dip is a great snack any time of day.

makes about 1 ½ cups

2 tightly packed cups baby spinach (one 6-ounce bag)

One 14-ounce can artichoke hearts, drained

1 scallion, trimmed and sliced

¼ cup grated Parmesan cheese

¼ cup jarred roasted red bell peppers (optional)

2 tablespoons light mayonnaise

Salt and freshly ground pepper, to taste

Squeeze of fresh lemon juice

1. Microwave, boil, or steam the spinach just until wilted, about 1 minute. Drain and squeeze as much liquid from the spinach as possible.
2. Place the cooked spinach, artichoke hearts, scallion, Parmesan cheese, bell peppers, if using, and mayonnaise in the bowl of a food processor and pulse to the desired consistency. Season with salt, pepper, and lemon juice. Refrigerate any leftovers.

▶ *Storage Tip:* This dip keeps for 2 days refrigerated.

APPROXIMATE NUTRITIONAL INFORMATION: Serving size: ¼ cup artichoke-spinach dip; Calories: 72 cals; Protein: 5 g; Carbohydrates: 9 g; Fat: 3 g; Fiber: 4 g; Sodium: 185 mg; Vitamin A: 5,246 IU; Vitamin C: 23 g; Diabetic Exchange: Fat 1, Vegetable 1.5

black bean dip

What's in this for baby and me? Vitamin C, folic acid, and fiber.

Here's a bean dip that's rich in **vitamin C**, **folic acid**, and **fiber**, and a good source of protein. It goes deliciously with whole wheat crackers, vegetables, and, of course, baked corn tortilla chips. Spread it on a burrito, use it in a sandwich instead of mayonnaise, or serve it at a party and watch it disappear.

makes about 1¾ cups

One 15.5-ounce can black beans, rinsed and drained

2 tablespoons chopped jarred roasted red peppers or pimentos (optional)

2 tablespoons water

1 tablespoon canola oil or olive oil

1½ tablespoons freshly squeezed lime juice, or to taste

2 tablespoons chopped fresh cilantro

½ teaspoon minced garlic (optional)

½ teaspoon ground cumin, or to taste

½ teaspoon salt, or to taste

A couple of drops of Tabasco

Combine all of the ingredients in the bowl of a food processor or blender and process until completely smooth, scraping down the sides of the bowl as needed. Adjust seasoning and serve; refrigerate leftovers.

▶ *Storage Tip:* This dip keeps for 2 days, refrigerated.

APPROXIMATE NUTRITIONAL INFORMATION: Serving size: ½ cup black bean dip; Calories: 146 cals; Protein: 7 g; Carbohydrates: 20 g; Fat: 5 g; Fiber: 7 g; Sodium: 359 mg; Vitamin C: 12 mg; Folic Acid: 120 mcg; Diabetic Exchange: Bread/Starch 1.5, Fat 1

vegetarian delights

～

THERE ARE ALMOST as many reasons for choosing a vegetarian lifestyle as there are vegetarians, and the definition of vegetarian varies from person to person. While *all* pregnant women need to focus on meal planning to meet their additional nutrient requirements, vegetarians, especially vegans, must pay special attention to fulfilling their protein, calcium, vitamin D, iron, vitamin B_{12}, and zinc needs. Most pregnant vegetarians do not need to drastically change their lifestyle or eating habits unless they were unhealthy to begin with. Be sure to inform your doctor that you are a vegetarian, describe your dietary restrictions and eating habits, and address any concerns you have regarding eating during pregnancy.

To optimize nutritional benefits, vegetarians and nonvegetarians alike should eat balanced meals that include a variety of foods. Eating a variety of healthy foods maximizes the body's ability to absorb nutrients, particularly calcium, iron, and zinc. Generally, a pregnant vegetarian will need to consume the following amounts from the basic food groups (for food suggestions and portion size see Food Groups and Serving Sizes for Pregnant Women, page 293).

FOOD GROUPS FOR A VEGETARIAN PREGNANCY[28]

Grain Group = 6 to 11 servings per day

Fruits = 2 to 4 servings per day

Vegetables = 3 to 5 servings per day

Protein Group = 3 servings per day

Milk and Dairy Group = 4 servings per day

Others (fats and sweets) = use sparingly

PROTEIN

MEETING THE PROTEIN requirements of pregnancy is usually not a problem for most vegetarians, although vegans who do not eat any dairy products might be challenged. Some vegetarian sources of protein include pasteurized cheese, low-fat cottage cheese, milk, low-fat yogurt, tofu (plain and enriched), tempeh, eggs, enriched soy beverages, cooked beans, soybeans, nuts, and nut butters (see Protein Sources, page 295, for a more complete list). Consult your doctor or dietitian if you feel you cannot meet your increased protein requirements during pregnancy, or if you are considering a protein supplement.

CALCIUM AND VITAMIN D

VEGETARIANS WHO EAT dairy products usually can meet their calcium and vitamin D requirements from milk, yogurt, and pasteurized cheeses. If your vegetarian diet excludes all dairy products, a calcium and vitamin D supplement will likely be advised. (For a list of Nondairy Calcium Sources, see page 297.) To ensure vitamin D production, vegans should try to get at least twenty to thirty minutes of direct sunlight on their hands and faces two to three times a week. Some good news is that vegetarians tend to absorb and retain more calcium from foods than non-vegetarians. However, calcium bioavailability, or the body's ability to absorb calcium, may be reduced by oxalic acid[29] (oxalates) and phytic acid[30] (phytates), found in certain plants and vegetables, and unrefined cereals.[31] This information is important to note because some vegetarian diets rely on large amounts of leafy greens and green vegetables for calcium intake.

IRON

IRON IS ESSENTIAL throughout pregnancy and iron deficiency occurs in vegetarian and nonvegetarian pregnancies alike. Some high-iron plant sources include blackstrap molasses, iron-fortified cereals, cooked beans (especially lima beans and soybeans), green leafy vegetables (such as spinach, Swiss chard, kale, and beet greens), lentils, baked potatoes (with skin on), tempeh, prune juice, and dried fruit (see Iron Sources, page 298, for a more complete list).

The tannins in leaf tea, coffee, calcium supplements, and certain foods high in phytic acid can limit iron absorption. To maximize iron absorption, vegetarians should try to consume iron-rich foods with foods high in vitamin C (see Vitamin C Sources, page 294). Also, vegetarians should opt for iron- and zinc-fortified soy products to minimize the inhibitory effect of phytic acid contained in certain soy products, such as soy flour, soy protein isolate, and tofu processed with calcium sulfate. (See Recommendations for Optimizing Iron and Zinc Bioavailability in Vegetarians, page 191.)

VITAMIN B$_{12}$

BECAUSE PLANTS DO not contain vitamin B$_{12}$, vegans may need to supplement their diets to ensure an adequate intake of B$_{12}$. Vegetarians who include eggs and dairy products in their diets are seldom at risk for a vitamin B$_{12}$ deficiency. Some good sources of vitamin B$_{12}$ include fortified soy beverages, milk products, fortified tofu and other fortified soy products, enriched breakfast cereal (see Cereals that Contain 100 Percent of the Daily Value of Vitamin B$_{12}$, page 302), and brewer's yeast (check with your doctor or dietitian before taking any brewer's yeast supplements).

ZINC

DAIRY PRODUCTS ARE among the best dietary sources of zinc for vegetarians. Vegans who do not consume any dairy products can obtain zinc from such sources as whole grains, legumes, brown rice, spinach, nuts, seeds, tofu, tempeh, fortified cereals, and wheat germ. As with iron, your body's ability to absorb zinc may be reduced by the presence of phytates, oxalates, fiber, calcium supplements, and soy proteins containing phytic acid. (See Recommendations for Optimizing Iron and Zinc Bioavailability in Vegetarians, page 191.)

sample menu for a vegan pregnancy

BREAKFAST
1 cup oatmeal with molasses
1 slice whole wheat toast
1 cup fortified soy beverage
½ cup calcium-fortified orange juice

MORNING SNACK
½ whole wheat bagel or bran muffin with nut butter or margarine
1 fruit

LUNCH
Veggie burger on whole wheat bun
1 cup cooked greens or green vegetable
1 fruit
1 cup fortified soy beverage

AFTERNOON SNACK
¾ cup ready-to-eat high-iron cereal with ½ cup berries
(or other high-vitamin C fruit)
1 cup fortified soy beverage or soy yogurt

DINNER
6 ounces tofu with 1 cup vegetables, stir-fried
1 cup brown rice
1 cup fortified soy beverage

BEDTIME SNACK
One 8-ounce container soy yogurt or fortified soy beverage
5 whole wheat crackers with 2 tablespoons nut butter

vegetarian delights

Light and Healthy Vegetable Ragout ▼

Three-Bean Vegetarian Chili ▼

Vegetarian Curry

Best-Ever Vegetarian Lasagna

Spaghetti with Herbed Tofu Balls and Tomato Sauce

Pasta with Tomatoes, Herbs, and Pasteurized Goat Cheese

Spinach-Cheese Quiche

Grilled or Roasted Marinated Vegetables ▼

Vegetarian Pad Thai

Homemade Tofu-Bean Burritos ▼

Cheese and Spinach Quesadillas

Old Bay Tofu Cakes with Cocktail Sauce

Sautéed Tofu and Portobello Mushrooms on a Bed of Greens ▼

Vegetarian Omelet for One

Lentil, Brown Rice, and Mushroom Pilaf

Swiss Chard or Spinach with Garlicky Soy Dressing ▼

Lima Beans with Artichoke Hearts and Dill

Okra and Tomatoes ▼

Classic Creamed Spinach

Simple and Tasty Brussels Sprouts ▼

Southern-Style Sweet Potato Casserole

Baked Acorn Squash with Molasses ▼

Annie Mozer's Greens ▼

▼ Vegan recipe

RECIPE NOTES

IF YOU ARE a vegetarian, you are sure to have fun with these vegetarian delights, not to mention the other eighty-five vegetarian recipes and thirty-one vegan recipes throughout the book. (Vegan recipes are designated by the ▼ symbol.) If you are not a vegetarian, trying a few of these dishes might just convince you that tofu can be quite tasty, or that eating a meat-free diet can be satisfying. The collection of recipes in *"Vegetarian Delights"* is designed to give you ideas for new recipes, and to put a healthy twist on some old favorites.

Most of the recipes are quick and easy. There are a few exceptions that are a bit more time-consuming and labor intensive—such as the Light and Healthy Vegetable Ragout, the Best-Ever Vegetarian Lasagna, and the Vegetarian Pad Thai. But the extra time and effort you put into these creations are well worth it. Also, after you've made these dishes the first time, and you are familiar with the ingredients and procedures, the next time will be quicker. Keep in mind that the different components of these dishes can be made in advance, leaving the assembly for the last minute. As with all cooking, choose the best fresh produce and ingredients you can find in your local grocery store, whole food store, health food store, or farmers' market. This is especially true for vegetarians who rely on fresh produce for the bulk of their diet.

A quick word about tofu. There are numerous varieties of tofu on the shelves today. Try several to see which works best for you. All of the recipes in this chapter call for extra firm tofu. Nasoya brand seems to hold up particularly well to stir-frying. Tofu is an excellent source of protein for young eaters. It is less of a choking hazard than many other protein sources and is easily digested, especially by anyone with lactose intolerance. So, vegetarian or not, if you've never tried tofu, don't be leery of it—buy it, cook with it, and you may just learn to love it!

Some notes about the recipes in this chapter:

- Most dairy products can be replaced with soy products, from soy milk to soy sour cream, and margarine can be substituted for butter. A few exceptions are mentioned in the recipes.
- Reduced-fat 2% milk can be substituted for whole milk.
- If you need to increase your calcium intake, choose calcium-fortified cheeses, including packaged grated cheddar cheese and Monterey Jack.
- If you need to watch your fat intake, use low-fat cheeses or those made with 2% milk, and use reduced-fat 2% milk.
- Check the expiration date on all packages of tofu and tempeh, and make sure that they are properly packaged. Try to avoid tofu sold out of tubs filled with water.
- Wash all greens and vegetables thoroughly, even if the package claims that they are prewashed (see Tips for Cleaning Fresh Produce, page 314).

- Use vegetarian bouillon cubes to add extra flavor to any dish (unless you need to watch your sodium intake).
- To save time, pick up as many ingredients as possible from a salad bar, such as shredded carrots, chopped onions, sliced mushrooms, and sliced red bell peppers.
- Try to avoid overcooking vegetables, a common mistake, especially when stir-frying. Keep in mind that the vegetables will continue to cook once removed from the heat.
- Frozen vegetables can be used, except where noted, if you are short on time.
- Don't be afraid to experiment and modify the recipes to suit your family's needs and tastes.

vegetarian staples to have on hand

Try to keep your pantry and freezer stocked with the following items:

▶ **Whole grain iron-, B$_{12}$-, and folic acid–fortified breakfast cereals**

▶ **Wheat germ**

▶ **Quick-cooking whole grain cereals**

▶ **Molasses**

▶ **Milk powder**

▶ **Whole wheat crackers**

▶ **Whole grains (such as barley, brown rice, bulgur wheat, and quinoa)**

▶ **Enriched pastas**

▶ **Tortillas**

▶ **Canned beans (pinto beans, kidney beans, soybeans, and chickpeas)**

▶ **Prepared vegetable soups**

▶ **Jarred or bottled tomato sauce**

▶ **V-8 juice, tomato juice, or other vegetable juices**

▶ **Calcium-fortified orange juice**

▶ **Nut spreads (including peanut butter and soy butter)**

▶ **Nuts and seeds**

▶ **Dried fruits**

▶ **Canned fruits in light syrup**

▶ **Frozen fruits**

▶ **Frozen vegetables**

▶ **Frozen fruit juice concentrates**

▶ **Frozen fortified waffles (preferably whole wheat)**

▶ **Main-course frozen foods, such as burritos, enchiladas, tamales, veggie burgers, pizza, and spinach lasagna**

pantry items for vegetarian delights

Fresh Produce
Acorn squash
Baby greens or lettuce
Baby spinach
Bok choy
Broccoli florets
Brussels sprouts
Carrots: regular and peeled baby
   carrots
Collard greens
Fresh herbs: basil, cilantro, dill, mint,
   oregano, and parsley
Garlic
Ginger
Green asparagus
Kale
Lemons
Limes
Mushrooms: button, cremini, porto-
   bello, and shiitake
Mustard greens
Okra
Onions: sweet (such as Vidalia), yel-
   low, and red
Purple eggplant
Red bell peppers
Red sweet potatoes
Scallions
Swiss chard
Tomatoes
Zucchini

Dairy and Soy Products
Cheddar cheese (grated)
Extra-firm tofu (15-ounce package
   drained weight)

Fontina cheese
Grade A large eggs
Gruyère cheese
Half-and-half (preferably ultra-pas-
   teurized)
Heavy cream
Milk: whole, reduced-fat 2% milk, or
   enriched plain soy beverages
Monterey Jack cheese (grated)
Parmesan cheese (grated)
Pasteurized feta cheese
Pasteurized goat cheese
Pasteurized part-skim low-moisture
   mozzarella cheese
Unsalted butter

Canned, Bottled, and Jarred Staples
Artichoke hearts packed in water or
   brine (14-ounce can)
Balsamic vinegar
Black beans (15.5-ounce can)
Black-eyed peas (15.5-ounce can)
Black olives (preferably pitted)
Canola oil
Canola oil cooking spray
Cocktail sauce
Crushed tomatoes (28-ounce can)
Dijon mustard
Fat-free low-sodium stock (any kind)
Hoisin sauce
Ketchup
Light or regular coconut milk (14-
   ounce can)
Light skim evaporated milk
Molasses

Olive oil
Peeled and diced tomatoes (14.5-ounce can)
Red kidney beans (16-ounce can)
Red wine vinegar
Reduced-fat stock (any flavor)
Rice vinegar (preferably seasoned)
Roasted red bell peppers
Salsa
Sesame oil (preferably toasted)
Soybeans (15-ounce can)
Soy sauce (regular or light)
Tomato juice or V-8 juice

Chinese rice noodles
Dried cranberries
Fajita-size tortillas (6-inch tortillas)
Flour: ubleached all-purpose, whole wheat, quick-dissolving
Green lentils
No-boil lasagna noodles
Nuts: peanuts, walnuts, pecans
Pad Thai rice noodles
Pasteurized instant nonfat dry milk
Rice: brown and/or white
Saltine crackers
Thin spaghetti, capellini, or linguine

Herbs and Spices
Basil
Chili powder
Dried oregano
Dried thyme
Ground allspice, cinnamon, or cloves
Ground cumin
Italian seasoning
Mild curry powder
Old Bay seasoning

Dry Staples
Bread crumbs (plain or seasoned)
Brown sugar
Burrito-size tortillas (10-inch tortillas)

Frozen Staples
9-inch pie crusts (preferably whole wheat)
Artichoke hearts (8 ounces)
Chopped spinach
Lima beans (8 ounces)

From the Salad Bar
Broccoli florets
Cauliflower florets
Diced onions
Roasted red bell peppers
Shredded carrots
Sliced mushrooms
Sliced red bell peppers

light and healthy vegetable ragout

What's in this for baby and me? Vitamins A and C.

THIS VERSATILE RAGOUT is perfect as a side dish, as a burrito filling with beans, rice, and cheese, in a sandwich, or over pasta or couscous with lots of fresh herbs and grated Parmesan cheese. It is an excellent source of **vitamins A** and **C** and a good source of fiber. Thinned with some tomato sauce or crushed tomatoes, the ragout turns into a fabulous sauce for vegetarian lasagna, or any other dish made with a tomato-based sauce. **Slow Cooker Instructions** follow.

serves 6 (makes about 8 cups)

⅓ cup olive oil or canola oil

1 medium onion, finely chopped

2 garlic cloves, minced

1 tablespoon dried oregano

2 large carrots, peeled and coarsely grated or shredded (about 1½ cups)

1 red bell pepper, cored, seeded, and cut into ¼-inch dice

1 medium (about 1 pound) purple eggplant, peeled and cut into ¼-inch dice (see Cooking Tip below)

Two 14.5-ounce cans diced tomatoes, drained

1¼ cups tomato juice or V-8 juice

1½ teaspoons sugar

1 medium zucchini, washed and cut into ¼-inch dice (optional)

One 14-ounce can quartered artichoke hearts (optional)

¼ cup chopped fresh basil or cilantro (optional)

Salt and freshly ground pepper, to taste

1. Heat the oil in a 6-quart nonreactive saucepan over medium-high heat. Add the onion and sauté for 3 minutes. Add the garlic, oregano, carrots, and red bell pepper and continue to sauté for 3 minutes, stirring frequently.
2. Add the eggplant and cook, stirring constantly, for 3 minutes. Add the tomatoes, tomato juice, and sugar, and stir, then reduce the heat and gently simmer, uncovered, for 15 minutes, stirring occasionally. Add the optional zucchini and artichoke hearts, stir, and cook for about 25 minutes, or until the vegetables are tender and the sauce has reached the desired consistency.
3. Add the basil, if desired, and season with salt and pepper. Serve immediately.

▶ *Timesaving Tip:* Because this recipe calls for a lot of chopped vegetables, see what you can pick up at a salad bar. You might find chopped onions, grated or shredded carrots, and chopped red bell peppers.

▶ *Cooking Tip:* Removing the moisture from the eggplant with salt is an optional step that requires 20 minutes to 1 hour. The advantage of this is that eggplant will not absorb as much oil, and it should also remove any bitterness. Place the diced eggplant in a colander on a large plate with a rim, sprinkle with 2 teaspoons salt, and toss gently. Allow the eggplant to stand for at least 20 minutes, or up to 1 hour. Rinse the eggplant quickly under cold water, then spread it out on a double thickness of paper towels. Cover with more paper towels and press firmly to extract as much water as possible.

▶ *Storage Tip:* This ragout keeps for 3 days refrigerated, and it can be frozen for up to 1 month.

▶ *Slow Cooker Instructions:*
1. Follow Step 1, then add the eggplant and cook, stirring constantly, for 3 minutes.
2. Transfer the contents of the skillet to the slow cooker and add the tomatoes, tomato juice, sugar, and optional zucchini. Cover and cook on high for 5 hours. *Note:* If you prefer a slightly thicker sauce, add 2 tablespoons quick-dissolving flour during the last 15 minutes of cooking. Finish the ragout as directed in Step 3.

▶ *Complete Meal Ideas:* Serve this ragout with:
   Pasta, rice, couscous, or any other grain
   3 ounces protein (you might want to make the Old Bay Tofu Cakes, page 186, and use the vegetable ragout instead of the cocktail sauce)
   Reduced-fat 2% milk or low-fat yogurt
   Fresh fruit

APPROXIMATE NUTRITIONAL INFORMATION: Serving size: 1 cup vegetable ragout; Calories: 146 cals; Protein: 3 g; Carbohydrates: 15 g; Fat: 9 g; Fiber: 4 g; Sodium: 553 mg; Vitamin A: 7,958 IU; Vitamin C: 60 mg; Diabetic Exchange: Fat 2, Vegetable 3

three-bean vegetarian chili

~

What's in this for baby and me? Protein, iron, vitamins A and C,
folic acid, and fiber.

THIS THREE-BEAN vegetarian chili is an excellent source of **protein**, **iron**, **vitamins A** and **C**, **folic acid**, and **fiber**, and a good source of calcium and B vitamins—all your nutrient bases are covered! For extra protein, add tofu sautéed with a dash of chili powder, or add frozen ground soy burger (see **Variation** below). Serve this chili over rice, quinoa, or couscous, or wrap it in tortillas. Some garnishes to pass at the table include grated cheddar cheese, Monterey Jack, or your favorite pasteurized cheese, thinly sliced romaine lettuce, thinly sliced scallions, and sliced black olives. **Slow Cooker Instructions** follow.

serves 6 (makes about 7 cups)

2 tablespoons olive oil or canola oil

1 small red onion, finely chopped

1 garlic clove, minced

1 tablespoon chili powder

2 teaspoons ground cumin

1 teaspoon dried oregano

1 red bell pepper, cored, seeded, and cut into small dice (optional)

8 ounces mushrooms (any kind), washed and thinly sliced (optional)

One 15.5-ounce can black beans, rinsed and drained

One 15.5-ounce can red kidney beans, rinsed and drained

One 15-ounce can soybeans (do not drain), or any other canned bean, rinsed and drained

One 14.5-ounce can diced tomatoes (do not drain)

1 cup water or low-sodium vegetable stock

A sprinkle or two of quick-dissolving flour, such as Wondra (optional)

1½ tablespoons balsamic vinegar, or to taste (optional)

½ cup chopped fresh cilantro, for garnish

1. Heat the olive oil in a 6-quart saucepan over medium-high heat. Add the onion and sauté for 3 minutes. Add the garlic, chili powder, cumin, and oregano and sauté for 30 seconds. Add the optional red bell pepper and mushrooms and sauté for 3 minutes.
2. Add the black beans, red kidney beans, soybeans, diced tomatoes, and water and bring to a boil. Reduce the heat to a gentle simmer and cook for 30 minutes, or until slightly thickened. If the chili is not thick enough for your taste after 30 minutes of cooking, add a dash or two of quick-dissolving flour and cook for 2 minutes longer.
3. Add the balsamic vinegar, if using, adjust the seasoning, and garnish with the cilantro. Serve immediately, with the accompaniments of your choice.

▶ *Variation:* Cut one 15-ounce package (drained weight) extra-firm tofu into ½-inch cubes and blot dry with paper towels. Sauté according to the instructions on page 189. Cover the sautéed tofu with foil and set aside. Add the tofu during the last 5 minutes of cooking in Step 2. You can also add frozen ground soy burger in Step 2 along with the beans. Feel free to add or substitute your favorite vegetables, and sauté them with the red bell pepper in Step 1.

▶ *Storage Tip:* This chili keeps for 5 days refrigerated, and it can be frozen for 1 month. Freeze in single-meal-size portions in zip-lock bags or plastic containers for lunch or dinner.

▶ *Slow Cooker Instructions: Use 1½ cups of water or vegetable stock instead of 1 cup.*
1. Follow Step 1 using a skillet instead of a saucepan.
2. Transfer the contents of the skillet to the slow cooker and add the black beans, kidney beans, soybeans, tomatoes, and water. Cover and cook on high for 5 hours. Add 2 tablespoons of quick-dissolving flour during the last 30 minutes of cooking. Finish the chili as directed in step 3.

▶ *Complete Meal Ideas:* Serve this chili with:
Rice, tortilla, or a whole wheat roll
Tossed salad (you might want to try romaine lettuce with the Caesar Salad
Dressing, page 143)
Reduced-fat 2% milk or low-fat yogurt
Fresh fruit that contains vitamin C

APPROXIMATE NUTRITIONAL INFORMATION: Serving size: 1 cup three-bean chili; Calories: 267 cals; Protein: 17 g; Carbohydrates: 34 g; Fat: 8 g; Fiber: 11 g; Sodium: 790 mg; Vitamin A: 1,820 IU; Vitamin C: 68 mg; Folic Acid: 151 mcg; Iron: 5 mg; Diabetic Exchange: Bread/Starch 1.5, Meat (Medium Fat) 1.5, Vegetable 2

vegetarian curry

What's in this for baby and me? Protein, iron, vitamins A and C, and folic acid.

THIS VEGETARIAN CURRY is an excellent source of **protein**, **iron**, **vitamins A** and **C**, and **folic acid**, and a good source of calcium and fiber—what more could you want? Have all of your ingredients ready (along with cooked rice or noodles) before you begin. Try to avoid overcooking the vegetables: they should be just crisp-tender, as they will continue cooking when removed from the heat. A surprising number of kids like a mild curry flavor and might enjoy this dish. By all means, use your family's favorite vegetables and consider omitting the cilantro and peanuts from the children's portions. This recipe can easily be halved.

serves 4 (makes about 7 cups)

2 tablespoons canola oil

2 tablespoons minced or grated fresh ginger, or to taste

1 garlic clove, minced

1 cup sliced baby carrots or shredded regular carrots

½ red bell pepper, quartered and thinly sliced

1 medium zucchini, washed, halved lengthwise, and thinly sliced

12–16 ounces asparagus, washed, tough ends trimmed, and cut into ½-inch slices (about 2 cups sliced asparagus), or broccoli florets, washed and ends trimmed

One 15-ounce package (drained weight) extra-firm tofu, drained, cut into ½-inch cubes, and blotted dry with paper towels

½ cup thinly sliced scallions

1 tablespoon plus 1 teaspoon mild curry powder, or to taste

One 14-ounce can light or regular coconut milk

1 tablespoon quick-dissolving flour (such as Wondra), to desired consistency

⅓ cup chopped fresh cilantro or basil

Juice of 1 lime, or to taste

Salt, to taste

½ cup dry-roasted peanuts or cashew nuts, coarsely chopped (optional)

1   In a large nonstick skillet or large wok, heat 1 tablespoon of the canola oil over medium high heat. Add the ginger and garlic and cook for 30 seconds. Add the carrots, bell pepper, zucchini, and asparagus and sauté for 3 minutes. Transfer the cooked vegetables to a serving dish, cover with foil, and set aside.

2   Add the remaining 1 tablespoon canola oil to the skillet and heat over medium-high heat. Add the tofu, scallions, and curry powder and sauté for 3 minutes. Add the coconut milk and cook for 3 minutes, or until hot. Sprinkle in the quick-dissolving flour and stir to mix. Add the reserved vegetables and mix gently, then stir in the cilantro and lime juice. Adjust the seasoning.

3   Transfer the curry to a serving bowl, garnish with the peanuts, if desired, and serve immediately.

▶ **Cooking Tip:** Regular coconut milk produces a creamier sauce.

▶ **Advance Preparation:** The curry can be made a day in advance. Reduce the cooking time of the vegetables to 2 minutes if the curry will be reheated in a microwave oven later. (The accompanying rice can be made up to 3 days in advance, or the rice noodles up to 1 day in advance.)

▶ **Timesaving Tip:** Pick up shredded carrots and other prepared vegetables from a salad bar. Convenient fresh vegetable stir-fry packs are available in some grocery stores. They usually come in 12-ounce packages and can be supplemented with your favorite vegetables—carrots, broccoli, and asparagus are among the healthiest. Sixteen-ounce bags of frozen stir-fry vegetables are also available in most grocery stores. Follow the package directions for stir-frying vegetables in oil.

▶ **Variation:** Nonvegetarians can substitute poultry, shrimp, seafood, or meat for the tofu; adjust the cooking time as necessary.

▶ **Diabetic Tip:** Omit the peanuts, to reduce the fat.

▶ **Complete Meal Ideas:** Serve this curry with:
    Rice, rice noodles, or quinoa
    Reduced-fat 2% milk or low-fat yogurt
    Fresh fruit that contains vitamin C

APPROXIMATE NUTRITIONAL INFORMATION: Serving size: 1¾ cups vegetarian curry; Calories: 422 cals; Protein: 19 g; Carbohydrates: 19 g; Fat: 31 g; Fiber: 5 g; Sodium: 465 mg; Vitamin A: 10,049 IU; Vitamin C: 52 mg; Folic Acid: 120 mcg; Iron: 7 mg; Diabetic Exchange: Fat 4, Meat (Medium Fat) 2, Vegetable 3

best-ever vegetarian lasagna

What's in this for baby and me? Protein, calcium, iron, vitamins A and C, folic acid, and fiber.

IT WOULD BE misleading to say that lasagna (vegetarian or not) is a quick and easy dish to prepare. While there are ways to make this family favorite less of a hassle (see **Time-saving Tip** below), the fact remains that it takes time to assemble and bake any lasagna. But the results are definitely worth the effort, especially with this nutrient-packed recipe! Best-Ever Vegetarian Lasagna is an excellent source of **protein**, **calcium**, **iron**, **vitamins A** and **C**, **folic acid**, and **fiber**, and a good source of B vitamins. Do not use the tofu if you plan to freeze the lasagna before baking.

serves 8

Tomato Sauce (makes 4 cups)
  2 tablespoons olive oil
  1 medium onion, finely chopped
  1 garlic clove, minced
  1 tablespoon dried basil or Italian seasoning
  1 tablespoon dried oregano
  One 28-ounce can crushed tomatoes
  2 tablespoons chopped fresh basil, oregano, or dill, or a combination (optional)
Vegetables
  1 tablespoon olive oil or canola oil
  1 pound mushrooms, preferably cremini, washed, trimmed, and thinly sliced

10 ounces baby spinach leaves, washed, or one 10-ounce package frozen chopped spinach, thawed and drained well

Enough no-boil (or oven-ready) lasagna noodles to fill a 13 x 9 x 2-inch pan

One 15-ounce package (drained weight) extra-firm tofu, thinly sliced and pressed (see Cooking Tip below) (optional)

4 cups shredded pasteurized part-skim low-moisture mozzarella cheese or Fontina cheese (about 1 pound)

6 tablespoons grated Parmesan cheese (optional)

1. To make the sauce, heat the olive oil in a large saucepan over medium-high heat. Add the onion and sauté for 3 minutes. Add the garlic, basil, and oregano and continue to sauté for 2 minutes. Add the crushed tomatoes, stir, and bring to a boil, then reduce the heat and simmer, uncovered, for 10 minutes. Stir in the fresh herbs and remove from the heat. The sauce should yield 4 cups; if not, add water (or tomato juice) to make 4 cups. Set aside.

2. To cook the vegetables, heat the olive oil in a large nonstick skillet over medium-high heat. Add the mushrooms and sauté for 5 minutes. Using a slotted spoon, transfer the mushrooms to a bowl, leaving behind any juices in the skillet. If using fresh spinach, add it to the skillet, in batches if necessary, and sauté until just wilted,

about 3 minutes. Add the spinach to the mushrooms and set aside. (If using frozen spinach, add it directly to the mushrooms.)

3. To assemble the lasagna, spread ¾ cup sauce over the bottom of an ungreased 13 x 9 x 2-inch pan. Place 3 or 4 no-boil lasagna noodles over the sauce (follow the instructions on your lasagna box—different brands require different preparation methods). Spread about one-third of the vegetables evenly over the noodles, followed by one-third of the tofu slices, if using, ¾ cup of the sauce, 1 cup of the mozzarella cheese, and 2 tablespoons of the Parmesan cheese (if using). Repeat the layering process of noodles, vegetables, tofu, sauce, and cheeses two more times. For the last layer, place 3 or 4 noodles on top of the cheese, then add the remaining sauce to cover the noodles, and top with the remaining mozzarella cheese. (See **Advance Preparation** below for make-ahead and freezing instructions at this point.)

4. To bake, adjust an oven rack to the middle position and preheat the oven to 375°F. Cover the pan with foil (lightly greased or sprayed with cooking oil spray) and bake for 45 minutes.

5. Remove the foil and bake for 15 minutes more, or until the top is nicely browned and a knife inserted into the middle of the lasagna indicates soft noodles. Remove the lasagna from the oven and let cool for 10 minutes before slicing.

▶ *Cooking Tip:* If adding tofu to this lasagna, drain it well, then slice it into ½-inch slices. Line a large plate with a triple thickness of paper towels, place the tofu slices on the plate, then using a second bunch of paper towels, blot the tofu to remove excess water. Repeat for the remaining slices.

▶ *Timesaving Tip:* Use frozen spinach or purchase fresh spinach in a microwaveable bag. After microwaving, drain the spinach and squeeze gently. Use presliced mushrooms from a package or a salad bar. Use store-bought high-quality pasta sauce (you will need 4 cups sauce).

▶ *Advance Preparation:* The sauce can be made up to 3 days in advance, covered, and refrigerated. After completing Step 3, the lasagna can be wrapped with plastic wrap and refrigerated overnight, or it can be frozen for up to 1 month. The frozen lasagna can be placed directly in the oven, but the cooking time will increase by about 15 to 20 minutes.

▶ *Storage Tip:* The cooked lasagna will keep for 3 days refrigerated and it can be frozen for up to 1 month. Use a microwave or conventional oven to reheat.

▶ *Complete Meal Ideas:* Serve this lasagna with:
    Tossed salad or a green vegetable (you might want to try the Vegetables with
        Lemon, Olive Oil, and Fresh Herbs, page 128.)
    Reduced-fat 2% milk or low-fat yogurt
    Fresh fruit that contains vitamin C

APPROXIMATE NUTRITIONAL INFORMATION: Serving size: one-eighth vegetarian lasagna; Calories: 371 cals; Protein: 24 g; Carbohydrates: 34 g; Fat: 16 g; Fiber: 7 g; Sodium: 526 mg; Vitamin A: 2,944 IU; Vitamin C: 19 mg; Folic Acid: 83 mcg; Calcium: 480 mg; Iron: 5 mg; Diabetic Exchange: Bread/Starch 2, Fat 1, Meat (Medium Fat) 2, Vegetable 1

spaghetti with herbed tofu balls and tomato sauce

~

What's in this for baby and me? Protein, calcium, iron, vitamins A and C, B vitamins, folic acid, and fiber.

A VEGETARIAN TWIST on meatballs, this spaghetti with herbed tofu balls and tomato sauce is an excellent source of **protein**, **calcium**, **iron**, **vitamins** A and **C**, **B vitamins**, **folic acid**, and **fiber**—how's that for a nutritional report card?

serves 4 (makes about 25 tofu balls and about 3½ cups tomato sauce)

12 to 16 ounces enriched thin spaghetti or linguine
½ tablespoon unsalted butter
Herbed Tofu Balls
   One 15-ounce package (drained weight)
      extra-firm tofu, drained, finely crumbled
      (use your hands or a fork), and blotted
      with paper towels
   ½ cup plain or seasoned breadcrumbs
   ⅓ cup finely grated Parmesan cheese
   3 large eggs, lightly beaten
   ¼ cup chopped fresh cilantro
   ¼ cup chopped fresh parsley

½ cup thinly sliced scallions
½ teaspoon salt
Freshly ground pepper, to taste
1 tablespoon canola oil
Tomato Sauce
   1 tablespoon canola oil or olive oil
   1 garlic clove, minced
   1 teaspoon dried oregano
   1 teaspoon Italian seasoning
   One 28-ounce can crushed tomatoes
   Additional chopped fresh cilantro and pars-
      ley, for garnish (optional)
   Grated Parmesan cheese, for the table

1. Cook the pasta according to the package directions; drain and return to the pot. Add the butter, stir, cover, and set aside in a warm place.
2. To make the herbed tofu balls, combine all of the ingredients except the oil in a bowl and mix until well blended. Using a rounded measuring tablespoon, scoop out mounds of the tofu mixture and place on 2 large plates, then form each portion into a ball.
3. Heat the canola oil in a large nonstick skillet over medium-high heat. Add half the tofu balls and sauté, turning several times, for about 7 minutes, or until light golden brown and heated through. Repeat with the remaining tofu balls. Transfer the tofu balls to a clean plate lined with a paper towel. Cover with foil to keep warm. (Do not rinse the skillet.)
4. To make the tomato sauce, heat the canola oil in the same skillet over medium heat. Add the garlic, oregano, and Italian seasoning and cook for 30 seconds. Add the

crushed tomatoes, stir, and simmer for 10 minutes, or until slightly thickened. Adjust the seasoning before serving.

5. To serve, place some of the pasta in a bowl, top with some of the tofu balls, and cover with sauce and chopped fresh herbs. Serve with Parmesan cheese.

▶ *Advance Preparation:* The tofu balls can be formed up to 4 hours in advance and refrigerated. The sauce can be made up to 2 days in advance, covered, and refrigerated. Add any fresh herbs at the last minute.

▶ *Timesaving Tip:* Use your favorite store-bought spaghetti sauce and fresh pasta, which has a shorter cooking time.

▶ *Variation:* You can doctor up this simple tomato sauce by sautéing the following in Step 3: ½ cup finely chopped onions, 8 ounces sliced cremini or button mushrooms, or ½ cup chopped red bell pepper before adding the garlic. You can also add sliced olives, caper berries, or fresh herbs to the finished sauce.

▶ *Complete Meal Ideas:* Serve this spaghetti with:
> Tossed salad or a green vegetable (you might want to try a tossed salad with the French-Style Tarragon Vinaigrette, page 141)
> Reduced-fat 2% milk or low-fat yogurt
> Fresh fruit that contains vitamin C

APPROXIMATE NUTRITIONAL INFORMATION: Serving size: one-fifth serving or 5 herbed tofu balls; Calories: 207 cals; Protein: 17 g; Carbohydrates: 12 g; Fat: 10 g; Fiber: .7 g; Sodium: 467 mg; Diabetic Exchange: Bread/Starch: 1, Meat (Medium Fat) 2

APPROXIMATE NUTRITIONAL INFORMATION: Serving size: 1 ¼ cups cooked spaghetti with ¾ cup tomato sauce; Calories: 355 cals; Protein: 12 g; Carbohydrates: 64 g; Fat: 7 g; Fiber: 7 g; Sodium: 555 mg; Vitamin A: 14,445 IU; Vitamin C: 18 mg; Folic Acid: 148 mcg; Iron: 5 mg; Diabetic Exchange: Bread/Starch 4, Fat 1.5

pasta with tomatoes, herbs, and pasteurized goat cheese

What's in this for baby and me? Protein, calcium, iron, vitamins A and C, B vitamins, and folic acid.

THIS NO-FUSS DISH, which is an excellent source of **protein**, **calcium**, **iron**, **vitamins A** and **C**, **B vitamins**, and **folic acid**, and a good source of fiber, is especially delicious in tomato season. The secret is adding a no-cook sauce to piping-hot pasta. For young eaters, substitute Parmesan cheese for the goat cheese.

serves 3 to 4

Fresh Tomato Sauce

2 large vine-ripened tomatoes, cut into small dice

3 tablespoons chopped fresh dill

3 tablespoons thinly sliced fresh basil

1 tablespoon olive oil, or to taste

2 teaspoons freshly squeezed lemon juice, or to taste

Salt and freshly ground pepper, to taste

8 ounces thin pasta, such as capellini or thin spaghetti

4 ounces pasteurized goat cheese, crumbled, or to taste (see Health Tip below)

1. Bring a large pot of water for cooking the pasta to a boil.
2. To make the sauce, combine all of the ingredients in a bowl and mix gently with a spoon. Adjust the seasoning and set aside.
3. Cook the pasta, drain, and immediately place it in individual serving bowls. Add the sauce and cheese and toss gently with 2 large forks until the sauce is well incorporated. Serve immediately.

▶ *Health Tip:* Use only pasteurized feta cheese (see Listeriosis Warning, page 107).

▶ *Complete Meal Ideas:* Serve this pasta with:
Tossed salad or a green vegetable (you might want to try the Spinach Salad with Mandarin Oranges and Toasted Almonds, page 138)
Reduced-fat 2% milk or low-fat yogurt
Fresh fruit

APPROXIMATE NUTRITIONAL INFORMATION: Serving size: one-third pasta dish (served over 1½ cups enriched cooked spaghetti); Calories: 527 cals; Protein: 22 g; Carbohydrates: 65 g; Fat: 20 g; Fiber: 5 g; Sodium: 141 mg; Vitamin A: 1,319 IU; Vitamin C: 18 mg; Folic Acid: 165 mcg; Diabetic Exchange: Bread/Starch 4, Fat 1, Meat (Medium Fat) 1.5

traditional classification of vegetarian diets

LACTO-OVOVEGETARIAN

Foods included: Fruits, grains, legumes, nuts, seeds, vegetables, milk and milk products, eggs
Foods excluded: Meat, poultry, and fish

LACTOVEGETARIAN

Foods included: Fruits, grains, legumes, nuts, seeds, vegetables, milk and milk products
Foods excluded: Meat, poultry, fish, eggs

OVOVEGETARIAN:

Foods included: Fruits, grains, legumes, nuts, seeds, vegetables, eggs
Foods excluded: Meat, poultry, fish, milk and milk products

VEGAN

Foods included: Fruits, grains, legumes, nuts, seeds, vegetables
Foods excluded: Meat, poultry, fish, eggs, milk and milk products

spinach-cheese quiche

What's in this for baby and me? Protein, calcium, and vitamin A.

PACKED WITH **protein**, **calcium**, and **vitamin A**, and a good source of iron, this spinach-cheese quiche is the perfect meal any time of day. You can play around with the filling, but try to avoid a hodgepodge of ingredients whose flavors cancel out each other—decide on a couple of flavors. See the **Variations** below for other filling possibilities. You can save time by purchasing a frozen crust (preferably whole wheat), but you will have to prebake it. The Homemade Whole Wheat Piecrust is simple to make and requires no prebaking. It does, however, have a higher fat content than store-bought varieties. The **Calcium Boost** offers a way to further increase the calcium in this quiche.

serves 4 to 6

One 9-inch piecrust, frozen or Homemade Whole Wheat Piecrust (recipe follows)
Spinach-Cheese Filling
   1¾ cups whole milk, soy beverage, half-and-half, or light skim evaporated milk
   2 large eggs plus 2 large egg yolks
   1 teaspoon Dijon mustard (optional)
   ½ teaspoon salt
   Freshly ground pepper, to taste

4 ounces (1 cup) grated cheddar, Monterey Jack, or Gruyère cheese
8 ounces frozen chopped spinach, thawed and squeezed dry, or fresh spinach (see Cooking Tip below for preparation instructions)
2 tablespoons thinly sliced scallions (optional)
2 tablespoons chopped fresh dill or parsley (optional)

1. Preheat the oven to 375°F. If using a store-bought piecrust, use the middle rack and prebake the crust according to package directions. If using the homemade piecrust, adjust oven rack to the lowest rung.
2. To make the filling, combine the milk, eggs, yolks, mustard, if using, salt, and pepper in a bowl and whisk until well blended.
3. Place half of the cheese in the bottom of the piecrust and top with half the spinach, half the scallions, and half the fresh herbs. Add half of the milk-egg mixture, then repeat this layering procedure with the remaining ingredients and the rest of the milk-egg mixture. (Note: If you are using bulky ingredients in your filling, you may not have room for all of the milk-egg mixture. Discard any extra mixture; do not overfill your quiche, or it may overflow in the oven.)
4. Bake a prebaked piecrust quiche for 25 to 30 minutes, or a homemade piecrust quiche for 50 to 60 minutes, or until the middle of the quiche is set. The quiche is done when the tip of a knife inserted in the center of comes out clean and an

instant-read thermometer reads 160°F. Remove the quiche from the oven and allow it to cool for 10 minutes on a cooling rack before serving. (Leftovers should be refrigerated and reheated in a microwave or conventional oven. Reheating in a microwave oven will cause the crust to become slightly soggy.)

homemade whole wheat piecrust

makes one 9-inch piecrust

¾ cup unbleached all-purpose flour	8 tablespoons (1 stick) unsalted butter, cut
¾ cup whole wheat flour	into small pieces
¼ teaspoon salt	1 large egg, slightly beaten

1. Combine both flours and the salt in a large bowl. Add the butter and rub in with your fingertips, or use a pastry blender, until the dough resembles small crumbs. Add the egg and stir with a fork until the dough holds together.
2. Flour your hands, then gather the dough and knead for a minute, or until it is smooth and soft. (Do not overwork the dough, or it will lose its flakiness. It is better to under-mix than to overmix.) Form the dough into a thick disk, cover with plastic wrap, and refrigerate for 20 minutes, or up to 2 days.
3. Roll out the dough on a piece of lightly floured parchment paper or plastic wrap (this prevents sticking). Transfer the dough to an ungreased 9-inch pie pan and crimp the edges or decorate with a fork. Prick the bottom of the pie with a fork and refrigerate for at least 15 minutes, or freeze for 10 minutes, before filling and baking.

▶ *Calcium Boost:* In a measuring cup combine ⅓ cup pasteurized instant nonfat dry milk with the whole milk. Mix until the milk powder has dissolved, then follow directions in Step 2.

▶ *Advance Preparation:* The egg mixture for the filling can be made one day in advance and refrigerated. The dough for the piecrust can be made up to 2 days in advance and refrigerated, or it can be frozen for up to 2 months. Thaw slightly before use; the dough should be cold.

▶ *Cooking Tip:* If using fresh spinach, remove the stems, wash the leaves, and then microwave, steam, or boil the spinach just until wilted. (Some grocery stores sell spinach packaged in microwaveable bags.) Drain, cool, and squeeze out as much liquid as possible, then coarsely chop.

▶ *Variation:* In addition to the cheese, use about 1 cup of a single filling or a mixture of any of these fillings per quiche. To prevent a soggy crust, be sure to thoroughly drain or dry all filling ingredients.

Asparagus: Cook until crisp-tender, drain well, and chop into ¼-inch pieces.

Broccoli florets: Cook until crisp-tender, drain well, pat dry with a paper towel, and chop.

Summer squash or zucchini: Quarter, thinly slice, and sauté; drain on paper towels.

Swiss chard or leeks: Thoroughly wash, slice, and boil, steam, or sauté until wilted and tender.

▶ *Health Tip:* If your doctor has restricted your fat intake, use low-fat cheddar cheese and reduced-fat 2% milk, "lite" skim evaporated milk, or nonfat dry milk for the filling.

▶ *Complete Meal Ideas:* Serve this quiche with:

Tossed salad, a vegetable, or vegetable soup (you might want to try the Gazpacho, page 90, or the Asparagus, Hearts of Palm, and Tomato Salad, page 134)

Reduced-fat 2% milk or low-fat yogurt

Fresh fruit, V-8 juice, or another source of vitamin C

APPROXIMATE NUTRITIONAL INFORMATION: Serving size: 1 slice (one-eighth) spinach cheese quiche (with a store-bought pie crust); Calories: 254 cals; Protein: 10 g; Carbohydrates: 16 g; Fat: 17 g; Fiber: 1 g; Sodium: 430 mg; Vitamin A: 2,639 IU; Calcium: 224 mg; Diabetic Exchange: Bread/Starch 1, Fat 2, Meat (High Fat) 1

APPROXIMATE NUTRITIONAL INFORMATION: Serving size: 1 slice (one-eighth) spinach cheese quiche with homemade whole wheat pie crust; Calories: 329 cals; Protein: 12 g; Carbohydrates: 21 g; Fat: 22 g; Fiber: 2 g; Sodium: 384 g; Vitamin A: 3,253 IU; Calcium: 231 mg; Diabetic Exchange: Bread/Starch 1.5, Fat 3, Meat (High Fat) 1

APPROXIMATE NUTRITIONAL INFORMATION: Serving size: 1 slice (one-eighth) homemade whole wheat pie crust (crust only); Calories: 198 cals; Protein: 4 g; Carbohydrates: 17 g; Fat: 13 g; Fiber: 2 g; Sodium: 83 mg; Diabetic Exchange: Bread/Starch 1, Fat 2.5

healthy additions to vegetarian cooking

Hard cheese (see Listeriosis Warning, page 107, for safe cheeses)

Low-fat cottage cheese

Part-skim ricotta cheese

Soy nuts

Tofu (plain or enriched)

Canned beans and peas

Hard-boiled eggs

Shredded carrots

Plain low-fat yogurt

Dried apricots and other dried fruits

Molasses

Sesame and pumpkin seeds

Nuts

Nut butters

V-8 or tomato juice

Diced or sliced red bell peppers

Enriched pasta

grilled or roasted marinated vegetables

What's in this for baby and me? Vitamins A and C.

Hɪɢʜ ɪɴ **vitamins A** and **C** and a good source of fiber, these vegetables are delicious as a side dish or main course. Use your favorite vegetables in place of ones listed below. Sautéing the onion and garlic separately brings out their sweetness more than grilling them does, but you can do either.

serves 6 (makes about 4 cups)

1 medium red bell pepper, washed, cored, seeded, and quartered

1 medium (about 8 ounces) purple eggplant, washed and cut into ½-inch slices (see Cooking Tip below)

2 medium (about 8 ounces) zucchini, washed and cut into ½-inch slices on the diagonal

8 ounces large button mushrooms or other large mushrooms, such as shiitake or portobello, washed and stems trimmed

1 tablespoon dried oregano

1 tablespoon dried basil or Italian seasoning

1 teaspoon salt

Freshly ground pepper, to taste

1 tablespoon freshly squeezed lemon juice

⅓ cup plus 2 tablespoons olive oil

1 medium sweet onion (preferably Vidalia), finely diced

2 garlic cloves, minced

One 14.5-ounce can diced tomatoes, drained

¼ cup chopped fresh basil or cilantro leaves, for garnish (optional)

1. Place the bell pepper, eggplant, zucchini, and mushrooms in a very large bowl (or in a large roasting pan if roasting). Add the oregano, basil, salt, pepper, lemon juice, and ⅓ cup of the olive oil, then gently toss until all the vegetables are well coated. Allow the vegetables to marinate at room temperature for 10 to 20 minutes.

2. Heat the remaining 2 tablespoons olive oil in a small nonstick skillet over medium-high heat. Add the onion and sauté, stirring occasionally, for 5 to 7 minutes, or until light golden. Add the garlic and sauté for 1 more minute. Add the canned tomatoes and cook just until heated; set aside. Cover to keep warm.

3. Preheat the grill (or see **Roasting Instructions** below). Grill the vegetables over medium-high heat for about 15 minutes, or until nicely browned and cooked through. Turn and move the vegetables around on the grill as necessary to promote even cooking and to avoid scorching.

4. Discard the marinade, then return the grilled vegetables to the bowl in which they were marinated. While they are still warm, chop the cooked vegetables into small dice.

5.   Place the diced vegetables in a serving bowl, add the reserved tomato mixture and the basil, and mix gently. Serve immediately.

▶ **Cooking Tip:** Removing the moisture from the eggplant with salt is an optional step that requires 20 minutes to 1 hour. The advantage of this is that it should remove any bitterness, and the eggplant will not absorb as much oil. Place the sliced eggplant in a colander on a large plate with a rim, sprinkle it with 2 teaspoons salt, and toss gently. Allow the eggplant to stand for at least 20 minutes, or up to 1 hour. Rinse the eggplant quickly under cold water, then spread it out on a double thickness of paper towels. Cover with more paper towels and press firmly to extract as much water as possible.

▶ **Roasting Instructions:** To roast the vegetables, preheat the oven to 475°F. Meanwhile, combine the prepared vegetables in a large roasting pan and marinate them as in Step 1. Roast the vegetables for 20 to 30 minutes, stirring them after 15 minutes of cooking. The vegetables are done when the eggplant and bell peppers are soft. Meanwhile, prepare the tomato mixture following the instructions in Step 2. Finish the vegetables as in Step 4.

▶ **Complete Meal Ideas:** Serve these vegetables with:
Enriched pasta, rice, couscous, or a whole wheat roll
3 ounces protein (you might want to try the Old Bay Tofu Cakes with Cocktail Sauce, page 186)
Reduced-fat 2% milk or low-fat yogurt
Fresh fruit

APPROXIMATE NUTRITIONAL INFORMATION: Serving size: ⅔ cup grilled or roasted vegetables; Calories: 196 cals; Protein: 3 g; Carbohydrates: 12 g; Fat: 16 g; Fiber: 3 g; Sodium: 620 mg; Vitamin A: 1,716 IU; Vitamin C: 67 mg; Diabetic Exchange: Fat 3, Vegetable 2

vegetarian pad thai

~

What's in this for baby and me? Protein, iron, vitamins A and C, folic acid and fiber.

THIS THAI-STYLE stir fry is packed with **protein**, **iron**, **vitamins A** and **C**, **folic acid**, and **fiber**, and it is a good source of calcium. Substitute your family's favorite vegetables for the ones called for, and for nonvegetarians, add any source of protein, such as shrimp or chicken. One large nonstick skillet will be used three times in this recipe and it does not need to be rinsed after each use. If a little sticking occurs, gently scrape the bottom of the pan using a wooden spoon or a Teflon utensil safe for nonstick surfaces. Don't be intimidated by the list of ingredients or the cooking steps. Most of the vegetables can be picked up at a salad bar, and after you've made this dish once, the steps will flow easily.

serves 4

6 ounces Pad Thai rice noodles

Sauce

  2 tablespoons hoisin sauce

  ¼ cup ketchup

  ¼ cup soy sauce

  ¼ cup warm water

  2 tablespoons seasoned rice vinegar

  2 tablespoons freshly squeezed lime juice

  2 tablespoons sugar

Stir-Fry

  2 tablespoons canola oil

  1 cup thinly sliced or shredded carrots

  12–16 ounces asparagus, washed, tough ends trimmed, and cut into 1-inch pieces (about 2 cups sliced asparagus)

2 cups broccoli florets, washed and cut into very small florets

One 15-ounce package (drained-weight) extra-firm tofu, drained, cut into ½-inch cubes, and blotted dry with paper towels

½ cup thinly sliced scallions

3 large eggs, lightly beaten

Garnishes

  ⅓ cup chopped fresh cilantro

  ⅓ cup chopped fresh mint (optional)

  ½ cup roasted peanuts, crushed or coarsely chopped

  1 lime, cut into wedges

1. Cook the noodles according to the package directions. Drain the cooked noodles, run them under cold water, drain again, and set aside.
2. To make the sauce, whisk together all of the ingredients in a small bowl. Set aside.
3. To make the stir-fry, heat 1 tablespoon of the canola oil in a large nonstick skillet over medium-high heat. Add the carrots, asparagus, and broccoli and sauté for 3 minutes. (Do *not* overcook; the vegetables will continue to cook off the heat.) Transfer the vegetables to a bowl, cover with foil, and set aside. (Do not rinse the skillet.)
4. Add 1½ teaspoons canola oil to the skillet and heat over medium-high heat. Add the tofu and sauté for 5 minutes, or until heated through and light golden brown.

Add *half* of the sauce and all the scallions to the skillet, stir, and cook for 1 minute, or until slightly thickened. Transfer to a bowl, cover with foil, and set aside. (Do not rinse the skillet.)

5. Add the remaining 1½ teaspoons canola oil to the skillet and heat over medium-high heat. Add the eggs and cook, stirring constantly, for 1 minute, or until set. (They will resemble scrambled eggs.) Add the remaining sauce and the reserved cooked noodles to the skillet, stir, and cook for 2 minutes.

6. To serve, transfer the noodles to individual serving bowls or a large serving dish. For individual servings, divide the reserved tofu and vegetables, then add the garnishes to each bowl. Or, make a bed of noodles in a large dish, and top with the tofu and the vegetables, followed by the garnishes. Serve immediately.

▶ *Advance Preparation:* The sauce can be made up to 3 days in advance. The whole dish may be made up to 12 hours in advance and reheated in a microwave just before serving.

▶ *Timesaving Tip:* Pick up shredded carrots, broccoli florets, and other prepared vegetables from a salad bar.

▶ *Health Tip:* If your doctor has restricted your sodium intake, use low-sodium or light soy sauce and go easy on the salt.

▶ *Complete Meal Ideas:* Serve this Pad Thai with:
   Reduced-fat 2% milk or low-fat yogurt
   Fresh fruit

APPROXIMATE NUTRITIONAL INFORMATION: Serving size: one-fourth vegetarian Pad Thai; Calories: 407 cals; Protein: 22 g; Carbohydrates: 41 g; Fat: 18 g; Fiber: 5 g; Sodium: 1,311 mg; Vitamin A: 10,044 IU; Vitamin C: 60 mg; Folic Acid: 153 mcg; Iron: 4 mg; Diabetic Exchange: Bread/Starch 2.5, Fat 1, Meat (Medium Fat) 2.5

homemade tofu-bean burritos

⌒

What's in this for baby and me? Protein, calcium, folic acid, and fiber.

A SIMPLE LUNCH or dinner you'll keep coming back to, these tofu-bean burritos are an excellent source of **protein**, **calcium**, **folic acid**, and **fiber**, and a good source of iron. The burrito filling can be made up to two days in advance, and you can fill and roll your burritos as needed. Some excellent brands of high-iron, organic sprouted-wheat burrito-size tortillas (such as Alvarado St. Bakery) and high-iron spinach tortillas are available on the market. Add your favorite ingredients to these burritos and serve them with salsa, avocados or Homemade Guacamole (page 145), sliced lettuce, reduced-fat sour cream, and/or jalapeño peppers.

serves 4 to 6 (makes about 4 cups filling)

1½ tablespoons canola oil

1 small onion, finely chopped

1 small garlic clove, minced

1½ teaspoons ground cumin

1½ teaspoons chili powder, or to taste

1½ teaspoons dried oregano

One 15-ounce package (drained weight) extra-firm tofu, cut into ½-inch cubes and blotted

dry with paper towels

One 15.5-ounce can black beans, rinsed and drained

6 large burrito-size (10-inch) tortillas

1½ cups (about 6 ounces) grated cheddar cheese, or Monterey Jack cheese, or a mixture

½ cup chopped fresh cilantro

1. Heat the canola oil in a large nonstick skillet over medium-high heat. Add the onion and sauté for 3 minutes, or until light golden. Add the garlic, cumin, chili powder, and oregano and sauté for 30 seconds longer.
2. Add the tofu and sauté for 3 minutes. Add the beans and sauté until heated through, about 3 minutes more. Cover with foil to keep warm and set aside.
3. To assemble the burritos, heat a large nonstick skillet over medium-high heat. Place a tortilla in the skillet and heat for 30 seconds on each side, or just until heated but not crisp. Place the warm tortilla on a work surface. Place ⅔ cup of the tofu-bean filling on the bottom third of the tortilla, and top with 3 tablespoons of the cheese and 1½ tablespoons cilantro. Make sure that the filling is neatly stacked and compressed, then fold the bottom edge over the filling, tuck in the sides, and roll up. Repeat with the remaining ingredients. Serve with your favorite garnishes.

▶ *Advance Preparation:* The filling can be made up to 2 days in advance. The burritos can be assembled up to 8 hours in advance. Place them on a plate, cover with a slightly dampened paper towel followed by plastic wrap and refrigerate. Reheat in a microwave oven before serving.

▶ *Complete Meal Ideas:* Serve these burritos with:
Lettuce and tomato, as part of the filling or as a side salad
Reduced-fat 2% milk or low-fat yogurt
Fresh fruit

APPROXIMATE NUTRITIONAL INFORMATION: Serving size: one tofu-bean burrito; Calories: 412 cals; Protein: 23 g; Carbohydrates: 40 g; Fat: 18 g; Fiber: 15 g; Sodium: 528 mg; Folic Acid: 86 mcg; Calcium: 304 mg; Diabetic Exchange: Bread/Starch 2.5, Fat 1, Meat (Medium Fat) 2

cheese and spinach quesadillas

What's in this for baby and me? Protein and calcium.

HIGH IN **protein** and **calcium**, and a good source of vitamin A, iron, and fiber, these quesadillas are as much fun to make as they are to eat. Fill them with roasted vegetables and cheese as a main course for lunch or dinner, or keep them simple for a snack. Serve with salsa, guacamole (recipe page 145) or avocado slices, or reduced-fat sour cream.

makes 1 quesadilla

2 fajita-size 6-inch tortillas (any flavor)
A heaping ⅓ cup grated cheddar cheese, Mon-
    terey Jack, or any other good melting
    cheese (see Health Tip below)
½ cup lightly packed baby spinach, washed

and stems trimmed, or ⅓ cup chopped
    frozen spinach, thawed, drained, and
    squeezed
1 tablespoon scallions, thinly sliced (optional)
1 tablespoon chopped fresh cilantro (optional)

1. Place 1 tortilla in a nonstick skillet over medium-high heat and heat until hot. Flip it over, and distribute the cheese, spinach, and optional ingredients evenly on top. Cover it with the second tortilla. Cook the quesadilla until the cheese begins to melt and the bottom is light golden, about 2 minutes, then flip and cook the other side until light golden.
2. Cut the quesadilla into quarters and serve with your favorite toppings.

▶ *Cooking Tip:* For a child-size portion, use one tortilla, add the desired amount of cheese (and any other fillings your child likes), and cook over medium-high heat until the cheese melts and the tortilla is light golden, then fold the tortilla in half, remove it from the skillet, and serve.

▶ *Variation:* Feel free to add your favorite ingredients to these quesadillas—olives, chopped jarred roasted red peppers, chopped cooked broccoli florets, or chopped cooked asparagus tips.

▶ *Health Tip:* Do not use soft Mexican cheese, such as queso fresco and asadero (see Listeriosis Warning, page 107).

▶ *Complete Meal Ideas:* Serve these quesadillas with:
    Tossed salad, tomato salad, or vegetable soup (you might want to try the Gazpa-
        cho, page 90, or the Creamy Asparagus-Artichoke Soup, page 68)
    Reduced-fat 2% milk or low-fat yogurt
    Fresh fruit, V-8 juice, or a source of vitamin C

APPROXIMATE NUTRITIONAL INFORMATION: Serving size: 1 cheese and spinach quesadilla; Calories: 257 cals; Protein: 12 g; Carbohydrates: 19 g; Fat: 15 g; Fiber: 2 g; Sodium: 393 mg; Diabetic Exchange: Bread/Starch 1, Fat 2, Meat (Medium Fat) 1

gas and tips for coping

Excess gas is a normal part of almost all pregnancies. It can be uncomfortable, and even embarrassing. Here are a few tips to help reduce excess gas:

- ▶ Reduce gas-producing foods in your diet as much as possible, or omit them. Some common culprits include beans, raw cucumber, raw peppers, raw cabbage, raw onion, cauliflower, and dried fruit.
- ▶ Get your body moving! Go for a walk after meals, or whenever you can. This will help keep your digestive tract functioning smoothly.
- ▶ Eat smaller meals more frequently.
- ▶ Chew foods well.
- ▶ Eat slowly.

old bay tofu cakes with cocktail sauce

What's in this for baby and me? Protein and vitamin C.

OLD BAY SEASONING isn't just for crab cakes anymore! These tofu cakes are a fabulous way to get **protein** and **vitamin C** into your diet, as well as a good amount of vitamin A, calcium, and iron. They double as delicious burgers on whole wheat buns with lettuce, sliced tomatoes, and pickles. If serving to children, you may want to replace the Old Bay seasoning with a milder spice—and don't forget to replace the cocktail sauce with ketchup! For an Asian twist, soy sauce goes nicely with these tofu cakes.

serves 6 (makes about 10 cakes)

One 15-ounce package (drained weight) extra-firm tofu, drained, finely crumbled (use your hands or a fork) and blotted dry with paper towels

½ cup plain or seasoned bread crumbs or finely crushed saltine crackers (about 12 crackers)

3 large eggs, lightly beaten

2 teaspoons Old Bay seasoning, or to taste

⅓ cup grated Parmesan cheese

⅓ cup chopped fresh cilantro, basil, or dill

¼ cup diced jarred roasted red peppers (optional)

1 tablespoon canola oil

Cocktail sauce or soy sauce, for the table

1. To make the tofu cakes, combine all of the ingredients except the oil (and cocktail sauce) in a bowl and mix until well blended. Using a ⅓-cup measuring cup, place portion sizes of the mixture on 2 large plates, then form each portion into a patty.
2. Heat the canola oil in a large nonstick skillet over medium-high heat. Add the cakes, in batches, and cook for about 3 to 4 minutes on each side, or until golden brown and heated through. If they are browning too quickly, reduce the heat. Serve hot with cocktail sauce.

▶ *Advance Preparation:* The tofu cakes can be shaped, covered, and refrigerated for up to 24 hours. Do not freeze them.

▶ *Complete Meal Ideas:* Serve these tofu cakes with:

Tossed salad, a green vegetable, or coleslaw (you might want to try romaine lettuce with the Caesar Salad Dressing, page 143)

Corn bread, a whole wheat roll, or pasta salad

Reduced-fat 2% milk or low-fat yogurt

Fresh fruit that contains vitamin C

APPROXIMATE NUTRITIONAL INFORMATION: Serving size: 2 tofu cakes; Calories: 229 cals; Protein: 16 g; Carbohydrates: 11 g; Fat: 13 g; Fiber: .5 g Sodium: 232 mg; Vitamin C: 17 mg; Diabetic Exchange: Bread/Starch 1, Fat 1, Meat (Medium Fat) 2

sautéed tofu and portobello mushrooms on a bed of greens

~

What's in this for baby and me? Protein.

THIS SALAD IS an excellent source of **protein**, and a good source of calcium, iron, vitamins A and C, folic acid, and fiber. Use your favorite bottled dressing, or make the French-Style Tarragon Vinaigrette on page 141. The tofu can be replaced with tempeh, sautéed as directed in Step 2. Serve this salad with hearty bread to mop up the dressing.

serves 2 to 3

1½ tablespoons canola oil

8 ounces portobellos, washed, trimmed, and
   thinly sliced (see Variation below)

1 small garlic clove, minced

Salt and freshly ground pepper, to taste

15 ounce package (drained weight) extra-firm
   tofu, drained, cut into strips, and blotted
   dry with paper towels

1 teaspoon dried oregano, or to taste

2 tablespoons balsamic vinegar, or to taste

One 10-ounce bag baby salad greens, washed
   and dried

¼ cup crumbled pasteurized feta cheese or
   pasteurized goat cheese (see Health Tip
   below), or to taste (optional)

¼ cup salad dressing, or to taste

1. Heat 1 tablespoon of the canola oil in a large nonstick skillet over medium-high heat. Add the mushrooms and sauté for 5 minutes. Add the garlic, season with salt and pepper, and sauté 1 minute longer. Transfer the mushrooms to a bowl and set aside.
2. Add the remaining 1½ teaspoons canola oil to the skillet and heat over medium-high heat. Add the tofu and oregano and sauté for 5 minutes. Add the balsamic vinegar and sauté for 1 minute longer. Return the reserved mushrooms to the skillet and sauté for 1 minute. Remove from the heat.
3. Place the salad greens in a serving bowl or on individual plates. Add the tofu-mushroom mixture and feta cheese, then drizzle the salad dressing over the entire salad. Season with salt and pepper and serve immediately.

▶ *Variation:* Replace the portobello mushrooms with cremini mushrooms, button mushrooms, or any other fresh mushrooms. Cut any large mushrooms in half and slice thinly.

▶ *Health Tip:* Use only pasteurized feta or pasteurized goat cheese (see Listeriosis Warning, page 107).

instructions for sautéing tofu

Sautéed tofu, seasoned or plain, adds protein and calcium to many dishes, including salads, chilis, stews, soups, and grain dishes. To sauté tofu, drain it well, then slice as called for in the recipe or as desired. Arrange it in an even layer on a large plate lined with a double thickness of paper towels. Using a second double thickness of paper towels, blot the tofu to remove as much moisture as possible.

Heat 1 tablespoon canola oil in a large nonstick skillet over medium-high heat. Add the tofu and any seasonings and sauté for five minutes, or until it is heated through and the surface is light golden. Remove the tofu from the skillet and drain on paper towels, or add it directly to another dish.

▶ *Complete Meal Ideas:* Serve this salad with:
Whole wheat roll or bread
Reduced-fat 2% milk or low-fat yogurt
Fresh fruit that contains vitamin C

APPROXIMATE NUTRITIONAL INFORMATION: Serving size: one-quarter sautéed tofu and portobello mushroom salad; Calories: 234 cals; Protein: 16 g; Carbohydrates: 11 g; Fat: 24 g; Fiber: 3 g; Sodium: 296 mg; Diabetic Exchange: Bread/Starch 1, Fat 3, Meat (Medium Fat) 2

vegetarian omelet for one

~

What's in this for baby and me? Protein, calcium, folic acid, and fiber.

Hɪɢʜ ɪɴ **protein, calcium, folic acid**, and **fiber**, and a good source of vitamin A and iron, this power-packed vegetarian dinner for one is a winner. The black beans can be replaced with your favorite beans, and any other ingredients you like can be added.

serves 1

2 large eggs

½ teaspoon unsalted butter, or canola oil cooking spray

½ cup canned black beans, rinsed, drained, and blotted dry with a paper towel

3 tablespoons grated cheddar cheese (or any cheese of your choice)

1 tablespoon chopped fresh cilantro (optional)

Salt and freshly ground pepper, to taste

Salsa, for the table

1. Whisk the eggs in a bowl, and set aside.
2. Melt the butter in a medium nonstick skillet over medium-high heat. Add the eggs and swirl to coat the bottom of the pan, then add the black beans, cheddar cheese, and cilantro. Gently tilt the skillet, using a spatula or wooden spoon to pull the cooked egg towards the center of the pan while allowing the raw egg to hit the hot skillet. Season with salt and pepper. Repeat this procedure until the egg is completely cooked. The whole process should take about 2 minutes.
3. Fold the omelet in half and cook about 30 seconds longer, or until the egg is no longer runny (the cheese will be runny), then transfer to a serving plate. Serve immediately, with the salsa.

▶ **Health Tip:** Be sure to cook your eggs *thoroughly* (both whites and yolks) during your pregnancy (see Eggs and Salmonella *enteritidis*, page 54). If your doctor has restricted your fat intake, use canola oil cooking spray for the skillet instead of butter, and use a reduced-fat grated cheese.

▶ **Complete Meal Ideas:** Serve omelet with:
    Whole wheat roll or bread
    Tossed salad
    Reduced-fat 2% milk or low-fat yogurt
    Fresh fruit that contains vitamin C

APPROXIMATE NUTRITIONAL INFORMATION: Serving size: one vegetarian omelet; Calories: 366 cals; Protein: 25 g; Carbohydrates: 21 g; Fat: 20 g; Fiber: 7 g; Sodium: 259 mg; Folic Acid: 179 mcg; Calcium: 226 mg; Diabetic Exchange: Bread/Starch 1.5, Fat 1, Meat (Medium Fat) 3

recommendations for optimizing iron and zinc bioavailability in vegetarians[32]

- ▶ Emphasize variety in your diet, especially foods that are micronutrient dense.

- ▶ Include plenty of sprouted lentils, chickpeas, and beans.

- ▶ Eat fermented soy foods (such as soy sauce, tempeh, and miso).

- ▶ Choose dried fruits for dessert.

- ▶ Eat plenty of fresh fruits and dark green leafy vegetables.

- ▶ Do not consume phytate-rich foods and calcium-rich dairy foods in the same meal.

- ▶ Do not consume calcium- and iron-rich foods in the same meal.

- ▶ Drink tea and coffee at times other than mealtime.

- ▶ Try to eat vitamin C–rich foods with iron-rich foods.

- ▶ Evaluate iron, zinc, calcium, and phytate intake on a regular basis.

- ▶ Use iron- and zinc-fortified foods if recommended by your doctor or nutritionist.

lentil, brown rice, and mushroom pilaf

What's in this for baby and me? Protein, folic acid, and fiber.

THIS LENTIL, BROWN rice, and mushroom casserole is an excellent source of **protein**, **folic acid**, and **fiber**, and a good source of iron. For a more intense mushroom flavor, mushroom broth can be used in place of vegetable stock.

serves 4 to 6

2 tablespoons unsalted butter

1 small onion, finely chopped

1 garlic clove, minced

8 ounces cremini or button mushrooms, washed, trimmed, and thinly sliced (optional)

1 teaspoon dried thyme

1 teaspoon dried oregano

¾ cup green lentils, picked over and rinsed

½ cup brown rice

½ teaspoon salt

4 cups vegetable stock

Grated Parmesan cheese, for the table

1. Preheat the oven to 350°F.
2. Melt the butter in a large nonstick skillet over medium-high heat. Add the onion and sauté for 3 minutes. Add the garlic, mushrooms, if using, thyme, and oregano and sauté for 1 minute more. Add the lentils and rice and sauté for 1 minute. Add the salt and stock and bring to a boil.
3. Carefully transfer the contents of the skillet to an 8 x 8 x 2-inch Pyrex baking dish. Bake for 2 hours, or until the rice and lentils in the center of the casserole are soft and the liquid is absorbed. Cover the dish with foil during the last 30 minutes of baking. Serve hot, with Parmesan cheese.

▶ *Variation:* Use long- or medium-grain white rice (not basmati or instant) and reduce the cooking time to about 1 hour.

▶ *Storage Tip:* This pilaf keeps for 5 days, refrigerated.

▶ *Complete Meal Ideas:* Serve this pilaf with:
   Green or yellow vegetable (you might want to try the Tomato and Mozzarella Salad with Fresh Basil, page 132)
   Reduced-fat 2% milk or low-fat yogurt
   Fresh fruit that contains vitamin C

APPROXIMATE NUTRITIONAL INFORMATION: Serving size:1 cup lentil, brown rice, and mushroom pilaf; Calories: 206 cals; Protein: 11 g; Carbohydrates: 30 g; Fat: 5 g; Fiber: 9 g; Sodium: 879 mg; Folic Acid: 110 mcg; Diabetic Exchange: Bread/Starch 2, Fat 1, Meat (Lean Fat) .5

sample menus for optimizing iron and zinc bioavailability[33]

~

INITIAL MENU	INITIAL MENU MODIFIED TO INCREASE IRON AND ZINC BIOAVAILABILITY
Breakfast	*Breakfast*
Wheat toast	Fortified breakfast cereal with raisins
English muffin	English muffin
Tea with milk	Herbal tea (see Herbal Teas to Avoid, page 49)
Apple	Orange juice
Lunch	*Lunch*
Vegetable salad	Sprouted bean and vegetable salad
Baked potato	Baked potato with low-fat cheese
Whole wheat bread and jelly	Whole wheat bread and peanut butter
Black coffee	Tomato juice
Dinner	*Dinner*
Tomato soup	Black bean soup
Noodles	Brown rice
Stir-fried vegetables	Tempeh with stir-fried vegetables
Strawberry yogurt	Orange-banana juice

swiss chard or spinach with garlicky soy dressing

⌇

What's in this for baby and me? Vitamins A and C.

Hɪɢʜ ɪɴ **vitamins A** and **C**, and a good source of iron and folic acid, Swiss chard or spinach with garlicky soy dressing is the perfect side dish for any main course. The dressing can be served with any other greens or a green vegetable such as broccoli or asparagus, or with sautéed eggplant.

serves 2 to 3 (makes about 1 ½ cups)

Garlicky Soy Dressing
1 tablespoon soy sauce
¼ teaspoon minced garlic (optional)
1 to 2 teaspoons brown sugar, or to taste
1 teaspoon canola oil
A drop or two of toasted sesame oil (optional)

10–12 ounces red or green Swiss chard (see Cooking Tip below) or one 10-ounce package baby spinach leaves, washed, stems trimmed
1 tablespoon canola oil

1. To make the sauce, combine the soy sauce, garlic, if using, and brown sugar in a small bowl. Stir until the sugar dissolves, then add the canola oil and sesame oil, stir, and set aside.
2. Heat the canola oil in a large nonstick skillet over medium-high heat. Add the Swiss chard and sauté just until wilted, about 3 minutes (if it does not fit in the pan all at once, you may need to sauté half of it, then add the rest after it has wilted). Transfer the cooked greens to a serving dish (after draining off any watery juices), add the reserved sauce, and mix gently. Serve hot or at room temperature.

▶ *Advance Preparation:* The sauce can be made up to 2 days in advance. The greens can be cooked up to 6 hours in advance, covered, and left at room temperature.

▶ *Cooking Tip:* To clean Swiss chard, trim the thick stems, then place the leaves in a large bowl or sink filled with water and gently rub the leaves with your fingers to dislodge any sand. Lift the greens out of the water and place them in a colander to drain. Wash the leaves a second time, or until no more sand remains. Slice the large leaves in half, then roll up a handful of leaves at a time and slice them about ½ inch thick.

▶ *Timesaving Tip:* Use frozen spinach. Cook it according to package directions and drain well.

APPROXIMATE NUTRITIONAL INFORMATION: Serving size: one-third Swiss chard with garlicky soy dressing; Calories: 83 cals; Protein: 2 g; Carbohydrates: 6 g; Fat: 6 g; Fiber: 2 g; Sodium: 477 mg; Vitamin A: 2,966 IU; Vitamin C: 17 mg; Diabetic Exchange: Fat 1, Vegetable 1

APPROXIMATE NUTRITIONAL INFORMATION: Serving size: one-third spinach with garlicky soy dressing: Calories: 87 cals; Protein: 3 g; Carbohydrates: 5 g; Fat: 7 g; Fiber: 2 g; Sodium: 409 mg; Vitamin A: 7,739 IU; Iron: 4 mg; Folic Acid: 139 mcg; Diabetic Exchange: Fat 1.5, Vegetable 1

lima beans with artichoke hearts and dill

~

What's in this for baby and me? Vitamin C and fiber.

Hɪɢʜ ɪɴ **vitamin C** and **fiber**, and a good source of protein, vitamin A, iron, and folic acid, this dish is the perfect complement to just about any main course. The fresh dill gives this salad a wonderful flavor. If serving this dish to young children, you might want to omit the dill in their portions, and refer to the lima beans as green M&M's.

serves 5 (makes about 2½ cups)

1 cup fat-free vegetable stock

8 ounces frozen lima beans (about 1¾ cups)

One 14-ounce can artichoke hearts, drained and cut into quarters, or one 8-ounce package frozen sliced artichoke hearts

½ cup half-and-half

1½ tablespoons quick-dissolving flour (such as Wondra), or to desired consistency

¼ cup chopped fresh dill

Salt and freshly ground pepper, to taste

Squeeze of fresh lemon juice, to taste

1. In a large saucepan bring the stock to a boil. Add the lima beans and artichoke hearts and return to a boil. Reduce the heat and simmer, covered, for 5 minutes.
2. Add the half-and-half and return to a simmer, then sprinkle in the flour, stir, and continue to simmer for 2 minutes. Add the dill and season to taste with salt and pepper and lemon juice. Serve warm.

▶ **Storage Tip:** This dish keeps refrigerated for 3 days. Do not freeze.

▶ **Health Tip:** If your doctor has restricted your fat intake, use 1½ cups stock and omit the half-and-half. The dish will be just as tasty but less creamy.

APPROXIMATE NUTRITIONAL INFORMATION: Serving size: ½ cup lima beans with artichoke hearts; Calories: 125 cals; Protein: 6 g; Carbohydrates: 20 g; Fat: 3 g; Fiber: 5 g; Sodium: 265 mg; Vitamin C: 14 mg; Diabetic Exchange: Bread/Starch 1, Fat 1, Vegetable 1

okra and tomatoes

~

What's in this for baby and me? Vitamin C.

Okra and tomatoes are an excellent source of **vitamin C**, and a good source of vitamin A, calcium, and fiber. This is delicious over rice, couscous, or quinoa, and for non-vegetarians it makes a lovely side dish for grilled meat, broiled chicken, or baked fish.

serves 4 (makes about 3 cups)

1 tablespoon olive oil

½ cup finely chopped onion

1 small garlic clove, minced

1 teaspoon Italian seasoning or dried oregano

10 ounces okra, washed, ends trimmed, and

cut into ½-inch slices

One 14.5-ounce can diced tomatoes (do not drain)

1 teaspoon sugar

Salt and freshly ground pepper, to taste

1. Heat the oil in a large saucepan over medium-high heat. Add the onion and sauté for 3 minutes, or until light golden brown. Add the remaining ingredients and bring to a boil, then reduce the heat, cover, and simmer gently for 30 to 35 minutes, or until the okra is tender.
2. Adjust the seasoning and serve.

▶ *Timesaving Tip:* One 10-ounce package sliced frozen okra, defrosted and drained, can be substituted for the fresh okra. Cook the okra according to the time listed on the package.

▶ *Variation:* Add your favorite vegetables, such as cubed zucchini, quartered canned artichoke hearts, or fresh green beans, with the okra.

▶ *Storage Tip:* This dish keeps for 3 days refrigerated, and it can be frozen for up to 1 month.

APPROXIMATE NUTRITIONAL INFORMATION: Serving size: one-quarter okra and tomatoes; Calories: 81 cals; Protein: 2 g; Carbohydrates: 11 g; Fat: 3 g; Fiber: 3 g; Sodium: 346 mg; Vitamin C: 30 mg; Diabetic Exchange: Fat .5, Vegetable 1

classic creamed spinach

⌒

What's in this for baby and me? Vitamins A and C, calcium, iron, and fiber.

CLASSIC CREAMED SPINACH is an excellent source of **vitamins A** and **C**, **calcium**, **iron**, and **fiber**, and a good source of protein—Popeye would approve!

serves 3 (makes about 1 ½ cups)

One 10-ounce package frozen chopped
   spinach, cooked and drained, or one 10–12
   ounce package fresh baby spinach
1 tablespoon unsalted butter
2 tablespoons finely chopped onion (preferably

a sweet onion such as Vidalia) (optional)
1 tablespoon all-purpose flour
½ cup whole milk or soy beverage
½ cup shredded Monterey Jack cheese
Salt and freshly ground pepper, to taste

1. If using fresh spinach, place about 2 cups of water in a large saucepan, add a pinch of salt, and bring to a boil. Add the spinach and cook for about 3 minutes, or just until wilted. Drain and cool, then squeeze dry, coarsely chop, and set aside.
2. Melt the butter in a large saucepan (you can use the same saucepan used to cook the fresh spinach) over medium-high heat. Add the onion, if using, and sauté for 3 minutes, or until lightly browned. Add the flour and continue to sauté for 30 seconds, then add the milk, stirring constantly, and cook, stirring, until smooth and slightly thickened, about 1 to 3 minutes.
3. Add the spinach and cheese and stir to heat through. Season, and serve immediately.

▶ *Timesaving Tip:* Use a microwaveable 10-ounce bag of baby spinach, available in many grocery stores. Cook according to the directions on the bag.

▶ *Storage Tip:* This dish keeps refrigerated for 3 days. Do not freeze.

▶ *Health Tip:* If your doctor has restricted your fat intake, replace the butter with margarine, use reduced-fat 2% milk, and either use a reduced-fat cheese or omit the cheese.

APPROXIMATE NUTRITIONAL INFORMATION: Serving size: ½ cup creamed spinach; Calories: 155 cals; Protein: 9 g; Carbohydrates: 5 g; Fat: 12 g; Fiber: 8 g; Sodium: 260 mg; Vitamin A: 5,395 IU; Vitamin C: 23 mg; Calcium: 259 mg; Iron: 6 mg; Diabetic Exchange: Fat 1, Meat (Medium Fat) 1, Vegetable 1

simple and tasty brussels sprouts

What's in this for baby and me? Vitamin C.

HIGH IN **vitamin C**, and a good source of vitamin A and folic acid, these tender, sweet Brussels sprouts are a great side dish. For some color and crunch, add toasted sliced almonds and dried cranberries to the sautéed sprouts.

serves 4 (makes about 2 cups)

10–12 ounces Brussels sprouts, washed, bottoms trimmed, loose or damaged outer leaves removed, and cut in half (or quarters, if they are very large)

1½ tablespoons unsalted butter
½ teaspoon sugar
Salt and freshly ground pepper, to taste

1. In a large saucepan, bring ½ cup water to a boil. Add the sprouts and cook for 8 minutes.
2. Drain the sprouts and return to the saucepan. Add the butter and sugar and sauté over high heat for 5 minutes, or until nicely browned. Season, transfer to a serving dish, and serve immediately.

▶ *Timesaving Tip:* Use whole frozen Brussels sprouts and cook according to package directions. Drain and sauté as described above.

APPROXIMATE NUTRITIONAL INFORMATION: Serving size: ¼ cup Brussels sprouts; Calories: 70 cals; Protein: 2 g; Carbohydrates: 7 g; Fat: 5 g; Fiber: 2 g; Sodium: 16 mg; Vitamin C: 44 mg; Diabetic Exchange: Fat 1, Vegetable 1.5

southern-style sweet potato casserole

⌒

What's in this for baby and me? Vitamin A and C.

THIS SWEET POTATO casserole, high in **vitamins A** and **C**, and a good source of protein and fiber, is a guaranteed crowd pleaser, particularly during the holidays. Canned sweet potatoes are a fine substitute for fresh, especially if time is scarce. Buy the vacuum-packed variety or those packed in light syrup rather than those in heavy syrup. (See **Timesaving Tip** for instructions on using canned sweet potatoes.) The amounts of brown sugar, molasses, and spices you add depend entirely your family's taste—they can be reduced or omitted. Omitting the nuts is a good idea if serving toddlers or small children. If you have a sweet tooth and don't need to worry about your calorie intake, see the **Variation** below for instructions for a truly decadent marshmallow topping. Adding marshmallows might also be a means to get your children to try this vitamin-packed dish.

serves 4 to 6

**Canola oil cooking spray or unsalted butter,
    for greasing the baking dish**
Sweet Potato Filling
    2 pounds (about 3 medium) red sweet
        potatoes, peeled and cut into large
        pieces of equal size
    ½ cup whole milk or soy beverage
    2 tablespoons unsalted butter
    1–2 tablespoons light brown sugar, or to
        taste (optional)
    2 tablespoons mild molasses, or to taste

    (optional)
    1 large egg
    ½ teaspoon ground cinnamon, cloves, or all-
        spice, or a mixture of any of these spices
    ¼ teaspoon salt
Nut Crumb Topping (optional)
    ¼ cup all-purpose flour
    ⅓ cup loosely packed light or dark brown
        sugar
    3 tablespoons unsalted butter
    ½ cup pecans or walnuts, or a mixture

1. Preheat the oven to 375°F. Grease an 8 x 8 x 2-inch baking dish or a 9-inch pie pan with canola oil cooking spray or butter.
2. To make the filling, place the potatoes in a large pot and add just enough water to cover the potatoes. Bring to a boil, then reduce heat and simmer for 20 to 25 minutes, or until the potatoes are soft. Drain.
3. Place the hot potatoes in a large bowl. Beat them with an electric mixer on low speed to break them up, then increase the speed to medium and beat for 1 to 2 minutes, or until fairly smooth. Add the remaining filling ingredients and mix on low speed until well blended and almost smooth, about 1 minute. Transfer the pureed potatoes to the prepared baking dish.

4. To make the optional nut crumb topping, combine the flour and brown sugar in a small bowl. Using a dull knife (such as a table knife) or your fingers, work in the butter until the dough has a crumb-like consistency. Mix in the pecans.
5. Distribute the topping evenly over the sweet potato casserole. Bake for 45 minutes, or until the casserole is heated through and the topping has set. If the topping has not set after 45 minutes, place the casserole under the broiler for a minute or two. Remove from the oven and serve immediately.

▶ *Timesaving Tip:* Substitute 2 pounds vacuum-packed or canned sweet potatoes or yams (in light syrup) for the fresh sweet potatoes. Drain, place the sweet potatoes in a large bowl, and proceed with Step 3. Omit the crumb topping.

▶ *Advance Preparation:* The filling can be prepared up to 1 day in advance; cover and refrigerate. The nut crumb topping can be made 2 to 5 days in advance; place it on the casserole just before baking.

▶ *Variation:* If you don't need to watch your calorie intake, a marshmallow topping is a decadent treat. To make the topping, cover the top of the baked casserole with mini marshmallows or large ones cut in half. Place the casserole under the broiler for a few seconds. Watch carefully to avoid burning the marshmallows.

▶ *Health Tip:* If your doctor has restricted your fat or calorie intake, use reduced-fat 2% milk and omit the butter, molasses, and sugar; do not use the nut crumb topping or marshmallow topping.

▶ *Diabetic Tip:* Do not use the nut crumb topping or marshmallow topping.

APPROXIMATE NUTRITIONAL INFORMATION: Serving size: one-eighth sweet potato casserole (without the marshmallows); Calories: 308 cals; Protein: 6 g; Carbohydrates: 43 g; Fat: 14 g; Fiber: 3 g; Sodium: 109 mg; Vitamin A: 19,707 IU; Vitamin C: 20 mg; Diabetic Exchange: Bread/Starch 3, Fat 3

baked acorn squash with molasses

~

What's in this for baby and me? Vitamin C and fiber.

Hᴵɢʜ ɪɴ **vitamin C** and **fiber**, and a good source of vitamin A and iron, this baked squash is a healthy and tasty side dish. The molasses and spices make it a sweet and homey dish that your kids will love too.

serves 4 (makes about 2 cups)

Canola oil spray for greasing the baking dish

1 large acorn squash (about 2 pounds), washed, sliced in half, and seeds removed

1 tablespoon brown sugar, or to taste

1 tablespoon mild molasses, or to taste

½ teaspoon ground cinnamon, cloves, or all-spice, or a mixture

1 tablespoon unsalted butter

Salt, to taste

1. Preheat the oven to 375°F. Line a baking dish with foil and lightly spray.
2. Place the squash cut-side down in the baking dish and bake for 40 to 50 minutes, or until tender. Check doneness by piercing the squash with the tip of a knife. Let cool slightly.
3. When cool enough to handle, scoop out the squash pulp from the shells with a large spoon and place it in a serving bowl. Add the remaining ingredients and mix gently. Reheat in a microwave oven before serving, if desired.

APPROXIMATE NUTRITIONAL INFORMATION: Serving size: ½ cup acorn squash; Calories: 150 cals; Protein: 2 g; Carbohydrates: 32 g; Fat: 3 g; Fiber: 8 g; Sodium: 10 mg; Vitamin C: 20 mg; Diabetic Exchange: Bread/Starch 2, Fat 1

annie mozer's greens

~

What's in this for baby and me? Calcium, vitamins A and C, and folic acid.

THESE SIMPLE AND tasty recipes will help you get **calcium**, **vitamins A** and **C**, and **folic acid** into your diet, not to mention iron and fiber.

collard greens with black-eyed peas and tomatoes

serves 4

2 tablespoons canola oil

1 medium onion, chopped

¾ pound fresh greens, washed, tough stems
    trimmed, and sliced into ½-inch strips

Salt, to taste

3 tablespoons red wine vinegar

A couple drops of Tabasco

One 15.5-ounce can black-eyed peas, rinsed
    and drained

2 vine-ripened tomatoes, diced

1. In a large nonstick skillet, heat the canola oil over medium-high heat. Add the onion and sauté for 3 minutes. Reduce the heat to medium, add the collard greens, and continue to sauté until wilted. (*Note:* You may need to add the collard greens in batches—as one batch wilts, add the next.)
2. Add 1 cup water and the salt and cook, uncovered, for 30 to 50 minutes, or until the collard greens are tender; add more water ¼ cup at a time as needed. Add the vinegar during the last 15 minutes of cooking.
3. Remove from the heat and add the Tabasco sauce, black-eyed peas, and tomatoes. Stir, adjust the seasoning, and serve.

APPROXIMATE NUTRITIONAL INFORMATION: Serving size: one-quarter collard greens with black-eyed peas and tomatoes; Calories: 191 cals; Protein: 8 g; Carbohydrates: 25 g; Fat: 8 g; Fiber: 8 g; Sodium: 343 mg; Vitamin A: 3,059 IU; Vitamin C: 32 mg; Folic Acid: 150 mcg; Diabetic Exchange: Fat 1, Vegetable 5

sautéed kale

serves 4

2 tablespoons canola oil
1 medium onion, chopped
¾ pound kale, washed, tough stems trimmed
  and sliced into ½-inch strips

Salt, to taste
3 tablespoons red wine vinegar

1. In a large nonstick skillet, heat the canola oil over medium-high heat. Add the onion and sauté for 3 minutes. Reduce the heat to medium, add the kale and salt, and continue to sauté until wilted. (*Note:* You may need to add the kale in batches—as one batch wilts, add the next.) Cook, uncovered, for about 15 minutes, stirring frequently. If the kale sticks to the skillet, add a little water, 2 tablespoons at a time. Add the vinegar during the last 5 minutes of cooking.
2. Adjust the seasoning and serve.

APPROXIMATE NUTRITIONAL INFORMATION: Serving size: one-quarter sautéed kale; Calories: 95 cals; Protein: 2 g; Carbohydrates: 7 g; Fat: 7 g; Fiber: 2 g; Sodium: 20 mg; Vitamin A: 6,294 IU; Vitamin C: 37 mg; Diabetic Exchange: Fat 1, Vegetable 1.5

sautéed mustard greens with dried cranberries

serves 4

2 tablespoons canola oil
1 medium onion, chopped
¾ pound mustard greens, washed, tough
  stems trimmed, and sliced into ½-inch

strips
Salt, to taste
3 tablespoons balsamic vinegar
¼ cup dried cranberries

1. In a large nonstick skillet, heat the canola oil over medium-high heat. Add the onion and sauté for 3 minutes. Reduce the heat to medium, add the mustard greens and salt, and continue to sauté until wilted. (*Note:* You may need to add the mustard greens in batches—as one batch wilts, add the next.) Cook, uncovered, for about 15 minutes, stirring frequently. If the mustard greens stick to the skillet, add a little water, 2 tablespoons at a time. Add the balsamic vinegar and dried cranberries during the last 5 minutes of cooking.
2. Adjust the seasoning and serve.

APPROXIMATE NUTRITIONAL INFORMATION: Serving size: one-quarter sautéed mustard greens with dried cranberries; Calories: 124 cals; Protein: 2 g; Carbohydrates: 14 g; Fat: 7 g; Fiber: 3 g; Sodium: 15 mg; Vitamin A: 2,578 IU; Vitamin C: 23 mg; Diabetic Exchange: Fat 1, Vegetable 3

bok choy and arugula with soy sauce

serves 5

1 tablespoon canola oil

2 tablespoons toasted sesame oil

1 medium onion, chopped

2 garlic cloves, minced

2¼ pounds bok choy, washed and cut into ½-inch slices (Note: Keep the thicker stem ends separate from the top leaves, as they will be cooked first.)

1 large bunch arugula, washed, and stems trimmed (about 3 cups leaves)

2 tablespoons soy sauce, or to taste

Freshly ground pepper, to taste

1. In a large nonstick skillet, combine the canola oil and sesame oil and heat over medium-high heat. Add the onion and sauté for 2 minutes. Add the garlic and sauté for 30 seconds. Reduce the heat to medium, add the white stems of the bok choy, and sauté for 3 minutes. Add the green leaves of the bok choy and the arugula and sauté for 5 minutes. If the skillet seems dry, add 2 tablespoons of water.
2. Add the soy sauce and sauté for 3 more minutes. Adjust the seasoning and serve.

APPROXIMATE NUTRITIONAL INFORMATION: Serving size: one-fifth bok choy and arugula with soy sauce; Calories: 115 cals; Protein: 4 g; Carbohydrates: 7 g; Fat: 9 g; Fiber: 4 g; Sodium: 486 mg; Vitamin A: 5,621 IU; Vitamin C: 57 mg; Folic Acid: 105 mcg; Diabetic Exchange: Fat 2, Vegetable 1

marvelous main courses

～

W E ALL LEAD hectic lives. Juggling family and career, or just family alone, is no
easy task. The stress is limitless, but most parents will agree that the joys of raising a family far outweigh the trials and tribulations one encounters along the way.

So, what's for dinner?

This is perhaps the most dreaded question of the day. Putting a hot meal on the table
at the end of a long day is a true challenge, even for the best home cooks. Menu planning is an art, and, depending on your organizational skills, time constraints, energy level,
and general taste preferences, meals can be planned in advance for the week, for the
day, or on the spur of the moment in the grocery store. Whatever your method, obstacles such as morning sickness (or all-day sickness), general fatigue, or the need for bed
rest can thwart even the best intentions to plan meals during pregnancy. This is where
restaurants and stores selling high-quality prepared and semi-prepared foods fit in. Read
labels carefully to make the healthiest choices possible. A ready-to-serve well-balanced
dinner can be as simple as a store-bought roasted chicken, a salad from the salad bar, V-
8 juice, and a glass of milk—all to go.

THINGS TO REMEMBER
WHEN YOU HAVE NO TIME TO COOK

- Healthy meals do not need to be hot, or fancy. An omelet, toast, green salad or green
  vegetable, milk or yogurt, and fruit is a complete breakfast, lunch, or dinner.
- Keep your freezer well stocked with high-protein frozen foods, frozen vegetables,
  and frozen dinners—both homemade and store-bought.
- V-8 juice or carrot sticks are an adequate substitute for a vegetable.
- Double your favorite recipes to have leftovers for future meals.

- Make meals on the weekends for busy weekdays.
- When grilling chicken, beef, or vegetables, cook extras and use the leftovers in salads, sandwiches, fajitas, or burritos.
- When choosing frozen foods or carryout foods, look for dishes that are low in fat and sodium and high in protein.
- Use easy-to-prepare, fallback recipes that you know your family likes. Don't try a new recipe when you're in a rush: frustration is the most likely outcome.
- Try using a slow cooker to have your meals ready when you get home.

EATING OUT

HECTIC WORK SCHEDULES, a heavy social calendar, or a necessary break from the kitchen are some of the reasons we eat out. If you maintain a nutritionally balanced diet when dining out, there is little reason to feel guilty. If, on the other hand, you continually order the greasiest dish on the menu, eat all the bread in the bread basket, and pig out at dessert, you need to reevaluate your eating habits, pregnant or not. Following are some tips to help you make healthy choices when dining out for breakfast, lunch, or dinner.

Tips for Eating in Restaurants

- Abstain from alcohol.
- Inform your waiter of any special dietary needs you have before you order.
- If your dish does not look good or taste good, don't be shy—send it back. After all, you're paying for it!
- Keep in mind your nutritional needs when ordering. Ask yourself: Did I get enough protein today, or should I have the chicken or fish? How am I doing in the fiber department? Vegetables? Calcium? Iron?
- Ask for all meat, poultry, and fish to be cooked well-done.
- Avoid greasy and fatty foods.
- Avoid dishes with lots of sauce or gravy, or ask for it on the side.
- Eat the healthy, whole grain breads and avoid highly salted or greasy breads. Don't add butter to your bread, because most restaurant foods contain more fat than home-cooked meals.
- Stay away from salads made with mayonnaise, especially at salad bars.
- Always survey a salad bar and make sure everything is clean and properly chilled. Choose a light salad dressing without mayonnaise, or, better yet, make your own from the oil and vinegar. Stay away from artificial foods such as bacon bits.
- Avoid high-calorie desserts. Opt for fresh fruit or fruit sorbet for dessert.

- Don't order dairy-based desserts that are served off a dessert cart without refrigeration.
- Avoid buying any food from street vendors, especially hot dogs.

It's a fact of life in our fast-paced society that at least at some time during pregnancy, you will probably eat in a fast food restaurant. It might be at a rest stop along the highway, or you might finally give in to your older children begging you for a "Happy Meal." Whatever the reason, fast food does not have to put you on a guilt trip as long as you make smart, healthy choices. The three major concerns with fast food are high calories, fat, and sodium. On average, 40 to 60 percent of the calories in fast foods come from fat. Frying, particularly deep-frying, is a major source of fat in foods like french fries, fish, and burgers. French fries, prepared sauces, and salad dressings are all extremely high in sodium. Following are a few tips to help you navigate the fast food lane (see Sample Smart Choice Fast Food Menus, page 233).

Tips for Choosing Fast Foods

- Try to select fast food restaurants or chains that offer salad bars, baked potatoes, baked chicken or fish, burritos, or grilled (not fried) meats and poultry.
- Do not order deep-fried foods. Opt for baked, broiled, or grilled items. Batter on chicken, fish, and onion rings acts as a sponge, absorbing large amounts of fat. Deep-fried chicken or fish could end up having three times the amount of fat of a plain grilled hamburger.
- Order your sandwiches without sauces. Add fresh fixings, such as lettuce, tomatoes, onions, and pickles, to them.
- Avoid bacon, sausages, pepperoni, and other processed meats that are high in fat, sodium, nitrites, and nitrates. Opt for a vegetarian pizza or a simple cheese pizza.
- Choose smart toppings for your baked potato. Use a minimal amount of sour cream, margarine, or butter, and opt for vegetable (broccoli or spinach) toppings, salsa, pasteurized cheese, or low-fat cottage cheese.
- Salad bars and packaged salads are excellent low-fat alternatives. However, you can quickly turn your low-fat salad into a high-fat nightmare by piling on the wrong toppings, such as creamy salad dressing. Because you can't control the amount of mayonnaise in them, try to avoid mayonnaise-based salads, such as macaroni and potato.
- Avoid croissant sandwiches, hot dogs, french fries, onion rings, and deep-fried fruit pies.
- Bean dishes, such as baked beans, chili with beans, and bean salad are all smart choices because they add protein, iron, and fiber to your diet.
- Avoid fruits in heavy syrup. Opt for fresh fruits if available.

- Do not use fast foods as snack foods or mini meals between your three main meals.
- Be more careful with your food choices for the rest of the day if you have eaten fast food. Try to fit in fresh fruits and vegetables (even V-8 juice) at some point.

Diabetics have unique eating challenges that can be difficult to keep track of, especially when dining out. If you were diabetic before pregnancy or have been diagnosed with gestational diabetes, the following tips should help you make healthy decisions when dining out. Be sure to seek the advice of your doctor, certified diabetes educator, or dietitian if you have any questions regarding certain meals or foods, or how they fit into your diabetic meal plan.

Tips for Diabetics Dining Out

- Remember your meal plan. If you have just received your diet plan or are on a new plan, carry a copy of it with you so you can make smart choices from a menu.
- Watch portion sizes. Some restaurants give you more-than-you-could-ever-eat portions, but this does not mean you have to clean your plate. Ask your waiter to modify your portion in accordance with your diet, or modify it yourself when your meal arrives, and take some home. Don't equate the cost of the dish with having to finish it.
- Avoid fats. Choose baked, grilled, or broiled dishes without added fat, gravy, or sauce; or ask that the gravy or sauce be served separately. (This applies to salad dressings as well.)
- Avoid all deep-fried foods, no matter how tempting they sound.
- Trim any visible fat from your meat. If your diet plan has only 1 fat exchange for your meal, use half a portion of butter and half a portion of salad dressing.
- Plan for your starch intake. If you choose the bread as an appetizer, be sure to count it against the starch exchanges in the rest of your meal.
- Always opt for fresh fruit for dessert. Ask your waiter for a piece of fresh fruit, even if it is not on the menu, or plan ahead and carry some fruit with you.
- Order the type of milk that fits your diet pattern.
- Remember your list of "free foods" for simple pleasures.

marvelous main courses

Spaghetti with Meat Sauce

Best-Ever American Meat Loaf

Flank Steak with Salsa Verde

Quick and Easy Chicken Curry

Chicken or Veal Cutlets with Mushroom-Caper Sauce

Mary Mulard's Baked Chicken

Marinated Grilled Chicken or Beef Fajitas

Moroccan-Style Chicken Stew

Chicken with Homemade Barbecue Sauce

Juicy Turkey Burgers

Homemade Chicken Tenders

Spice-Rubbed Pork Chops

Marinated Grilled or Broiled Lamb Chops

Sautéed Shrimp with Pasta

Shrimp and Vegetable Stir-Fry

Crab Cakes with Red Bell Pepper Sauce

Sautéed Salmon on a Bed of Greens with Citrus Vinaigrette

Roasted Salmon with Papaya Salsa

Tilapia Mediterranean Style

RECIPE NOTES

IF YOU ARE pregnant with your first child, enjoy your final days of cooking and eating dinner (or any meal, for that matter) in peace. Soon you will have a newborn demanding to be fed while you are trying to cook or eat. Or you might already have a toddler clinging to your leg, crying, just because it's late-afternoon-meltdown time. These obstacles get in the way of preparing dinner, not to mention the fact that you're exhausted after putting in a full day's work at the office or at home.

There is no right or easy solution to getting dinner on the table. The best advice is to try to plan meals for a couple of days at a time and to shop for those meals in one trip. Also, try to cook meals in segments, whenever you have a free minute. (See How to Make Dinner Ahead, page 213). Side dishes, such as enriched pasta, rice, or couscous, and vegetables can all be cooked ahead and reheated in a microwave at mealtime.

Some notes about the recipes in this chapter:

- Buy the freshest ingredients you can find. Use them promptly to maximize their vitamin and nutrient content. Check all expiration dates. (See Food Safety Tips on Meat, Poultry, and Seafood, page 304)
- Buy high-quality meats and poultry on sale and freeze them. Whenever possible and affordable, choose minimally processed, all-natural meats and poultry that are antibiotic-, hormone-, and preservative-free.
- Fish and shellfish are generally best if prepared on the day they are purchased.
- Use an instant-read thermometer to avoid any doubt about whether something is cooked well-done or not. Cook and eat all of your food well-done during pregnancy.
- Avoid cross-contamination from juices of meat, poultry, and seafood. Keep raw meat, poultry, and seafood away from other foods, and after cutting or handling them, wash your hands, the cutting board, knife, and countertops with hot soapy water, or use an anti-bacterial spray cleanser.
- Marinating food is an extra step, but it greatly improves the taste of any dish.
- Discard all marinades, rubs, or sauces that have come in contact with raw foods, and do not use them to baste foods on the grill or under the broiler.
- Place all cooked foods on clean plates or serving platters.
- Salt to taste, but be cautious when adding salt to dishes that contain high-sodium ingredients, such as olives, anchovies, or canned vegetables or beans.
- All of the sauces, marinades, and rubs in this book can be used with any meat, poultry, or seafood.

- Allow meat and poultry to rest for five minutes after cooking. It will be juicier and more tender if the meat relaxes.
- Slice cooked meats and poultry with a sharp knife against the grain on a slight angle. This particularly applies to flank steak, skirt steak, and chicken breasts.
- Be sure to clean your grill every time you use it. Nothing is worse than a beautiful piece of salmon or steak that tastes like a dirty grill.
- If broiling anything, watch it very carefully. Never leave the broiler unattended.
- Slow cooker instructions are given in some of the recipes.
- Freeze dishes in meal-size portions in zip-lock bags or small plastic containers. Label and date everything.
- Remove the child's portion of a dish before adding spices, fresh herbs, or anything that your child may not like.
- Adjust any of the recipes to suit your family's eating habits and tastes.

HOW TO MAKE DINNER AHEAD

- *Spaghetti with Meat Sauce:* Cook the meat sauce ahead; freeze. Cook the pasta ahead. Microwave to reheat
- *Best-Ever American Meat Loaf:* Form and bake the meat loaf ahead; microwave to reheat.
- *Flank Steak with Salsa Verde:* Marinate the flank steak up to two days in advance. Make the salsa verde ahead; freeze. The flank steak is best just off the grill, but it can be grilled a bit ahead.
- *Quick and Easy Chicken Curry:* Marinate the chicken and vegetables; cook ahead. Make the rice ahead; microwave to reheat.
- *Chicken or Veal Cutlets with Mushroom-Caper Sauce:* Cook ahead. Make the noodles ahead. Microwave to reheat.
- *Mary Mulard's Baked Chicken:* Assemble the casserole up to six hours before baking; refrigerate.
- *Marinated Grilled Chicken or Beef Fajitas:* Marinate the chicken or beef up to two days in advance. Grill, broil, or sauté in advance. Cook the onions and bell peppers up to two days in advance. Microwave to reheat.
- *Moroccan-Style Chicken Stew:* Cook ahead (use a slow cooker); freeze. Microwave to reheat.
- *Chicken with Homemade Barbecue Sauce:* Make the barbecue sauce ahead. Marinate the chicken up to two days ahead. Bake the chicken and grill or broil at the last minute.
- *Juicy Turkey Burgers:* Form the burgers ahead. Cook the burgers ahead. Microwave to reheat.
- *Homemade Chicken Tenders:* Bake the tenders ahead; freeze. Use a conventional oven or microwave to reheat.
- *Spice-Rubbed Pork Chops:* Make the spice rub ahead. Marinate the pork chops ahead. The pork chops are best cooked just before serving, but they can be made ahead and reheated in a microwave or conventional oven.
- *Marinated Grilled or Broiled Lamb Chops:* Make the marinade ahead. Marinate the lamb chops up to two days in advance. The lamb chops are best cooked just before serving, but they can be made ahead and reheated in a microwave or conventional oven.
- *Sautéed Shrimp with Pasta:* Make the shrimp ahead. Make the pasta ahead. Microwave to reheat.
- *Shrimp and Vegetable Stir-Fry:* Prepare all of the vegetables and cook the rice up to one day ahead. Stir-fry at the last minute.
- *Crab Cakes with Red Bell Pepper Sauce:* Make the red bell pepper sauce up to three days ahead. Form the crab cakes ahead; cook ahead. Microwave to reheat.
- *Sautéed Salmon on a Bed of Greens with Citrus Vinaigrette:* Make the vinaigrette up to three days ahead. Sauté the salmon ahead. Mix the salad ahead, but dress it at the last minute.

- *Roasted Salmon with Papaya Salsa:* Make the papaya salsa up to three hours ahead. Cook the salmon ahead. Microwave to reheat.
- *Tilapia Mediterranean Style:* Cook ahead and microwave to reheat. Or, make just the sauce ahead (the herbs will lose their bright green color but this does not affect the taste) and cook the fish just before serving. Make the rice ahead.

pantry items for marvelous main courses

Fresh Produce
Avocados
Baby greens
Broccoli florets
Carrots: regular and peeled baby carrots
Cherry tomatoes
Fresh herbs: basil, cilantro, dill, mint, parsley, rosemary, thyme
Garlic
Ginger
Lemons
Limes
Mushrooms: button or cremini
Navel oranges
Onions: sweet (such as Vidalia), yellow, red
Papayas
Red bell peppers
Scallions
Shallots
Snow peas
Zucchini

Meats, Poultry, and Fish
Beef skirt steak
Boneless, skinless chicken breasts
Chicken tenders
Flank steak
Ground turkey
Jumbo lump crabmeat or back fin crabmeat, or a combination
Lamb chops (about 1½ inches thick)
Lean ground beef
Meat loaf mixture of beef, pork, and veal
Medium shrimp
Pork chops (about 1 inch thick)
Roasted chicken or cooked chicken
Skinless chicken parts (bone-in)
Skinned salmon fillet
Skin-on salmon fillet
Thin-sliced chicken cutlets
Tilapia
Veal cutlets

Dairy and Soy Products
Grade A large eggs
Half-and-half (preferably ultra-pasteurized)
Heavy cream (preferably ultra-pasteurized)
Parmesan cheese (grated)
Part-skim ricotta cheese
Plain low-fat yogurt
Swiss cheese
Unsalted butter
Whole milk

Canned, Bottled, and Jarred Staples
Anchovy fillets or anchovy paste
Canola oil
Canola oil cooking spray
Capers (small or medium)
Chickpeas (7¾-ounce can)
Condensed chicken soup (any kind) (10¾-ounce can)
Dijon mustard
Fat-free low-sodium stock (any kind) (14.5-ounce can)
Fish sauce
Hoisin sauce
Honey
Kalamata olives or other brine-cured black olives (preferably pitted)

Ketchup
Light mayonnaise
Mandarin oranges in light syrup or
juice (8-ounce can)
Olive oil
Peeled and diced tomatoes
(14.5-ounce can)
Rice vinegar (seasoned)
Sesame oil (toasted)
Soy sauce (regular or light)
Tomato paste
Tomato sauce (15-ounce can)
Worcestershire sauce

Dry Staples
Bread crumbs (plain or seasoned)
Enriched all-purpose flour (preferably
unbleached)
Enriched linguine and spaghetti
(thin or regular)
Enriched medium egg noodles
Fajita-size tortillas (6- or 7-inch)
Light or dark raisins
Nuts: cashew nuts, roasted peanuts

Quick-dissolving flour (such as Won-
dra or Pillsbury Shake and Blend)
Saltine crackers
Sugar: brown and white

Herbs and Spices
Chili powder
Dried oregano
Dried tarragon
Garlic powder
Ground allspice, cinnamon, and/or
cloves
Ground cumin
Ground ginger
Italian seasoning
Mild curry powder
Old Bay seasoning

From the Salad Bar
Diced onions
Broccoli florets
Sliced mushrooms
Sliced red bell peppers

e. coli warning

Escherichia coli O157:H7 is a bacterium, usually found in undercooked contaminated ground beef, that causes food-borne illness. Other known means of infection are drinking unpasteurized milk and juice, swimming in or drinking sewage-contaminated water, and consuming sprouts, lettuce, and salami. The poor hygiene of infected persons (or caretakers of those persons) suffering from diarrhea can also spread the bacteria.

Escherichia coli O157:H7 can be found on a small number of cattle farms and can live in the intestines of healthy cattle. Meat can become contaminated during slaughter, and organisms can be thoroughly mixed into the beef when it is ground. Contaminated meat looks and smells normal. Bacteria present on the cow's udders or on equipment may get into raw milk, causing contamination. The symptoms of infection are usually severe bloody diarrhea and abdominal cramps, but symptoms are not always present. Fever is uncommon, and the illness usually runs its course in five to ten days.

Here are a few tips to prevent infection.[38]

- Cook all ground beef and hamburger thoroughly. Because beef can turn brown before disease-causing bacteria are killed, use an instant-read thermometer to check that ground beef has reached the well-done stage of 160°F. Wash the thermometer in between each test of the meat.
- Keep raw meat separate from uncooked foods. Wash hands, counters, and utensils with hot soapy water after touching raw meat.
- Never put cooked hamburgers or ground beef back on the plate that held the raw patties.
- Drink only pasteurized milk, juice, or cider.
- Wash fruits and vegetables thoroughly, especially those that will not be cooked.
- Avoid alfalfa sprouts.
- Drink municipal water that has been treated with chlorine and other disinfectants, or drink bottled water.
- Avoid swallowing lake or pool water while swimming.
- Make sure that persons with diarrhea, especially children, wash their hands, to reduce the risk of spreading infection, and that anyone washes his or her hands after changing soiled diapers.

spaghetti with meat sauce

What's in this for baby and me? Protein, vitamins A and C, and folic acid.

HIGH IN **protein**, **vitamins A** and **C**, and **folic acid**, and a good source of iron, this simple and tasty meat sauce is sure to become a dinner staple. Simmering the meat in milk or half-and-half softens it and gives the finished dish a slightly creamy consistency. Feel free to add your favorite sauce ingredients and omit any of the items that your children might not like, such as the mushrooms, red bell peppers, or fresh herbs. One and one-half cups of cooked enriched spaghetti is an excellent source of **protein** and **folic acid**, and a good source of iron, B vitamins, and fiber—now you do the math! Be sure to top your spaghetti with lots of Parmesan cheese for calcium.

serves 6 to 8 (makes about 8 cups sauce)

2 tablespoons olive oil

1 onion, finely diced (optional)

1 garlic clove, minced (optional)

2 teaspoons dried oregano

2 teaspoons dried Italian seasoning

1 pound lean ground beef

1 cup whole milk or half-and-half

8 ounces mushrooms (any kind), washed, stems trimmed, and thinly sliced (optional)

1 small red bell pepper, washed, cored, seeded, and cut into small dice (optional)

One 15-ounce can tomato sauce

One 14.5-ounce can diced tomatoes (do not drain)

Salt and freshly ground pepper, to taste

Enriched spaghetti or your favorite pasta (see headnote), cooked according to package directions

3–4 tablespoons chopped fresh basil, parsley, or dill, for garnish (optional)

Grated Parmesan cheese, for the table (optional)

1. In a large heavy-based nonreactive saucepan, heat the olive oil over medium-high heat. Add the onion and sauté for 3 minutes. Add the garlic, oregano, and Italian seasoning and sauté for 1 minute longer.

2. Crumble the ground beef into the saucepan and sauté for 5 minutes, stirring and breaking up any large lumps of meat with the back of a wooden spoon. Add the milk (see **Cooking Tip** below), mushrooms, and bell pepper and simmer gently for 30 minutes, or until most of the liquid has evaporated.

3. Add the tomato sauce and diced tomatoes and simmer for 30 minutes longer, or until the sauce has thickened to the desired consistency. (Cook the pasta while the sauce is simmering.)

4. Adjust the seasoning, add the basil, and serve over the spaghetti. Pass the cheese at the table.

▶ **Cooking Tip:** It is essential to use very fresh milk or half-and-half. You will probably see a little bit of separation as the milk or half-and-half cooks, this is normal.

▶ **Timesaving Tip:** Use jarred pasta sauce.

▶ **Storage Tip:** The meat sauce keeps 3 days refrigerated, and it can be frozen for up to 1 month.

▶ **Diabetic Tip:** Reduce the portion size of cooked spaghetti to 3⁄4 cup per serving.

▶ **Complete Meal Ideas:** Serve this spaghetti with:

> Green salad or a green vegetable (you might want to try a green salad with the
>   Caesar Salad Dressing, page 143)
> Reduced-fat 2% milk or low-fat yogurt
> Fresh fruit that contains vitamin C

APPROXIMATE NUTRITIONAL INFORMATION: Meat Sauce: Serving size: 1 cup; Calories: 248 cals; Protein: 19 g; Carbohydrates: 11 g; Fat: 15 g; Fiber: 2 g; Sodium: 627 mg; Vitamin A: 1,489 IU; Vitamin C: 45 mg; Diabetic Exchange: Bread/Starch: .5, Fat 1.5, Meat (Medium Fat) 2

APPROXIMATE NUTRITIONAL INFORMATION: Spaghetti: Serving size: 1 1⁄2 cups cooked spaghetti; Calories: 296 cals; Protein: 10 g; Carbohydrates: 60 g; Fat: 1 g; Fiber: 4 g; Sodium: 2 mg; Folic Acid: 147 mcg; Diabetic Exchange (values per 3⁄4 cup serving): Bread/Starch: 2

best-ever american meat loaf

What's in this for baby and me? Protein.

MEAT LOAF IS to American cuisine what Norman Rockwell is to American art. Both conjure up images of family gatherings and happy times. Make this meat loaf using only beef, or use a combination of beef, pork, and veal. If your kids object to green things in their meat loaf, leave out the herbs. You can't beat meat loaf for a powerful dose of **protein**, and a good dose of iron and vitamin C. Served hot with mashed potatoes or sweet potatoes, or eaten cold in a sandwich with some good mustard and baby pickles, meat loaf is just plain good!

serves 11

**Canola oil or canola oil cooking spray for
  greasing the baking pan**
Glaze (optional)
  ¼ cup ketchup
  1 tablespoon molasses
  1 teaspoon seasoned rice vinegar
Meat Loaf
  **2 pounds lean ground beef (preferably
    chuck) or a meat loaf mix of pork, veal,
    and beef (sold in many grocery stores)**
  2 large eggs, lightly beaten
  ⅔ cup thinly sliced scallions (optional)

¼ cup chopped fresh parsley (optional)
¼ cup chopped fresh dill (optional)
1 teaspoon dried oregano
1 tablespoon Worcestershire sauce
2 teaspoons Dijon mustard
**¾ cup finely crushed saltine crackers
    (about 18 crackers) or 1 cup plain bread
    crumbs**
1½ teaspoons salt
**½ teaspoon freshly ground pepper, or a
    couple drops of Tabasco sauce**
½ cup plain low-fat yogurt or whole milk

1. Preheat the oven to 350°F. Line a large baking pan with foil and lightly grease it.
2. To make the optional glaze, mix all of the ingredients in a measuring cup or a small bowl; set aside.
3. To make the meat loaf, combine all of the ingredients in a large bowl and mix with a fork or your hands (wet your hands first to reduce sticking) until well blended. (See the **Cooking Tip** below for checking the seasoning of the meat loaf mixture.) Form the meat loaf mixture into a large ball and transfer it to the baking pan. Using your hands, form it into an oval-shaped loaf approximately 10 inches long and 2½ inches high. Using the back of a spoon, evenly "frost" the meat loaf with the glaze, if using.
4. Bake for 1 hour and 25 to 30 minutes, or until completely cooked: an instant-read thermometer should read 160°F, and the juices should run clear when the center of the loaf is pierced with a knife or skewer. Remove the meat loaf from the oven and allow it to rest for 15 minutes before slicing.

▶ **Cooking Tip:** To check the seasoning before baking, spray a small skillet with canola oil cooking spray and cook about 1 tablespoon of the meat loaf mixture until well-done. Taste the cooked meat, and adjust the seasoning in remaining meat mixture if necessary.

▶ **Advance Preparation:** The meat loaf can be assembled up to 6 hours before baking and refrigerated. The baking time may increase by 10 to 15 minutes.

▶ **Storage Tip:** The meat loaf keeps 3 days refrigerated. It does not freeze well.

▶ **Health Tip:** Be sure to wash your hands thoroughly with warm water and soap for at least 20 seconds after handling the raw meat.

▶ **Complete Meal Ideas:** Serve this meat loaf with:
  Mashed potatoes, baked potatoes, or sweet potatoes (you might want to try the Southern-Style Sweet Potato Casserole, page 200)
  Green salad or green vegetable (try one of Annie Mozer's Greens, pages 203–205, or the Classic Creamed Spinach, page 198)
  Reduced-fat 2% milk or low-fat yogurt
  Fresh fruit that contains vitamin C

APPROXIMATE NUTRITIONAL INFORMATION: Serving size: one 4.5-ounce serving (about one-eleventh of the meat loaf); Calories: 300 cals; Protein: 27 g; Carbohydrates: 8 g; Fat: 17 g; Fiber: .5 g; Sodium: 499 mg; Diabetic Exchange: Bread/Starch .5, Meat (Medium Fat) 3.5

flank steak with salsa verde

What's in this for baby and me? Protein and vitamin C.

NOTHING BEATS FLANK steak for a tender, priced-right, lean cut of beef that is high in **protein** and provides a good dose of iron. The key to a truly great flank steak is marinating it, for as long as possible, before grilling. The salsa verde, an excellent source of **vitamin C**, is a take on an Argentinean herb-and-garlic sauce called *chimichurri* that can also be served with poultry or fish, as well as meat. Like pesto, salsa verde can be frozen.

serves 4

One 1½-pound flank steak
Marinade
  ¼ cup soy sauce
  1 teaspoon canola oil
  2 teaspoons seasoned rice vinegar or freshly squeezed lime juice
  1 tablespoon Worcestershire sauce
  1 garlic clove, minced
  1 tablespoon minced fresh ginger, or 1 teaspoon ground ginger (optional)
  1 tablespoon chopped fresh rosemary (optional)

Salsa Verde (makes ⅓ cup) (optional)
  1½ cups packed fresh cilantro leaves
  3 anchovy fillets or 1 teaspoon anchovy paste (optional)
  1½ tablespoons small or medium capers
  1 garlic clove
  1½ tablespoons freshly squeezed lemon juice, or to taste
  ¼ cup olive oil
  Freshly ground pepper, to taste

1. Remove any visible fat from the flank steak. Using a fork, pierce the steak all over, then place it in a 1-gallon zip-lock bag or in a shallow pie dish and set aside.
2. To make the marinade, combine all of the ingredients in a small bowl or measuring cup and mix well. Add the marinade to the flank steak, turning to make sure that it is completely covered with the marinade, and refrigerate for at least 1 hour, or up to 48 hours.
3. To make the salsa verde, combine all of the ingredients in the bowl of a food processor and process until pureed and the sauce is slightly emulsified, scraping down the sides of the bowl as needed. Transfer to a serving bowl, cover with plastic wrap, placing it directly against the surface of the sauce (this is to prevent discoloration), and refrigerate.
4. Preheat the grill. Have a serving platter ready for the cooked flank steak. Grill the flank steak for 12 to 15 minutes, or until well-done; an instant-read thermometer should read 160°F. Transfer the meat to the platter and allow it to rest for 5 minutes for the juices to re-distribute and the meat to relax.

5. To serve, using a sharp knife held on a diagonal slant, on a chopping board with gutters to catch juices, slice the flank steak against the grain into ½-inch slices. Place the slices on the serving platter and serve immediately, with the salsa verde.

▶ *Health Tip:* Discard all leftover marinade—do not use it to baste the flank steak on the grill. Place the finished flank steak on a clean serving platter.

▶ *Advance Preparation:* The flank steak should marinate for at least 1 hour, and up to 48 hours.

▶ *Storage Tip:* The cooked flank steak and salsa verde keep 3 days refrigerated. The salsa verde can be frozen for up to 1 month.

▶ *Complete Meal Ideas:* Serve this steak with:
> Potatoes, rice, pasta salad, or cornbread (you might want to try the Noodles with Spinach, Red Peppers, and Sesame Dressing, page 122, or the Pink Potato Salad, page 130)
> Green vegetable or green salad
> Reduced-fat 2% milk or low-fat yogurt
> Fresh fruit that contains vitamin C (if you are not using the salsa verde)

APPROXIMATE NUTRITIONAL INFORMATION: Flank steak: Serving size: 4 ounces; Calories: 259 cals; Protein: 35 g; Carbohydrates: 0; Fat: 12 g; Fiber: 0; Sodium: 75 mg; Diabetic Exchange: Meat (Lean) 5

APPROXIMATE NUTRITIONAL INFORMATION: Salsa verde: Serving size: 2 tablespoons; Calories: 90 cals; Protein: .9 g; Carbohydrates: 1 g; Fat: 9 g; Fiber: .4g; Sodium: 143 mg; Vitamin C: 15 mg; Diabetic Exchange: Fat 2

quick and easy chicken curry

~

What's in this for baby and me? Protein and vitamins A and C.

A QUICK AND easy curry dish loaded with flavor and packed with **protein** and **vitamins A** and **C**. Feel free to replace the red peppers with another vegetable, such as small broccoli florets or sliced zucchini, and the chicken with shrimp. Serve over basmati rice or rice noodles, if desired.

serves 3

1 pound chicken tenders, cut into ½-inch slices
    on the diagonal
1 red bell pepper, cored, seeded, quartered,
    and cut into ¼-inch strips
1 medium sweet onion (such as Vidalia),
    halved and thinly sliced
1 tablespoon mild curry powder
1 tablespoon sugar

3 tablespoons canola oil
1 tablespoon fish sauce or soy sauce
3 scallions, trimmed and sliced into large
    pieces
¼ cup chopped fresh cilantro, or to taste
Freshly squeezed lime juice, to taste
Lime wedges for the table

1. Combine the chicken, red bell pepper, onion, 2 tablespoons of the canola oil, curry powder, sugar, and fish sauce in a bowl. Mix until well combined, then allow to marinate, covered and refrigerated, for at least 30 minutes, or overnight.
2. Heat the remaining 1 tablespoon canola oil in a large nonstick skillet over medium-high heat. Add *half* of the chicken mixture, and *half* of the scallions and sauté for about 5 to 7 minutes, or until the chicken is cooked. (*Note*: Use a splatter screen to reduce cleanup.) Transfer the cooked chicken to a serving bowl and cover with foil to keep warm. Reheat the skillet, add the remaining chicken mixture and scallions, and repeat the procedure.
3. Garnish with the cilantro and a squeeze of fresh lime juice. Serve immediately, with the lime wedges.

▶ *Variation:* Substitute 1 pound peeled medium or large raw shrimp for the chicken. Allow them to marinate for at least 30 minutes, and up to 3 hours. The cooking time will be closer to 5 minutes than 7.

▶ *Advance Preparation:* The chicken should marinate for at least 30 minutes, and up to 12 hours, and the shrimp for at least 30 minutes, and up to 3 hours.

▶ *Storage Tip:* This chicken curry keeps 3 days refrigerated, and it can be frozen for up to 1 month.

▶ *Complete Meal Ideas:* Serve this curry with:

    Rice, rice noodles, quinoa, or soba noodles

    Green vegetable or green salad (you might want to try the Vegetables with
        Lemon, Olive Oil, and Fresh Herbs, page 128)

    Reduced-fat 2% milk or low-fat yogurt

    Fresh fruit

APPROXIMATE NUTRITIONAL INFORMATION: Serving size: 7 ounces chicken curry dish; Calories: 236 cals; Protein: 25 g; Carbohydrates: 8 g; Fat: 11 g; Fiber: 1 g; Sodium: 397 mg; Vitamin A: 1,824 IU; Vitamin C: 66 mg; Diabetic Exchange: Bread/Starch .5, Meat (Medium Fat) 3

smart choice frozen foods

The frozen foods market is expanding daily to meet the needs of busy people. Many whole foods stores stock their shelves with high-quality frozen foods, ranging from vegetarian lasagna and ravioli to hearty beef stews. Usually these "in-house" prepared frozen foods contain fewer preservatives and less sodium than the big-name brands carried by large-chain grocery stores. When choosing frozen foods, look for foods containing the highest amount of protein (usually about 10 grams) and the least amount of fat per serving. Reduced-fat frozen dinners are good options, and frozen vegetarian dishes tend to be lower in fat. While frozen foods are convenient, they can be expensive—read labels carefully, because a few pennies more might buy you extra protein and less fat. Also, if you are on a reduced-sodium diet, keep in mind that most frozen foods have a high sodium content.

chicken or veal cutlets with mushroom-caper sauce

What's in this for baby and me? Protein.

HIGH IN **protein** and a good source of vitamins A and C and iron, this tasty dish is sure to become a favorite. Feel free to change the sauce ingredients according to your family's tastes. Older kids might like the capers, younger kids might object to green things, or vice versa—and you can always serve the chicken or veal without the sauce. Have your rice or wide egg noodles ready before making the recipe. The heavy cream is optional, but it adds a velvety smoothness to the sauce. Do not substitute milk or half-and-half, because they tend to curdle in the sauce.

serves 4

¼ cup all-purpose flour, for dredging the cutlets

½ teaspoon salt

12 to 16 ounces boneless, skinless thin-sliced chicken breast cutlets or thin-sliced veal cutlets (if cutlets are not available, see Cooking Tip below for instructions on using boneless, skinless chicken breasts)

1½ tablespoons canola oil

2 tablespoons unsalted butter

8 ounces mushrooms (any kind), washed, stems trimmed, and thinly sliced

One 14.5-ounce can fat-free low-sodium stock

2–3 tablespoons drained small or medium capers, or to taste

¼ cup heavy cream (optional)

1 tablespoon quick-dissolving flour (such as Wondra), to desired consistency

¼ cup chopped fresh parsley or dill or 1 teaspoon dried tarragon (optional)

1 to 2 tablespoons freshly squeezed lemon juice, or to taste

Salt and freshly ground pepper, to taste

1. Have 2 large plates ready, one for the floured cutlets and the other for the cooked cutlets. Combine the flour and salt in a shallow dish or pie pan. Coat one cutlet at a time with flour, shake off any excess, and place on one of the plates; set aside.
2. Heat 1 tablespoon of the canola oil in a large nonstick skillet over medium-high heat until hot. Add half the chicken cutlets, and cook, turning only once, for about 3 minutes on each side, or until lightly browned and thoroughly cooked. (*Note:* The cooking time will depend on the thickness of the cutlets.) Transfer the cutlets to the clean plate, and cover loosely with foil. Add the remaining canola oil to the skillet, heat it, and cook the remaining cutlets. Transfer the cutlets to the plate. (Do not rinse the skillet.)
3. Melt the butter in the same skillet over medium-high heat. Add the mushrooms, if using, and sauté for 3 minutes. Add the stock and bring to a boil. Reduce the

heat to low, add the capers and the heavy cream, if using, and simmer gently for 2 minutes. Stir in the quick-dissolving flour and simmer for 2 minutes more. Add the chicken cutlets to the skillet and simmer until they are hot, about 3 to 5 minutes more.

4. Add the chopped parsley and lemon juice, adjust the seasoning, and serve immediately.

▶ **Cooking Tip:** If cutlets are not available, use boneless, skinless chicken breasts. Cut each breast horizontally in half, then pound each piece between two sheets of plastic wrap until ⅛ inch thick.

▶ **Storage Tip:** The cutlets and sauce keep for 3 days refrigerated. They do not freeze well. You may need to add a bit of water or stock to thin the sauce when reheating it.

▶ **Complete Meal Ideas:** Serve these cutlets with:
  Egg noodles, orzo, or rice
  Green vegetable or green salad (you might want to try to Spinach Salad with
    Mandarin Oranges and Toasted Almonds, page 138)
  Reduced-fat 2% milk or low-fat yogurt
  Fresh fruit that contains vitamin C

APPROXIMATE NUTRITIONAL INFORMATION: Serving size: one-quarter of the chicken cutlets with mushroom-caper sauce; Calories: 353 cals; Protein: 36 g; Carbohydrates: 5 g; Fat: 20 g; Fiber: 1 g; Sodium: 594 mg; Diabetic Exchange: Meat (Lean) 5

APPROXIMATE NUTRITIONAL INFORMATION: Serving size: one-quarter of the veal cutlets with mushroom-caper sauce; Calories: 483 cals; Protein: 34 g; Carbohydrates: 5 g; Fat: 36 g; Fiber: 1 g; Sodium: 597 mg; Diabetic Exchange: Fat 1, Meat (Medium Fat) 5

mary mulard's baked chicken

~

What's in this for baby and me? Protein and calcium.

BAKED CHICKEN DOES not get much easier or tastier than this! Loaded with **protein** and **calcium**, and a good source of vitamin A, this dish takes ten minutes to prepare and about fifty minutes to bake. Serve it with elbow noodles or your kid's favorite pasta, and watch it disappear.

serves 6

1½ pounds (about 4) boneless, skinless
    chicken breasts
8 ounces (about 4 thick slices) Swiss cheese
One 10¾-ounce can condensed chicken soup

¼ cup water
¾ cup herb-seasoned stuffing mix or corn
    bread stuffing, coarsely crushed

1. Preheat the oven to 350°F.
2. Place the chicken breasts in an ungreased 8 x 8 x 2-inch baking dish. Cover them with the cheese slices; set aside.
3. In a small bowl, mix the chicken soup with the water until almost smooth. Pour the soup evenly over the chicken and top with the stuffing mix. Bake for 50 to 60 minutes, or until an instant-read thermometer inserted into the center (through the side) of a chicken breast reads 170°F.

▶ *Storage Tip:* The chicken keeps refrigerated for 3 days. It does not freeze well.

▶ *Complete Meal Ideas:* Serve this chicken with:
    Noodles, rice, or couscous
    A salad or vegetable (you might want to try the Asparagus, Hearts of Palm, and
        Tomato Salad, page 134)
    Reduced-fat 2% milk or low-fat yogurt
    Fresh fruit

APPROXIMATE NUTRITIONAL INFORMATION: Serving size: one-sixth baked chicken; Calories: 401 cals; Protein: 48 g; Carbohydrates: 10 g; Fat: 18 g; Fiber: .5 g; Sodium: 634 mg; Diabetic Exchange: Bread/Starch .5, Meat (Medium Fat) 6

toxoplasmosis warning

~

Toxoplasmosis is an infection caused by the parasite *Toxoplasma gondii*, which can be transmitted by eating undercooked infected meat, or by handling soil or cat feces that contain the parasite. Others sources of infection may be raw goat's milk and raw eggs. Insects, such as flies and cockroaches, that have been in contact with cat feces can contaminate food as well.[35]

Swelling of the lymph nodes or flu-like symptoms (fever, fatigue, and sore throat) may be present, although most adults have no symptoms.[36] If a woman contracts toxoplasmosis for the first time during her pregnancy (active infection only occurs once in a lifetime, although the parasite remains in the body indefinitely), there is a 40 percent chance that her unborn child will also become infected. The risk and severity of the baby's infection depend partly on the timing of the mother's infection. Unborn children infected in early pregnancy are the most likely to suffer severe effects, which may include blindness, deafness, hydrocephalus (water on the brain), seizures, and mental retardation. Tests can determine whether an unborn child is infected, and medications can prevent or reduce severity of effects in unborn children. Toxoplasmosis can also result in miscarriage or stillbirth.

The March of Dimes suggests that pregnant women take the following precautions to prevent toxoplasmosis. [37]

▶ Don't empty your cat's litter box; have someone else do this.

▶ Don't feed your cat raw or undercooked meat.

▶ Keep your cat indoors to prevent it from hunting birds or rodents.

▶ Don't eat raw or undercooked meat, especially lamb or pork. Meat should be cooked to an internal temperature of 160°F throughout.

▶ If you handle raw meat, wash your hands immediately with soap. Never touch your eyes, nose, or mouth with potentially contaminated hands.

▶ Wash all raw fruits and vegetables before you eat them.

▶ Wear gloves when gardening, since soil may contain the parasites from cats. Keep your hands away from your mouth and eyes, and wash your hands thoroughly when finished. Keep gardening gloves away from food products.

▶ Avoid children's sandboxes, as cats may use them as a litter box.

marinated grilled chicken
or beef fajitas

~

What's in this for baby and me? Protein, iron, and vitamins A and C and folic acid.

GRILLED *FAJITAS*, AN excellent source of **protein**, **vitamins A** and **C**, and **folic acid**, and a good source of calcium, iron, fiber, and B vitamins, are the perfect summertime meal. They can be as plain or elaborate as you wish, and since everyone assembles their own, everyone is guaranteed to be happy. Some topping ideas include: grated cheese (such as cheddar or Monterey Jack), guacamole (store-bought or homemade) or sliced avocado, diced vine-ripened tomatoes, shredded lettuce, sliced pitted black olives, jalapeño peppers, sprigs of fresh cilantro, salsa, reduced-fat sour cream or plain yogurt, and lime wedges. If you are short on time, the beef or chicken can be sliced before marinating (see **Timesaving Tip** below), then broiled, grilled, or sautéed. For a delicious fajita filling, vegetarians can grill marinated portobello mushrooms, vegetables, or extra-firm tofu (see **Variation** below). Any leftover beef, chicken, vegetables, or tofu can be made into delicious sandwiches, quesadillas (see Cheese and Spinach Quesadillas, page 184), or tacos.

serves 4

Marinade
 2 tablespoons canola oil
 2 tablespoons seasoned rice vinegar or
  freshly squeezed lime juice
 2 tablespoons Worcestershire sauce
 1 large garlic clove, crushed
 ½ teaspoon ground cumin
 1 teaspoon chili powder

1¼ to 1½ pounds beef skirt steak or boneless skinless chicken breasts (cut horizontally in half), or cutlets or a mixture
1 tablespoon canola oil
2 large bell peppers (any color), washed, cored, seeded, and cut into strips
1 sweet onion (such as Vidalia), thinly sliced
Twelve 7-inch flour tortillas

1. For the marinade, combine all of the ingredients in a small bowl, mix well, and set aside. (*Note*: If you plan to marinate the beef or chicken in a bowl rather than a zip-lock bag, use a large bowl to make the marinade.) Using a fork, pierce the beef (or chicken) all over to allow the marinade to seep in, then place it in a 1 gallon zip-lock bag. Add the marinade, seal (or cover with plastic wrap), and refrigerate for at least 30 minutes, or overnight.
2. Heat the canola oil in a large skillet over medium-high heat. Add the pepper and onion and sauté for 10 minutes. Remove from the heat, cover, and set aside.

3. *To grill* the beef or chicken, preheat the grill. The chicken will take longer to cook than the beef, so if you are serving both, start the chicken first. Have a clean platter ready for the cooked meat. Grill the chicken for approximately 10 to 12 minutes on each side, or until the juices run clear when the chicken is pierced with the tip of a knife and an instant-read thermometer inserted into the center (through the side) of the chicken breast reads 170°F. Grill the beef for approximately 6 to 8 minutes on each side, or until an instant-read thermometer inserted into the center of the meat reads 160°F. Transfer to the platter.

   To broil the beef or chicken, preheat the broiler. Arrange the beef or chicken in a broiler pan lined with foil. Broil the chicken for approximately 12 minutes on each side, the beef for approximately 7 minutes on each side (refer to the well-done temperatures above). Transfer to the platter.
4. While the meat is cooking, heat the tortillas according to package directions. You can also heat them on the grill just before serving by toasting them for a minute or two on each side. Wrap the tortillas in foil to keep them warm.
5. Using a sharp knife and a chopping board with gutters to catch any juices, slice the cooked beef or chicken, against the grain, about ¼ inch thick on the diagonal, and serve immediately. Place all of your chosen toppings, including the pepper-onion mixture, in small bowls on the table.

▶ *Timesaving Tip:* Cut the beef or chicken into ¼-inch strips before marinating. This will cut the marinating time down to about 15 minutes, as the flavor will be more quickly absorbed into the meat. A grill rack might be necessary for the grill, but the strips can also be broiled or sautéed.

▶ *Variation:* You can replace the beef or chicken with peeled fresh large shrimp. Marinate for about 30 minutes, then grill, broil, or sauté for just a couple of minutes on each side—shrimp cook quickly. For vegetarian fajitas, marinate tofu, portobello mushrooms, or your favorite vegetables in the marinade for about 30 minutes, then grill or broil to desired tenderness. Slice into strips before serving.

▶ *Advance Preparation:* The beef or chicken should marinate for at least 30 minutes, and up to 12 hours. The sautéed pepper-onion mixture can be made 2 days in advance, covered, and refrigerated; reheat in a microwave oven.

▶ *Health Tip:* Discard all leftover marinade—do not use it to baste the beef or chicken on the grill or under the broiler. Place the finished beef or chicken on a clean serving platter. If your doctor has restricted your sodium intake, use only 1 tablespoon Worcestershire sauce and don't use olives as a topping. To reduce the fat, use low-fat cheese and low-fat or nonfat sour cream or yogurt as toppings.

▶ *Storage Tip:* The fajitas keep refrigerated for 3 days. They do not freeze well.

▶ *Complete Meal Ideas:* Serve these fajitas with:

Green salad (you might want to try romaine lettuce with the Sun-Dried Tomato and Basil Dressing, page 142)

Reduced-fat 2% milk or low-fat yogurt

Fresh fruit that contains vitamin C

APPROXIMATE NUTRITIONAL INFORMATION: Chicken Fajitas: Serving size: one-sixth of the fajitas (including chicken, flour tortilla, and filling); Calories: 402 cals; Protein: 35 g; Carbohydrates: 40 g; Fat: 10 g; Fiber: 3 g; Sodium: 377 mg; Vitamin A: 2,281 IU; Vitamin C: 77 mg; Folic Acid: 95 mcg; Diabetic Exchange: Bread/Starch 2.5, Meat (Lean) 4

APPROXIMATE NUTRITIONAL INFORMATION: Beef Fajitas: Serving size: one-sixth of the fajitas (including beef, flour tortilla, and filling); Calories: 460 cals; Protein: 31 g; Carbohydrates: 40 g; Fat: 19 g; Fiber: 3 g; Sodium: 384 mg; Vitamin A: 2,261 IU; Vitamin C: 77 mg; B Vitamins: Thiamine: .4 mg, Riboflavin: .3 mg, Niacin: 7 mg; Folic Acid: 99 mcg; Iron 5 mg; Diabetic Exchange: Bread/Starch 2.5, Meat (Medium Fat) 3.5

sample smart choice fast food menus

BREAKFAST
English muffin with an egg
¾ cup fortified cereal with skim milk
8 ounces orange juice
8 ounces reduced-fat 2% milk
8 ounces decaf coffee or tea (optional)

LUNCH OR DINNER
Grilled chicken sandwich, plain roast beef sandwich,
or grilled hamburger/cheeseburger
2 cups prepared salad or salad from the salad bar
About 2 tablespoons reduced-fat salad dressing
8 ounces reduced-fat 2% milk

SAMPLE SALAD
2 cups spinach or dark green lettuce
A large spoonful of beans (kidney or chickpeas)
2–4 tablespoons tuna or chopped egg
1 cup vegetables
¼ cup reduced-fat salad dressing
1 slice whole wheat bread or 2 crackers
8 ounces reduced-fat 2% milk

moroccan-style chicken stew

~

What's in this for baby and me? Protein and vitamins A and C.

THIS FLAVOR-PACKED chicken stew can be made on the stove top or in a slow cooker (See **Slow Cooker Instructions** below). It is an excellent source of **protein** and **vitamins A** and **C**, and a good source of iron, folic acid, and fiber. You can play around with the seasonings and vegetables—adjusting amounts, and adding or omitting anything to suit your family's taste. Vegetarians can substitute tofu for the chicken and add more vegetables. Couscous, quinoa, rice, or tiny pasta (such as orzo or *acini di pepe*) mixed with a pat of butter or olive oil is the perfect side dish and can be cooked while the stew is simmering. Don't be intimidated by the long ingredient list—there are only three cooking steps.

serves 6 to 8

¼ cup canola oil

1 tablespoon ground cumin

1 teaspoon ground ginger

½ teaspoon ground allspice, cinnamon, or cloves, or a mixture

2 pounds boneless, skinless chicken breasts or chicken tenders, cut into 1-inch cubes

1 medium onion (preferably a sweet onion like Vidalia), chopped

4 carrots, peeled and sliced, or 1½ cups sliced baby carrots

One 14.5-ounce can diced tomatoes, drained

½ cup fat-free low-sodium stock or water

1 tablespoon tomato paste

1 tablespoon sugar

About 1 cup (one 7¾-ounce can) chickpeas (optional)

1 medium zucchini, washed and diced, or one 8½-ounce can artichoke hearts, drained and quartered (optional)

1 cup light or dark raisins (optional)

1–2 teaspoons quick-dissolving flour (such as Wondra), to desired consistency

1 teaspoon salt

Freshly ground pepper, to taste

3 tablespoon chopped fresh parsley or cilantro, for garnish

1. Combine the canola oil, cumin, ginger, and allspice, in a 6-quart heavy-based non-reactive saucepan or Dutch oven and heat over medium-high heat for 30 seconds, or just until the spices give off their aroma. Add the chicken and sauté for 3 minutes, turning to cook on all sides. Add the onion and sauté for 3 minutes. Add the carrots, diced tomatoes, stock, tomato paste, and sugar and bring to a boil. Reduce the heat and simmer gently, covered, for 20 minutes.
2. Add the chickpeas, zucchini, and raisins, if using, and continue to simmer for 15 minutes, or just until the zucchini is tender. During the last 5 minutes of simmering, add the flour (adjust the amount to desired consistency) and stir gently.

3.   Add the salt and pepper, garnish with the parsley, and serve immediately.

▶ **Slow Cooker Instructions:** *Use ¼ cup chicken stock instead of ½ cup. Ideally, you should use chicken meat on the bone, such as skinless chicken thighs or breast meat on the bone, as it tends to dry out less than boneless chicken breasts during cooking.*

1.   Using a large nonstick skillet instead of a saucepan, follow the instructions for Step 1 and cook the onions with the chicken. Transfer the contents of the skillet to a slow cooker, then add the carrots, diced tomatoes, stock, tomato paste, and sugar. Cover and cook on low for 6 to 8 hours, or on high for 4 to 6 hours.

2.   Up to one hour and at least 30 minutes before turning the slow cooker off, add the chickpeas, zucchini, raisins, and quick-dissolving flour.

3.   Once cooked, season with salt and pepper, garnish with parsley, and serve immediately, or bring to room temperature, cover, and refrigerate or freeze.

▶ **Storage Tip:** This stew keeps for 3 days refrigerated, and it can be frozen for up to 1 month. To prevent scorching, reheat over medium heat or in a microwave oven.

▶ **Complete Meal Ideas:** Serve this stew with:
  Couscous, quinoa, or brown rice
  Green salad or vegetable (if you did not use many vegetables in the stew)
  Reduced-fat 2% milk or low-fat yogurt
  Fresh fruit that contains vitamin C

APPROXIMATE NUTRITIONAL INFORMATION: Serving size: One-tenth of the Moroccan-style chicken stew; Calories: 288 cals; Protein: 29 g; Carbohydrates: 23 g; Fat: 9 g; Fiber: 3 g; Sodium: 333 mg; Vitamin A: 5,332 IU; Vitamin C: 13 mg; Diabetic Exchange: Bread/Starch: 1.5, Meat (Lean) 3

chicken with homemade barbecue sauce

What's in this for baby and me? Protein.

HOMEMADE BARBECUE SAUCE is like homemade salad dressing. Once you've discovered how much better it is than the bottled stuff, there's no going back! For optimal flavor, marinate the chicken overnight or as long as 2 days. This recipe calls for baking the chicken completely *before* grilling or broiling it to ensure that is it fully cooked. Grilling or broiling caramelizes the sauce and adds to the flavor. Any cut of chicken, which is high in **protein**, can be used. Boneless, skinless breast meat cooks the fastest but it is the least juicy. Skinless thighs or breasts on the bone or drumsticks are good choices. Garnish the chicken with chopped fresh cilantro and lime wedges, if desired.

serves 6

Barbecue Sauce
½ cup ketchup
2 tablespoons molasses
⅓ cup soy sauce
½ teaspoon ground ginger (optional)

¼ teaspoon ground cloves, allspice, or cinnamon, or a mixture
1 garlic clove, minced
2 tablespoons minced fresh ginger
2½ pounds skinless chicken parts (see head-note above)

1. To make the barbecue sauce, combine all of the ingredients in a small bowl, mix well, and set aside. (*Note*: If you plan to marinate the chicken in a bowl rather than a zip-lock bag, make the barbecue sauce in a large bowl.)
2. Remove any visible fat from the chicken pieces. Using a fork, pierce the chicken all over to allow the marinade to seep in. Place the chicken in a 1-gallon zip-lock bag (or in the bowl), add the barbecue sauce, seal (or cover with plastic wrap), and refrigerate for at least 2 hours, or up to 48 hours.
3. To cook the chicken, preheat the oven to 400°F.
4. Transfer the chicken with all of the sauce to a large baking dish. Bake for 30 minutes, or until an instant-read thermometer inserted into the center (through the side) of the breast meat or thigh reads 170°F for white meat, 180°F for dark meat, and the juices run clear when the chicken is pierced with a knife. Remove from the oven.
5. Before grilling or broiling, have a platter ready for the barbecued chicken. Grill the chicken, turning to cook on all sides, over high heat for about 5 minutes, or until the sauce is caramelized. Or, to broil, remove about half of the sauce from the pan and discard it, then place the chicken under the broiler and cook, turning once, for a couple of minutes on each side.

▶ *Advance Preparation:* Marinate the chicken for at least 2 hours, or up to 48 hours.

▶ *Health Tip:* Discard all leftover marinade—do not use it to baste the chicken on the grill or under the broiler.

▶ *Storage Tip:* The barbecued chicken keeps for 3 days refrigerated. It does not freeze well.

▶ *Complete Meal Ideas:* Serve this chicken with:
> Potato, enriched pasta, or couscous salad (you might want to try the Couscous Salad with Chickpeas and Vegetables, page 124, or the Asian-Style Pasta and Vegetable Salad, page 116)
> Green vegetable or a green salad
> Reduced-fat 2% milk or low-fat yogurt
> Fresh fruit

APPROXIMATE NUTRITIONAL INFORMATION: Serving size: 4 ounces roasted chicken (breast meat); Calories: 187 cals; Protein: 35 g; Carbohydrates: 0 g; Fat: 4 g; Fiber: 0 g; Sodium: 84 mg; Diabetic Exchange: Meat (Very Lean) 5

APPROXIMATE NUTRITIONAL INFORMATION: Serving size: 1 tablespoon homemade barbecue sauce; Calories: 49 cals; Protein: 2 g; Carbohydrates: 11 g; Fat: 0 g; Fiber: .3 g; Sodium: 1,050 mg; Diabetic Exchange: Other Carbohydrate 1

juicy turkey burgers

～

What's in this for baby and me? Protein.

TURKEY BURGERS DON'T get any better than this! The ricotta cheese keeps the burgers moist and the fresh herbs add a burst of flavor. Serve these burgers, with or without buns, accompanied by the usual lineup of burger fixin's and condiments, or with the Salsa Verde (page 222), Papaya Salsa (page 254), Red Bell Pepper Sauce (page 250), or Sun-Dried Tomato Dressing (page 142). For young children, cut up the burgers and serve them with lots of ketchup. These burgers are an excellent source of **protein**, and a fine source of calcium and iron.

makes 4 burgers

1 pound ground turkey

½ cup part-skim ricotta cheese

½ teaspoon salt

2 teaspoons Worcestershire sauce (optional)

2 teaspoons Dijon mustard (optional)

1 tablespoon freshly squeezed lemon juice

2 tablespoons chopped fresh cilantro or parsley (optional)

1 tablespoon canola oil, or canola oil cooking spray

1. Combine all of the ingredients except the canola oil in a bowl and mix until well blended. If the mixture is too pasty or sticky, add 1 tablespoon water. (*Note:* The consistency should be softer than a burger made with ground beef, but firm enough to hold its shape.) Divide the turkey mixture into 4 portions, form each portion into a patty, and place on a large plate.
2. If panfrying, heat the canola oil in a large nonstick skillet over medium heat. If grilling, before preheating the grill, position a piece of foil over the grill rack and poke holes in it. (This will prevent the burgers from sticking to the grill and falling apart.) Just before cooking the burgers, generously spray the foil with canola oil cooking spray. Add the burgers to the skillet or grill and cook for 6 minutes, or until the underside is dark brown. Flip the burgers and cook on the second side for about 6 minutes, or until the center of the burgers is completely opaque and an instant-read thermometer inserted into the center (through the side of the burger) reads 165° to 170°F.
3. Remove from the skillet or grill and serve immediately.

▶ *Advance Preparation:* The burgers can be formed, covered, and refrigerated up to 4 hours in advance.

▶ *Variation:* Substitute ground chicken for the turkey.

▶ **Storage Tip:** These turkey burgers keep for 3 days refrigerated. They do not freeze well.

▶ **Complete Meal Ideas:** Serve these burgers with:
>Whole wheat bun or enriched pasta or potato salad (you might want to try the Best-Ever Tabbouleh Salad, page 126, or the Asparagus, Hearts of Palm, and Tomato Salad, page 134)
>Green salad or tomato salad
>Reduced-fat 2% milk or low-fat yogurt
>Fresh fruit

APPROXIMATE NUTRITIONAL INFORMATION: Serving size: one 5-ounce turkey burger; Calories: 316 cals; Protein: 35 g; Carbohydrates: 3 g; Fat: 18 g; Fiber: 0 g; Sodium: 498 mg; Diabetic Exchange: Fat 1, Meat (Lean) 5

salt and high-sodium foods

It is a common misconception that salt intake should be restricted during pregnancy. An adequate sodium intake is essential for maintaining fluid balance and regulating electrolytes (sodium, potassium, and chloride). It is usually advisable to *salt to taste* unless otherwise advised. Consult your doctor or nurse if you are concerned about your salt intake and its effects on your blood pressure. Look for low-sodium labels on food products if you need to reduce your salt intake.

POPULAR HIGH-SODIUM FOODS

MEATS AND FISH: Bacon; sausage; bologna; salami; ham; corned beef; hot dogs; canned meats; sardines; tuna fish; smoked meat, chicken, or fish; frozen prepared dinners

SNACK FOODS: Salted chips, pretzels, tortilla chips and corn chips; salted popcorn; nuts and seeds; salted crackers; rolls or breads with salt toppings; french fries; pickles; olives; fast food

SEASONINGS: Salt, sea salt, "lite" salt; seasoned salt (such as onion and garlic salt); Accent; soy sauce; barbecue sauce; ketchup and mustard; packaged sauces and gravies

OTHER: Canned or packaged soups, broths, and bouillons; processed and prepared foods; canned vegetables; cottage cheese; soft drinks; tomato juice or V-8 juice; pickles

homemade chicken tenders

~

What's in this for baby and me? Protein, iron and B vitamins.

ANYONE WITH KIDS knows what a staple meal chicken tenders are. These homemade chicken tenders are an excellent source of **protein**, **iron**, and **B vitamins**, and a good source of calcium and folic acid. Some of the store-bought brands are quite good, but if you have the time and energy, why not make your own? The tenders can be sautéed or baked and eaten right away, or frozen for later. Grown-ups might like these tenders in a Caesar salad (see Caesar Salad Dressing, page 143), or accompanied by a more sophisticated dipping sauce than ketchup, such as store-bought mango chutney or cocktail sauce. To avoid getting your hands completely caked with flour, egg, and bread crumbs, keep one hand wet and one dry while you work, as explained in the recipe steps, or work with two forks.

makes about 20 to 25 chicken tenders

1¼ pounds chicken tenders or boneless skinless chicken breasts
½ cup all-purpose flour
1 cup plain or seasoned bread crumbs
⅓ cup finely grated Parmesan cheese
A pinch of Old Bay seasoning, Italian herbs, or

dried oregano (optional)
2 large eggs
Canola oil cooking spray if baking the chicken
 tenders, or 1–3 tablespoons canola oil if
 sautéing the tenders

1. Cut packaged chicken tenders in half. Or, if using boneless breasts, cut one lengthwise into 3 strips, then cut each strip on the diagonal into 2- to 2¼-inch strips. (Don't worry too much about the size and shape.) Place the tenders in a bowl and set aside.
2. Place the flour in a shallow pie dish or plate with sides; set aside. Combine the bread crumbs, Parmesan cheese, and seasonings in a shallow pie dish or a plate with sides and mix well; set aside. Place the eggs in a bowl and beat; set aside.
3. Set up your work station as follows: chicken tenders, flour, egg, bread crumb mixture, and 2 large plates. Using your *dry* hand, place about half of the tenders in the flour, tossing gently to coat all sides. Transfer the tenders in batches to the egg and coat them with egg using your other *(wet)* hand, then transfer them to the bread crumbs. Using your *dry* hand, cover the tenders with bread crumbs, pressing gently so they adhere, then place the breaded tenders on the plates. Repeat this procedure with the remaining tenders. (Discard all leftover flour, bread crumbs, and egg.)

4. *To bake,* preheat the oven to 450°F. Just before baking, preheat a baking sheet for 3 minutes (this helps the tenders brown evenly). Remove it from the oven and spray it generously with canola oil cooking spray. Arrange the tenders on the baking sheet, and lightly spray them with canola oil. Bake for 20 minutes, or until thoroughly cooked, turning once.

   To panfry, heat 1 tablespoon canola oil in a large nonstick skillet over medium-high heat. Without crowding, place half of the tenders in the skillet and cook for about 7 to 9 minutes, turning once or twice, until browned and crisp on both sides and fully cooked. Transfer to a clean plate lined with paper towels to drain. Use a big wad of paper towels to wipe out the skillet, then repeat the pan frying procedure with the remaining tenders. (If you use a small skillet, you may need to cook the tenders in 3 batches.) Serve immediately.

▶ **Storage Tip:** These chicken tenders keep for 3 days refrigerated, and they can be cooked then frozen for up to 1 month.

▶ **Complete Meal Ideas:** Serve these chicken tenders with:
   Potato salad, enriched pasta salad, or rice (you might want to try the Pink Potato Salad, page 130, or the Asian-Style Pasta and Vegetable Salad, page 116, or the Couscous Salad with Chickpeas and Vegetables, page 124)
   Green salad or green vegetable
   Sliced tomatoes or yellow vegetable
   Reduced-fat 2% milk or low-fat yogurt
   Fresh fruit that contains vitamin C

APPROXIMATE NUTRITIONAL INFORMATION: Serving size: about 5 homemade chicken tenders; Calories: 445 cals; Protein: 47 g; Carbohydrates: 26 g; Fat: 16 g; Fiber: .8 g; Sodium: 399 mg; B Vitamins: Thiamine: .3 mg, Riboflavin: .4 mg, Niacin: 19 mg; Iron: 4 mg; Diabetic Exchange: Bread/Starch 1.5, Meat (Lean) 6

spice-rubbed pork chops

~

What's in this for baby and me? Protein.

THIS SPICE RUB can be used with any type of meat, poultry, or fish. Don't be put off by the number of steps in this recipe—they include instructions for both grilling or broiling the pork chops. Pork is an excellent source of **protein** and a good source of B vitamins.

makes four 4-ounce chops

Spice Rub

1 teaspoon Italian seasoning

½ teaspoon chili powder

½ teaspoon garlic powder or 1 small garlic clove, crushed

½ teaspoon ground ginger

½ teaspoon ground cumin

2 teaspoons canola oil

1 pound pork chops (about 4 chops)

1. To make the spice rub, combine the ingredients in a small bowl or measuring cup, mix well, and set aside.
2. Trim any visible fat from the pork chops. Smear one side of the pork chops with half of the spice rub. Using a fork, pierce the meat all over to allow the spices to seep in, and repeat on the other side. Place the pork chops in a 1-gallon zip-lock bag, seal, and refrigerate for at least 1 hour, or up to 48 hours.
3. *To grill* the pork chops, preheat the grill. Have a clean plate ready for the cooked meat. Grill the pork chops for approximately 7 minutes on each side (depending on their thickness), or until an instant-read thermometer inserted into the center of the meat close to the bone reads 160°F.

   To broil the pork chops, preheat the broiler and line a shallow baking pan, or a baking sheet with sides, with foil. Arrange the pork chops in the pan and broil for approximately 5 to 7 minutes on each side (see above for well-done temperature). Watch carefully to prevent burning.

▶ *Advance Preparation:* Rub the spices into the pork chops from 1 to 48 hours in advance; bag and refrigerate.

▶ *Health Tip:* Discard any extra spice rub. Place the finished pork chops on a clean serving platter.

▶ *Storage Tip:* These pork chops keep for 3 days refrigerated. They do not freeze well.

▶ *Complete Meal Ideas:* Serve these pork chops with:

Baked or boiled potatoes, rice, or enriched pasta (you might want to try the Pasta Salad with Basil Pesto, page 121, or the Roasted Beets with Walnuts and Baby Greens, page 133)
Green salad or green vegetable
Sliced tomatoes or yellow vegetable
Reduced-fat 2% milk or low-fat yogurt
Fresh fruit

APPROXIMATE NUTRITIONAL INFORMATION: Serving size: one 4-ounce pork chop; Calories: 267 cals; Protein: 32 g; Carbohydrates: 0 g; Fat: 15 g; Fiber: 0 g; Sodium: 64 mg; Diabetic Exchange: Meat (Lean) 4.5

salt substitutes to spice up your food

Here are a few tips to help take the salt out of your diet without sacrificing taste:

- ▶ Add fresh or dried leafy herbs (such as basil, parsley, dill, tarragon, and chervil) to salads, vegetables, dips, seafood, and poultry.
- ▶ Rosemary, thyme, basil, oregano, and marjoram (fresh or dried) are wonderful additions to meats, poultry, fish, and vegetables such as carrots and potatoes. These herbs also work well on pizza and in pasta sauces.
- ▶ Use dried spices (such as nutmeg, allspice, and cumin) to enhance flavors. For example, add a dash of nutmeg to creamed spinach or a dash of cumin to a cauliflower gratin.
- ▶ Use curry powder to enhance vegetables, meats, fish, and poultry and to liven up dips, marinades, and mayonnaise.
- ▶ Use freshly squeezed lemon juice to flavor vegetables such as broccoli and asparagus (the acid in the lemon will probably discolor the vegetables) and on meats such as veal and lamb.
- ▶ Garlic is a great flavor booster for meats, poultry, fish, sauce, marinades, and salad dressings.
- ▶ Fresh ginger is a delicious addition to stir-fried dishes and marinades. Lemongrass adds a strong Asian flavor to curries, soups, and marinades.
- ▶ Use a touch of Parmesan cheese on soups and salads. Parmesan cheese does contain salt; however, it is also high in calcium.
- ▶ Go nuts. Add your favorite unsalted nuts (preferably toasted) to pasta, rice, and vegetable dishes. For example, toasted sliced almonds are wonderful with green beans, and toasted pine nuts combined with fresh herbs transform a bland rice dish into a flavorful creation.
- ▶ Use pepper instead of salt. A dash of Tabasco sauce is another option, if you can handle the heat.

marinated grilled or broiled lamb chops

What's in this for baby and me? Protein.

SIMPLE AND DELICIOUS, these lamb chops are an excellent source of **protein** and a good source of iron. The combination of garlic, lemon, olive oil, and rosemary is a traditional flavoring for many Greek and Italian dishes. These chops require no sauce, but a squeeze of lemon and a sprinkle of chopped fresh parsley add the perfect finishing touch. This marinade and garnish also works beautifully with chicken.

serves 4

1½ pounds lamb chops, about 1½ inches thick

Marinade

  2 garlic cloves, minced

  3 tablespoons freshly squeezed lemon juice

  1 to 2 tablespoons chopped fresh rosemary, mint, or thyme

1 tablespoon olive oil

Lots of freshly ground pepper

2 tablespoons freshly squeezed lemon juice, for garnish (optional)

¼ cup chopped fresh parsley, for garnish (optional)

Salt, to taste

1. Trim any visible fat from the lamb chops, then, using a fork, pierce the meat all over to allow the marinade to seep in. Place the lamb chops in a 1-gallon zip-lock bag. Add the garlic, lemon juice, chopped rosemary, olive oil, and pepper to the bag and squish it around to make sure that the chops are completely covered with the marinade. Seal the bag and refrigerate for at least 1 hour, or up to 24 hours.

2. *To grill* the lamb chops, preheat the grill. Have a clean plate ready for the cooked meat. Grill the lamb chops approximately 7 minutes on each side (depending on their thickness), or until an instant-read thermometer inserted into the center of the meat close to the bone reads 160°F.

   To broil the lamb chops, preheat the broiler and line a shallow baking pan, or a baking sheet with sides, with foil. Arrange the lamb chops in the pan and broil for approximately 5 to 7 minutes on each side (see above for well-done temperature). Watch carefully to prevent burning.

3. Arrange the cooked lamb chops on the plate and sprinkle with the optional lemon juice, a dash of salt, and chopped parsley.

▶ *Advance Preparation:* Marinate the lamb chops for at least 1 hour, or up to 24 hours.

▶ *Health Tip:* Discard all excess marinade. Place the cooked lamb chops on a clean serving plate.

▶ *Complete Meal Ideas:* Serve these lamb chops with:

> Tabbouleh, couscous, or enriched pasta (you might want to try the Best-Ever Tabbouleh Salad, page 126, or the Couscous Salad with Chickpeas and Vegetables, page 124)
>
> Green salad or green vegetable
>
> Sliced tomatoes or yellow vegetable
>
> Reduced-fat 2% milk or low-fat yogurt
>
> Fresh fruit that contains vitamin C

APPROXIMATE NUTRITIONAL INFORMATION: Serving size: one 4-ounce lamb chop; Calories: 245 cals; Protein: 34 g; Carbohydrates: 0 g; Fat: 11 g; Fiber: 0 g; Sodium: 95 mg; Diabetic Exchange: Meat (Lean) 4.5

sautéed shrimp with pasta

⌒

What's in this for baby and me? Protein, iron, vitamin C, and folic acid.

THIS QUICK AND easy shrimp and tomato combination is delicious served over any type of pasta, from thin spaghetti or penne to fresh basil- or saffron-flavored pasta. If you cannot find fresh peeled and deveined shrimp, or you don't have the time to clean shrimp, use peeled frozen shrimp, or substitute salmon (see **Variations** below). This dish is high in **protein**, **iron**, **vitamin C**, and **folic acid**, and a good source of calcium, fiber, and B vitamins.

serves 4

12 to 16 ounces enriched linguine or thin
    spaghetti

2 tablespoon plus 1 teaspoon olive oil

1 small onion, finely diced

1 garlic clove, minced

1¼ pounds medium-size shrimp, peeled and
    deveined (for cleaning instructions, see
    Cooking Tip below)

One 14.5-ounce can diced tomatoes (do not
    drain)

1 teaspoon grated lemon zest (from about 1
    lemon) (optional)

1 tablespoon freshly squeezed lemon juice, or
    to taste

¼ cup chopped fresh basil, cilantro, dill, or a
    mixture

Salt and freshly ground pepper, to taste

Grated Parmesan cheese, for the table

1. Cook the pasta according to the package directions; drain. Place it back in the hot pot, stir in 1 teaspoon of the olive oil (to prevent sticking), and set aside in a warm place.

2. Heat the remaining 2 tablespoons olive oil in a large nonstick skillet over medium-high heat. Add the onion and sauté for 2 minutes, then add the garlic and sauté for 30 seconds. Add the shrimp and cook for 3 minutes, turning the shrimp once. Gently stir in the diced tomatoes, lemon zest, if using, and lemon juice and sauté for 1 minute longer.

3. Add the herbs, then season with salt and pepper. Serve immediately, over the pasta. Pass the Parmesan cheese at the table.

▶ *Cooking Tip:* To clean shrimp, start by removing the shell from the body of the shrimp by holding the underside of the shrimp with your thumb and pulling the shell off with your other hand in an upward motion. When you reach the tail, carefully pull off the hard shell. (*Note:* Remove the tail shell gently—if you pull too hard, you could rip the shrimp in half.) To devein the shrimp, make a very shallow incision from the top end to the middle of the outer curve of the shrimp to expose the dark vein. Using your fingers, pull out the vein and discard.

limitations on certain fish consumption

Most fish is safe and healthy to eat during pregnancy. However, certain types of fish can be contaminated with high levels of mercury or industrial pollutants (such as poly-chlorinated biphenyls or PCBs), which can harm the fetus's brain, resulting in developmental delays. The U.S. Food and Drug Administration recommends that pregnant women, or women who could become pregnant, eat no more than one meal per month of swordfish or shark, two large predatory fish that are known to contain high levels of mercury. Other types of fish that may be contaminated by mercury, as well as by PCBs, include bluefish and striped bass, and freshwater fish (such as salmon, pike, trout, and walleye) from contaminated lakes and rivers.

Pregnant women should also avoid raw fish, especially shellfish (oysters and clams), which can be polluted with raw sewage and can contain harmful microorganisms that can lead to severe gastrointestinal illness. *All* fish and shellfish should be *thoroughly cooked* to kill any disease-causing bacteria or parasites. Consumers should check with their state or local health departments for specific advice about fish from local waters. Consult your physician regarding any additional or specific seafood or shellfish restrictions.[34]

▶ *Variation:* Cook frozen shrimp according to the package directions. Drain well and pat dry with paper towels. To make this dish with salmon, use 1 pound skinned salmon fillet (ask your fishmonger to skin the salmon if necessary). Cut the fillet lengthwise in half, then slice each strip into 1/2-inch-wide rectangles.

▶ *Storage Tip:* The shrimp and tomato sauce will keep refrigerated for 2 days. This dish does not freeze well.

▶ *Complete Meal Ideas:* Serve this shrimp and pasta with:
> Green salad or green vegetable (you might want to try the Romaine Lettuce with Olive Oil–Lemon Dressing, page 144, or one of Annie Mozer's Greens, pages 203–205)
> Reduced-fat 2% milk or low-fat yogurt
> Fresh fruit that contains vitamin C

APPROXIMATE NUTRITIONAL INFORMATION: Serving size: one-quarter of the shrimp sauce with 1½ cups of enriched pasta; Calories: 474 cals; Protein: 35 g; Carbohydrates: 65 g; Fat: 7 g; Fiber: 5 g; Sodium: 597 mg; Vitamin C: 21 mg; Folic Acid: 156 mcg; Iron: 7 mg; Diabetic Exchange: Bread/Starch 4, Meat (Lean) 3.5

shrimp and vegetable stir-fry

~

What's in this for baby and me? Protein, iron, and vitamins A and C.

THE KEY TO successful stir-frying, for any recipe, is to have all the ingredients prepped and ready *before* you begin. Also, it's best not to sauté the vegetables for more than 5 minutes, because they will continue to cook off the heat. Serve this stir-fry over rice, high-protein quinoa (see page 118 for cooking instructions), or quick-cooking Chinese rice noodles—all of which can be made in advance. The chopped fresh cilantro and cashew nuts added just before serving give the dish a wonderful taste and crunch, but they should be omitted for young eaters who don't like green things in their food and who could choke on the nuts. This stir-fry is an excellent source of **protein**, **iron**, and **vitamins A** and **C**, and a good source of calcium, B vitamins, folic acid, and fiber. This recipe can be halved to serve two.

serves 4 (makes about 8 cups)

Marinade

    2 tablespoons soy sauce

    2 tablespoons hoisin sauce

    2 tablespoons water

    1 garlic clove, minced

    1 tablespoon minced fresh ginger

    1¼ pounds medium shrimp, peeled and deveined (for cleaning instructions, see Cooking Tip below)

Stir-Fry Sauce

    1 tablespoon hoisin sauce

    3 tablespoons water

    2 tablespoons soy sauce

    1 teaspoon cornstarch

    1 teaspoon brown sugar

1 tablespoon canola oil

A few drops of toasted sesame oil (optional)

1 tablespoon minced fresh ginger

1 garlic clove, minced

1 cup sliced or grated carrots

¾ cup fresh snow peas, washed, and ends trimmed

1½ cups fresh broccoli florets, washed and ends trimmed

½ red bell pepper, washed and thinly sliced

1 cup sliced zucchini or yellow squash

3 scallions, trimmed and thinly sliced

⅓ cup cashew nuts, coarsely chopped (optional)

¼ cup chopped fresh cilantro (optional)

Cooked rice or noodles, to serve with the stir-fry

1. To make the marinade, combine all of the ingredients in a medium-size bowl and whisk. Add the shrimp, cover, and refrigerate for at least 15 minutes, or up to 12 hours.
2. To make the stir-fry sauce, combine all of the ingredients in a small bowl and whisk until the cornstarch is completely dissolved; set aside.
3. To cook the stir-fry, heat the canola oil and optional sesame oil in a very large nonstick skillet or large nonstick wok over medium-high heat. Add the ginger and garlic and sauté for 30 seconds. Add the carrots, snow peas, broccoli florets, red bell pepper, and zucchini and cook, stirring occasionally, for 5 minutes, or until crisp-tender.

Keep a cover or a piece of foil over the skillet or wok when you are not stirring; if the vegetables stick to the pan, add 1 tablespoon water. Transfer the cooked vegetables to a serving bowl and cover with foil to keep warm. (Do not rinse the skillet.)

4. Reheat the skillet over medium-high heat. Add the shrimp, and its marinade, and the stir-fry sauce, stir, cover, and cook for 3 minutes. Add the scallions and cook 1 minute more. Transfer the contents of the skillet to the serving bowl containing the vegetables, gently mix, and garnish with the cashew nuts and cilantro, if desired. Serve immediately, with the rice.

▶ *Cooking Tip:* To clean shrimp, start by removing the shell from the body of the shrimp by holding the underside of the shrimp with your thumb and pulling the shell off with your other hand in an upward motion. When you reach the tail, carefully pull off the hard shell. (*Note:* Remove the tail shell gently—if you pull too hard, you could rip the shrimp in half.) To devein the shrimp, make a very shallow incision from the top end to the middle of the outer curve of the shrimp to expose the dark vein. Using your fingers, pull out the vein and discard.

▶ *Advance Preparation:* Marinate the shrimp for at least 15 minutes, or up to 3 hours. The stir-fry sauce can be made 1 day in advance, covered, and refrigerated, and the vegetables can be prepared up to 3 days in advance and refrigerated.

▶ *Variation:* The shrimp can be replaced with chicken strips, beef strips (use thin-sliced beef rib eye Delmonico steak), scallops, or any other source of protein. For vegetarians, one 15-ounce package (drained weight) extra-firm tofu, cut into ½-inch cubes and blotted dry with paper towels, can be used in place of the shrimp. Use your favorite vegetables, equal to 6 to 7 cups (about 1 to 1¼ pounds). Try to cut all of the vegetables about the same size so they require the same cooking time.

▶ *Timesaving Tip:* Convenient fresh vegetable stir-fry packs are available in some grocery stores. They usually come in 12-ounce packs and can be supplemented with your favorite vegetables—carrots, broccoli, and asparagus are among the healthiest. Avoid fresh bean sprouts (see E. coli Warning, page, 217). Sixteen-ounce bags of frozen stir-fry vegetables are also available in most grocery stores. Follow the package directions for stir-frying vegetables in oil.

▶ *Health Tip:* If your salt intake has been restricted, use low-sodium soy sauce, use less hoisin sauce, and omit the cashew nuts.

▶ *Complete Meal Ideas:* Serve this stir-fry with:
    Rice, rice noodles, or quinoa
    Reduced-fat 2% milk or low-fat yogurt
    Fresh fruit

APPROXIMATE NUTRITIONAL INFORMATION: Serving size: 2 cups shrimp and vegetable stir-fry; Calories: 301 cals; Protein: 30 g; Carbohydrates: 21 g; Fat: 11 g; Fiber: 3 g; Sodium: 1,377 mg; Vitamin A: 10,807 IU; Vitamin C: 79 g; Diabetic Exchange: Fat .5, Meat (Medium Fat) 2.5

crab cakes with red bell pepper sauce

What's in this for baby and me? Protein and vitamin C.

WHEN YOUR BUDGET allows for a splurge, there is nothing better than these home-made crab cakes laced with fresh herbs and served with a creamy red bell pepper sauce. The crab cakes are an excellent source of **protein** (and a good source of folic acid), and the red bell pepper sauce is high in **vitamin C** (and a good source of vitamin A). If red bell peppers aren't your thing, other sauces in this book, such as the Salsa Verde (page 222), Papaya Salsa (page 254), or Sun-Dried Tomato Dressing (page 142) are excellent alternatives—and, of course, store-bought cocktail sauce always works. Any leftover crab cakes can be eaten cold with a salad or made into delectable sandwiches. The recipes for both the sauce and the crab cakes can be cut in half for a smaller yield.

makes 7 crab cakes

Red Bell Pepper Sauce (makes about 1 cup)
- **1 large red bell pepper, washed, cored, seeded, and coarsely diced**
- **¾ cup half-and-half**
- **Salt and freshly ground pepper, to taste**

Crab Cakes
- **8 ounces jumbo lump crabmeat, picked over to remove any shells (see Cooking Tip below)**
- **8 ounces back fin crabmeat, picked over to remove any shells**

- **½ cup plain bread crumbs**
- **2 tablespoons finely chopped scallions or fresh chives**
- **¼ cup chopped fresh dill, cilantro, or basil, or a mixture, or to taste**
- **2 teaspoons grated lemon zest (optional)**
- **2 teaspoons Dijon mustard (optional)**
- **2 large eggs, lightly beaten**
- **2 tablespoons light mayonnaise**
- **2 tablespoons canola oil**
- **Lemon or lime wedges, for the table**

1. To make the sauce, combine the bell pepper and half-and-half in a small nonreactive saucepan. Bring to a boil, reduce the heat, and simmer about 15 minutes, or until the peppers are tender. Cool, then puree in a food processor or blender until smooth. Adjust the seasoning, cover, and set aside.

2. To make the crab cakes, combine all of the crab cake ingredients in a bowl. Mix gently until well incorporated. To form the crab cakes, use a ⅓-cup measuring cup to portion out each crab cake, then form it into a patty and place it on a large plate. Cover and refrigerate until ready to cook.

3. Heat the canola oil in a large nonstick skillet over medium-high heat. Add 3 crab cakes (avoid overcrowding) and cook on one side for about 3 minutes, or until golden brown. Carefully flip and cook the other side for about 3 minutes, or until golden brown and thoroughly heated. (*Note:* You may need to adjust the heat if the crab

cakes are browning too quickly.) Transfer the cooked crab cakes to a serving plate and cover loosely with foil to keep warm. Cook the remaining crab cakes, and serve immediately with the red bell pepper sauce and lemon wedges.

▶ *Cooking Tip:* One pound of jumbo lump or back fin crabmeat (which equals about 2 cups of crabmeat) can be used in place of 8 ounces of each. Generally, back fin crabmeat needs to be picked over more carefully, as it contains more bits of shell.

▶ *Advance Preparation:* The crab cakes can be formed up to 12 hours in advance covered and refrigerated. The red bell pepper sauce can be made 1 day in advance, covered, and refrigerated.

▶ *Health Tip:* If your doctor has restricted your fat intake, use light skim evaporated milk instead of half-and-half in the red bell pepper sauce.

▶ *Storage Tip:* The crab cakes and red bell pepper sauce keep for 3 days refrigerated. Neither freezes well.

▶ *Complete Meal Ideas:* Serve these crab cakes with:
    Corn on the cob, potato salad, or pasta salad
    Green salad or green vegetable (you might want to try some baby greens with the
        French-Style Tarragon Vinaigrette, page 141)
    Reduced-fat 2% milk or low-fat yogurt
    Fresh fruit

APPROXIMATE NUTRITIONAL INFORMATION: Serving size: One crab cake (about 3 ounces); Calories: 163 cals; Protein: 15 g; Carbohydrates: 6 g; Fat: 8 g; Fiber: .2 g; Sodium: 288 mg; Diabetic Exchange: Bread/Starch .5, Fat .5, Meat (Lean) 2

APPROXIMATE NUTRITIONAL INFORMATION: Serving size: 2 tablespoons red bell pepper sauce; Calories: 33 cals; Protein: .7 g; Carbohydrates: 2 g; Fat: 3 g; Fiber: .2 g; Sodium: 10 mg; Vitamin C: 28 mg; Diabetic Exchange: Fat .5

sautéed salmon on a bed of greens with citrus vinaigrette

~

What's in this for baby and me? Protein, vitamins A and C, folic acid, B vitamins, and fiber.

THIS MAIN-COURSE salmon salad is an excellent source of **protein**, **vitamins A** and **C**, **folic acid**, **B vitamins**, and **fiber**, and a good source of iron—WOW! The leftover dressing is delicious on spinach salad, or any other greens or vegetables. This recipe calls for cutting the salmon into strips before cooking it, but feel free to grill, bake, or broil a whole salmon fillet instead and serve it alongside your salad drizzled with some of the citrus vinaigrette.

serves 2

Citrus Vinaigrette (makes about ⅔ cup)
   Juice of 1 lemon
   Juice of 1 orange
   1 tablespoon plus 1 teaspoon honey
   1 teaspoon finely chopped shallots
     (optional)
   1 teaspoon Dijon mustard
   ⅛ teaspoon ground ginger
   A couple drops of toasted sesame oil
   ⅓ cup plus 2 tablespoons canola oil
Salmon

12 ounces skinned salmon fillet, cut lengthwise in half, then cut into 1-inch-wide strips
1 tablespoon soy sauce
1 tablespoon canola oil
3–4 cups baby greens, washed and well dried
1 avocado, peeled, pitted, and sliced (optional)
1 cup cherry tomatoes, washed (optional)
2 tablespoons chopped fresh cilantro (optional)

1. To prepare the citrus vinaigrette, combine the citrus juices (they should equal ⅔ cup, if not add more of either juice) and 1 tablespoon of the honey in a small saucepan and bring to a boil. Reduce the heat and simmer for 10 minutes, or until reduced by half (to ⅓ cup).

2. Transfer the reduced citrus juice to a small bowl or measuring cup and add the remaining honey, the shallots, if using, mustard, and ginger. Mix well, then add the sesame oil and canola oil and whisk until emulsified; set aside.

3. To cook the salmon, combine the salmon with the soy sauce and canola oil in a bowl and mix gently. Have a plate for the cooked salmon ready. Heat a large non-stick skillet over medium-high heat until hot. Add the salmon and cook for 2 minutes on each side, or until cooked through and light golden brown on the outside; use a splatter screen if you have one. (*Note*: The cooking time will depend on the thickness of the salmon. The flesh should flake easily and the interior should be fully cooked.) Transfer the cooked salmon to the plate; set aside.

4. To assemble the salad, combine the baby greens, and optional avocado, cherry tomatoes, and cilantro with ¼ cup of the vinaigrette in a bowl and toss gently. Divide the salad between two plates, place the sautéed salmon around the salad, and drizzle with just a bit more citrus vinaigrette. Serve immediately.

▶ *Timesaving Tip:* Use your favorite bottled dressing instead of the citrus vinaigrette and use smoked salmon (about 3 to 4 ounces) instead of cooking fresh salmon.

▶ *Variation:* Use 8 to 12 ounces fresh shrimp, peeled and drained (see Cooking Tip on page 246 for instructions), or scallops in place of the salmon. Adjust the cooking time as needed to thoroughly cook the shellfish.

▶ *Storage Tip:* The salmon keeps for 2 days refrigerated, and the citrus vinaigrette keeps for 5 days refrigerated.

▶ *Complete Meal Ideas:* Serve this salad with:
    Whole wheat roll or bread
    Reduced fat 2% milk or low-fat yogurt
    Fresh fruit that contains vitamin C

APPROXIMATE NUTRITIONAL INFORMATION: Serving size: one-half serving of the sautéed salmon and the salad (about 6 ounces of salmon); Calories: 482 cals; Protein: 34 g; Carbohydrates: 10 g; Fat: 35 g; Fiber: 5 g; Sodium: 480 mg; Vitamin A 1,736 IU; Vitamin C: 29 mg; Folic Acid: 164 mcg; B Vitamins: Thiamine: .6 mg, Riboflavin: .3 mg, Niacin: 13 mg; Diabetic Exchange: Bread/Starch .5, Fat 2, Meat (Medium Fat) 4.5

roasted salmon with papaya salsa

What's in this for baby and me? Protein and vitamins A and C.

REFRESHINGLY LIGHT, COLORFUL, and delicious—this combination of salmon and papaya is heavenly. The roasted salmon is an excellent source of **protein** and a good source of vitamin C, folic acid, and B vitamins, and the papaya salsa is rich in **vitamins A and C**. If papaya does not appeal to you, use your favorite fruits in place of the ones called for—try peaches, nectarines, grapes, apricots, plums, pineapple, mango, and avocado. The raw red onion and red bell pepper are optional because they can cause indigestion in some people. The marinade for the salmon is also optional, but it gives it a wonderful depth of flavor. It can be used to marinate any type of fish. For more flavor, add some crushed garlic (about 1 teaspoon) and minced fresh ginger (about 1 tablespoon) to the marinade. This recipe can be halved to serve two.

serves 4

1½ pounds salmon filet, skin left on

Marinade

   2 tablespoons soy sauce

   1 tablespoon canola oil

   Freshly ground pepper, to taste

Papaya Salsa (makes about 2½ cups)

   1 small papaya, peeled, seeded, and finely diced (about 1 cup diced papaya)

   ⅓ cup finely diced red bell pepper

(optional)

½ cup quartered cherry tomatoes

¼ cup finely diced red onion (optional)

2 tablespoons chopped fresh cilantro or mint

One 8-ounce can mandarin oranges in light syrup, drained and sliced

1 tablespoon freshly squeezed lime juice or seasoned rice vinegar, or to taste

1. To marinate the salmon fillet, place it in a 1-gallon zip-lock bag. Add the soy sauce, canola oil, and pepper, swish it around, and seal the bag. Refrigerate for at least 30 minutes, or up to 8 hours.
2. To make the papaya salsa, mix all of the ingredients in a bowl. Cover and refrigerate until ready to serve. (*Note:* The salsa is best if allowed to sit for 30 minutes before serving, to allow the flavors to develop. It can be made up to 3 hours in advance.)
3. To bake the salmon, preheat the oven to 450°F. Line a baking sheet with sides, or a baking pan, with aluminum foil. (Do not grease the foil; see **Cooking Tip** Below.)
4. Place the salmon on the baking sheet, skin side down, leaving the marinade juices behind. Bake the salmon, uncovered, for 12 to 15 minutes, or until fully cooked. The flesh should flake easily and the interior should be fully cooked. Serve immediately, with the papaya salsa.

▶ **Health Tip:** Discard all leftover marinade.

▶ **Cooking Tip:** If you do *not* grease the foil the salmon skin will stick to it and the salmon fillets can be separated from the skin easily. You might need to cut the salmon fillet (not the skin) down the center to facilitate removing it.

▶ **Storage Tip:** The salmon keeps for 2 days refrigerated. The papaya salsa becomes a little mushy after 8 hours, but the taste is unaffected.

▶ **Complete Meal Ideas:** Serve this baked salmon with:

> Couscous, quinoa, or enriched pasta (you might want to try the Quinoa Salad, page 118, or the Noodles with Spinach, Red Peppers, and Sesame Dressing, page 122)
> Green salad or green vegetable
> Reduced-fat 2% milk or low-fat yogurt
> Fresh fruit

APPROXIMATE NUTRITIONAL INFORMATION: Serving size: about 6 ounces baked salmon; Calories: 385 cals; Protein: 39 g; Carbohydrates: 0 g; Fat: 24 g; Fiber: 0 g; Sodium: 564 mg; Diabetic Exchange: Meat (Medium Fat) 5

APPROXIMATE NUTRITIONAL INFORMATION: Serving size: 1/2 cup papaya salsa; Calories: 55 cals; Protein: .8 g; Carbohydrates: 14 g; Fat: .2 g; Fiber: 2 g; Sodium: 7 mg; Vitamin A: 1,276 IU; Vitamin C: 54 mg; Diabetic Exchange: Fruit 1

tilapia mediterranean-style

What's in this for baby and me? Protein and Vitamin C.

THIS QUICK, EASY, and beautiful-on-the-plate Mediterranean dish works well with just about any kind of fish, including red snapper, sole, or cod (see Limitations on Certain Fish Consumption, page 247). The tilapia is an excellent source of **protein**, and the tomato sauce is a great source of vitamin C. This recipe can be cut in half to serve two people. If your kids like olives, they might be willing to give this a try.

serves 4

2 tablespoons olive oil

1 garlic clove, minced

1 cup pitted kalamata olives or other brine-cured black olives, chopped

15 ounces (about 3 cups) cherry tomatoes, halved

⅓ cup chopped fresh parsley

¼ cup chopped fresh basil (optional)

2 tablespoons freshly squeezed lemon juice, or to taste

Salt and freshly ground pepper, to taste

1½ pounds tilapia fillets

1. Heat 1 tablespoon of the olive oil in a large nonstick skillet over medium-high heat. Add the garlic and sauté for 30 seconds. Add the olives, cherry tomatoes, parsley, basil, if using, and lemon juice and cook for 2 minutes, or until the cherry tomatoes are soft and their skin wrinkled. Adjust the seasoning, transfer to a heatproof bowl, cover, and set aside. (Do not rinse the skillet.)
2. Have a serving platter ready. Heat the remaining 1 tablespoon olive oil in the skillet over medium-high heat. Add half the fish, season the fish with salt and pepper, and cook for 3 minutes on each side, turning once, or until cooked through. Transfer the cooked fish to the serving platter and cover with aluminum foil. Repeat this procedure with the remaining fish, making sure to reheat the skillet before adding the second batch of fish.
3. Ladle the reserved sauce over the fish and serve immediately.

▶ **Storage Tip:** This tilapia Mediterranean-style keeps 2 days, refrigerated. It does not freeze well.

▶ **Complete Meal Ideas:** Serve this tilapia with:
   Rice, enriched pasta, couscous
   Green salad or green vegetable (you might want to try the Vegetables with Lemon, Olive Oil, and Fresh Herbs, page 128)
   Reduced-fat 2% milk or low-fat yogurt
   Fresh fruit

APPROXIMATE NUTRITIONAL INFORMATION: Serving size: one-fourth tilapia Mediterranean style (about 6 ounces of tilapia); Calories: 110 cals; Protein: 11 g; Carbohydrates: 4 g; Fat: 6 g; Fiber: .9 g; Sodium: 148 mg; Diabetic Exchange: Meat (Medium Fat) 1.5

salmonellosis warning

Salmonellosis is a food-borne illness caused by the bacteria *salmonella*, which can be acquired from infected animals (usually poultry, swine, and cattle), raw milk and raw milk products, undercooked or raw eggs and egg products (see eggs and *Salmonella Enteritidis*, page 54), and contaminated water. Fecal-oral transmission from person to person, especially in infants, is another cause of salmonella poisoning. Certain pets, such as turtles, tortoises, iguanas, chicks, dogs, cats, and rodents, can also carry the bacteria in their intestines.

The symptoms of gastrointestinal infection usually include fever, nausea and vomiting, abdominal cramping, and diarrhea, which may be bloody. Other complications, such as enteric (typhoid) fever or extra-intestinal infections (infection that has spread outside the intestines), may occur. Following are a few tips to help prevent infection:[39]

- ▶ Avoid raw eggs or food that contains raw or partially cooked eggs.
- ▶ Avoid raw (unpasteurized) milk and any food that contains raw milk or raw milk products.
- ▶ Thoroughly cook all poultry and meat (see Well-Done Temperature Guide, page 303). Wash instant-read thermometers in between tests of foods that require further cooking.
- ▶ Keep raw meat separate from uncooked foods. Wash hands, counters, and utensils with hot soapy water after touching raw meat.
- ▶ Consume only safe drinking water or bottled water, especially when traveling to underdeveloped countries.
- ▶ Wash hands thoroughly after touching any of the pets mentioned above.
- ▶ Make sure that persons with diarrhea, especially children, wash their hands to reduce the risk of spreading infection, and that anyone washes his or her hands after changing soiled diapers.
- ▶ Avoid swallowing lake or pool water while swimming.

sweet treats:
desserts and snacks

〜

DESSERTS

DESSERT MAY BE the least essential part of the meal, but for many people it is the most satisfying. If you have a sweet tooth, pregnancy-induced or preexisting, curtailing your sugar intake may be one of your biggest challenges during pregnancy. One thing to keep in mind is that not all sweets are sticky, gooey, high fat, and fabulously rich. A bowl of fresh fruit or canned or jarred fruit, a serving of sorbet or frozen yogurt, applesauce, raisins, or a glass of juice can satisfy the urge for something sweet and provide some nutrients at the same time.

It is the empty, high-fat calories (such as pastries, doughnuts, and candy) that a pregnant woman should try to avoid. One of the best ways to eliminate these nonessential items from your diet is to keep them out of your shopping cart. This is admittedly difficult if you have young children or a husband who also has a sweet tooth, but in the long run, it is better for the entire family to avoid such items and to develop healthy eating habits.

While homemade desserts and snacks are best (because you can control what goes into them), lack of time, energy, or the desire to bake or cook can keep them off your list of things to do. When buying desserts and snacks, read labels carefully and try to choose those that have the most nutritional value per calorie. Try not to let desserts or snacks take the place of high-nutrient foods, especially if you are diabetic or if you need to watch your calorie intake. The bottom line is that you should enjoy your pregnancy, and you should also enjoy eating during your pregnancy. We all need to indulge at times, and as long as it is done in *moderation*, and not on a daily basis, a dessert that has some nutritional benefits is a well-deserved treat, pregnant or not!

SNACKS

THE BIGGEST DANGER with snacks is turning them into mini meals. Generally, pregnant women should consume three meals and two or three snacks a day. It is important always to remember portion sizes and to try to choose the most nutrient-dense snacks possible. Incorporating protein into your snack, such as having crackers and cheese, satisfies hunger and at the same time helps fulfill your protein requirements.

Your biggest snack challenge might be young children who seem to be in constant need of a snack. While you are doling out Goldfish, pretzels, or animal crackers, you might find yourself mindlessly putting handfuls in your mouth too. This goes with the territory of being a tired, overworked, and hungry mom who probably eats lunch standing up and considers her toddler's leftovers part of her own meal. While you are pregnant, try to choose the healthiest snacks for yourself and your children. Below is a list of snacks and snack combinations to get you started in the right direction.

Healthy Snacks to Have on Hand

Milk and Dairy: Low-fat yogurt, pasteurized cheese, string cheese, low-fat cottage cheese, smoothies, frozen yogurt

Fruit and Vegetables: Fresh fruit, fresh vegetables, vegetable soups, raisins, dates, figs, prunes, dried apricots, individual fruit cups in light syrup, mandarin orange slices in juice or light syrup, applesauce or other fruit sauces, juice boxes, all-fruit Popsicles, Jell-O fruit cups fortified with vitamin C

Grains and Seeds: Whole wheat crackers, rice cakes, graham crackers, cereal bars, granola bars, oatmeal cookies, popcorn, reduced-salt pretzels, whole grain pita bread, whole grain bagels, instant oatmeal, fortified dry cereal, muffins, bagels, baked potato

Protein: Pasteurized cheese, low-fat cottage cheese, peanut butter, hummus, bean dips, hard-boiled eggs or a small helping of leftovers from the night before

▶ *Some Ideas for Healthy Snack Combinations*
   1 to 2 ounces pasteurized cheese with 4 whole wheat crackers
   1 hard-boiled egg or egg salad with 4 whole wheat crackers
   ¼ cup low-fat cottage cheese with fruit or 4 whole wheat crackers
   ⅓ cup hummus with 1 pita bread or 4 whole wheat crackers
   ⅓ cup bean dip with 4 whole wheat crackers or vegetables
   Celery or apple slices with 2 tablespoons peanut butter
   1 cup low-fat yogurt with granola or fresh fruit, or both
   Half a peanut butter or nut butter sandwich
   1 cup fortified dry cereal with ½ cup reduced-fat 2% milk
   Fresh vegetables with ¼ cup healthy dip or salsa

sweet treats: desserts and snacks

Peach and Blackberry Cobbler

Apple-Blueberry Granola Crisp

Strawberry Whole Wheat Short Cake

No-Bake Fresh Strawberry-Raspberry Pie

Low-Fat Frozen Raspberry Pie

Reduced-Fat Ricotta Cheese Cake

Pumpkin Pie

Carrot Cake with Cream Cheese Frosting

Angel Food Cake with Lemon Drizzle

Vanilla Flan with Fresh Berries

Orange, Blueberry, and Date Salad with Frozen Yogurt

Patricia Terry's Pumpkin Bread

Fruit-Filled Granola ▼

Rhubarb Sauce ▼

▼Vegan recipe

RECIPE NOTES

SOME DESSERTS ARE associated with seasons, others with holidays, and still others with celebrations. What would summer be without fresh fruit cobblers, or Thanksgiving without pumpkin pie? But don't limit yourself to these dessert stereotypes. Use frozen or canned fruit to create a satisfying soul-warming crisp or cobbler in December, and serve pumpkin pie in the middle of June.

Portion control and *moderation* are essential when it comes to sweets of any kind for anybody—not just pregnant women! One small slice of pie or cake, a small serving of crisp or cobbler with a modest scoop of ice cream or frozen yogurt, or a small slice of angel food cake should not make you feel guilty in the slightest. If you are craving sweets, and you have some time and energy, this collection of homemade treats should serve you well. Enjoy!

Some notes about the recipes in this chapter:

- Avoid the temptation to taste any batter that contains raw egg (see Eggs and *Salmonella Enteritidis,* page 54).
- If you are making a custard-type dessert that contains eggs, be sure that the eggs are fully cooked. An instant-read thermometer should read 160°F.
- When measuring dry ingredients, level them off with the back of a knife or another straight edge.
- Use a liquid measure (Pyrex measuring cup) to measure wet ingredients and a dry measure (stainless steel or plastic cups) for dry ingredients.
- Factor in the need for advance planning and cool-down times. Some recipes require chilling or freezing, some need to sit overnight, and others need to cool completely before serving.
- Use your favorite fruits in the cobbler and crisp recipes.
- Use frozen fruit or canned fruit in juice or light syrup in place of fresh fruit if you are in a hurry or if fresh fruit is not in season.
- Buy bags of already chopped walnuts and other nuts to save time and energy.
- You can substitute margarine for unsalted butter.
- All-purpose flour should ideally be enriched and unbleached.
- You can substitute soy beverages and other soy products for dairy products.
- Use "old-fashioned" rolled oats (not quick cooking) in any recipe that calls for oats.
- You can substitute nondairy topping (some brands are reduced-fat) for whipped cream.
- Wherever indicated use 9-ounce graham cracker pie shells "with 2 extra servings" to avoid overspill.
- Line the baking sheet with foil before placing pie dishes or other things on it to bake.
- Since all oven temperatures vary, be sure to pay close attention to cooking times and judge the doneness according to your oven's performance, not the exact time given in a recipe.

- Modify the recipes to suit your dietary needs and your family's tastes.
- You will notice that only six of the recipes in this chapter have diabetic exchange values. We decided to omit the values because it is important not to substitute a low-nutrient food for a high-nutrient food if you are diabetic or if you have gestational diabetes.

PLANNING AHEAD FOR SWEET TREATS:
DESSERTS AND SNACKS

▶ *Best eaten the day they are made:*

Peach and Blackberry Cobbler
Apple-Blueberry Granola Crisp
Strawberry Whole Wheat Shortcake
No-Bake Fresh Strawberry-Raspberry Pie
Pumpkin Pie
Angel Food Cake with Lemon Drizzle
Orange Blueberry, and Date Salad with Frozen Yogurt

▶ *Can be made up to 6 hours ahead or the night before:*

No-Bake Fresh Strawberry-Raspberry Pie
Low-Fat Frozen Raspberry Pie
Reduced-Fat Ricotta Cheesecake
Carrot Cake with Cream Cheese Frosting
Vanilla Flan with Fresh Berries
Orange Blueberry, and Date Salad with Frozen Yogurt

▶ *Can be made up to 3 days ahead:*

Reduced-Fat Ricotta Cheesecake
Pumpkin Pie
Carrot Cake with Cream Cheese Frosting
Vanilla Flan with Fresh Berries
Patricia Terry's Pumpkin Bread
Rhubarb Sauce

▶ *Can be frozen for up to 1 month:*

Carrot Cake with Cream Cheese Frosting (freeze unfrosted)
Patricia Terry's Pumpkin Bread

▶ *Can be kept in an airtight container at room temperature for up to 5 days:*

Fruit-Filled Granola

pantry items for sweet treats: desserts and snacks

⁓

Fresh Produce
Blackberries
Blueberries
Carrots
Granny Smith Apples
Lemons
Mint
Navel Oranges
Peaches
Raspberries
Rhubarb
Strawberries

Dairy
Reduced-fat or fat-free cream cheese or Neufchâtel
Grade A large eggs
Low-fat or nonfat plain yogurt
Part-skim ricotta cheese
Reduced-fat or nonfat dairy sour cream
Unsalted butter
Whole or reduced-fat milk 2%

Dry Staples
9-inch store-bought ready-made pie crusts (preferably whole wheat) and/or frozen pie crusts
9-inch store-bought reduced-fat graham cracker pie crusts
9-ounce capacity store-bought graham-cracker crusts "with 2 extra servings"
Baking powder
Baking soda
Cake flour
Chopped walnuts and/or pecans

Cornstarch
Cream of tartar
Dark or light raisins
Dried apricots
Dried banana slices
Dried cherries
Dried pitted dates
Enriched all-purpose flour (preferably unbleached)
Granulated sugar
Kellogg's Healthy Choice Low Fat Granola without Raisins
Light or dark brown sugar
Plain or vanilla-flavored meringue cookies (such as Miss Meringue)
Powdered sugar
"Old-fashioned" rolled oats (not quick cooking)
Sliced almonds
Whole wheat flour

Spices and Flavorings
Ground cinnamon
Ground ginger
Ground nutmeg
Pumpkin pie spice mix
Pure vanilla extract

Canned, Bottles, and Jarred Staples
Applesauce
Canola oil
Canola oil cooking spray
Crushed pineapple (8-ounce can)
Honey

Lite evaporated skim milk (12-ounce can)

Mandarin orange segments in light syrup or juice (15-ounce can)

Maple syrup

Molasses

Nonfat sweetened condensed milk (14-ounce can)

Solid pack pumpkin (not pumpkin pie mix) (15-ounce can)

Yellow cling peaches in light syrup (29-ounce can)

Frozen Staples

Blackberries

Blueberries

Fat free non-dairy whipped topping (12-ounce container)

Frozen yogurt or ice cream

Peaches

Raspberries (12-ounce bag)

From the Salad Bar

Grated carrots (not shredded)

reduced-fat ricotta cheesecake

～

What's in this for baby and me? Protein.

THIS REDUCED-FAT cheesecake is loaded with **protein**, and it is a good source of calcium. Topped with sliced fresh fruit or berries, some Diabetic-Friendly Strawberry-Raspberry Syrup (page 38) or Rhubarb Sauce (page 287), it is delicious.

Makes one 9-inch cheesecake; serves 8

One 9-ounce store-bought graham cracker crust "with 2 extra servings" or one 9-inch store-bought reduced-fat graham cracker crust

One 8-ounce package fat-free or reduced-fat cream cheese or Neufchâtel

1 cup part-skim ricotta cheese

⅓ cup sugar

1 large egg

½ cup nonfat plain yogurt or reduced-fat or nonfat dairy sour cream

1 teaspoon pure vanilla extract

1. Preheat the oven to 350°F. Place the graham cracker crust on a baking sheet lined with foil.
2. Place the cream cheese and ricotta cheese in a large bowl and beat with an electric mixer on medium speed until creamy. Add the sugar and continue to beat for 30 seconds. Add the egg, yogurt, and vanilla extract and beat until well blended.
3. Pour the filling into the graham cracker crust. Bake for 45 minutes, or until the center of the cheesecake is almost firm (it will firm up as it cools). Remove the cheesecake from the oven, and let cool to room temperature, then refrigerate for at least 4 hours before serving. (Refrigerate leftovers.)

APPROXIMATE NUTRITIONAL INFORMATION: Serving size: one-eighth of the reduced-fat ricotta cheesecake; Calories: 211 cals; Protein: 10 g; Carbohydrates: 27 g; Fat: 7 g; Fiber: 0 g; Sodium: 299 mg; Diabetic Exchange: Bread/Starch 2, Fat 1

artificial sweeteners during pregnancy

Are artificial sweeteners, such as saccharin and aspartame (Equal and NutraSweet), safe during pregnancy? Saccharin can cross the placenta to the baby and since no one is sure if this is a problem or not, it should be avoided. Aspartame is composed of the amino acids aspartate and phenylalanine. Aspartame seems to be of little concern for pregnant women, because these two amino acids are found in most of the protein we eat. It is unlikely that eating or drinking an average amount (such as one can of diet soda or one serving of aspartame-sweetened dessert per day) would be harmful.[40] Consult your doctor for specific recommendations regarding artificial sweeteners.

peach and blackberry cobbler

What's in this for baby and me? Vitamin C and fiber.

WHEN FRESH PEACHES are in season and you've got the time to peel and slice them, by all means use them in this recipe (see **Cooking Tip** below for instructions on peeling fresh peaches). Off-season, or if you are short on time, use frozen or canned peaches. The blackberries, or blueberries if you prefer, can be fresh or frozen. This cobbler is an excellent source of **vitamin C** and **fiber**, and a good source of vitamin A, calcium, folic acid, and B vitamins. The cobbler dough can be used to cover any 9-inch baking dish of fruit.

makes one 9-inch cobbler; serves 8

Cobbler Dough
- ¾ cup all-purpose flour
- ¾ cup whole wheat flour
- 2 teaspoons baking powder
- ¼ cup sugar
- Pinch of salt
- 6 tablespoons unsalted butter, cut into pieces
- ¾ cup whole or reduced-fat 2% milk
- 1½ teaspoons pure vanilla extract

Peach and blackberry filling
- 1½ pounds peaches (about 5) washed, pitted, peeled, and sliced (see variations below)
- 8 ounces (about 2 cups) fresh blackberries or blueberries, washed, or 2 cups frozen berries
- ⅓ cup sugar
- 2 tablespoons all-purpose flour or 1½ tablespoons cornstarch
- ½ teaspoon ground cinnamon (optional)

1. Preheat oven the to 425°F. Have a 9-inch baking dish ready.
2. To make the dough, combine the whole wheat and all-purpose flours, baking powder, sugar, and salt in a large bowl and stir to mix. Add the butter, then, using your fingers, rub the mixture until it resembles coarse meal. Stir in the milk and vanilla just until the dough comes together; set aside.
3. To prepare the filling, combine all of the ingredients in a large bowl and mix until well blended. (*Note:* You do not need to thaw the frozen fruit before baking. If using frozen fruit, your baking time will increase by about 10 to 15 minutes.) Transfer the filling to the baking dish, then drop heaping spoonfuls of the cobbler dough over the fruit, leaving some empty spaces for the fruit to show through.
4. Bake for 12 minutes, then reduce the heat to 400°F and continue to bake for 30 to 35 minutes, or until the peaches are tender when pierced with the tip of a knife and the juices are bubbling. Remove the cobbler from the oven and allow to cool slightly before serving. (Refrigerate leftovers.)

▶ *Cooking Tip:* To peel fresh peaches, bring a pot of water to a rapid boil. Have a bowl filled with ice water ready to stop the cooking process. Add the whole peaches to the boiling water and cook for 30 seconds, then immediately plunge them into the ice water. Cool for about 1 minute, then drain and peel.

▶ *Variations:* An equal amount of all-purpose flour can be substituted for the whole wheat flour. One pound sliced frozen peaches or one 29-ounce can yellow sliced cling peaches in light syrup may be substituted for the fresh peaches. Drain the canned peaches. If you are using canned peaches and have extra space in your baking dish, add a few more blackberries or blueberries.

APPROXIMATE NUTRITIONAL INFORMATION: Serving size: one-eighth peach-blackberry cobbler; Calories: 290 cals; Protein: 4 g; Carbohydrates: 48 g; Fat: 10 g; Fiber: 5 g; Sodium: 114 mg; Vitamin C: 13 mg

apple-blueberry granola crisp

What's in this for baby and me? Folic acid and fiber.

WARM FROM THE oven, topped with a scoop of frozen yogurt, ice cream, or whipped cream, nothing beats this super-crunchy crisp. Rich in **folic acid** and **fiber**, the crisp is also a good source of iron and vitamins A, C and the Bs. The granola topping can be used to cover any 8-or 9-inch baking dish of fruit—peaches or nectarines combined with berries are particularly good.

makes one 9-inch crisp; serves 8

Apple-Blueberry Filling
   4 large Granny Smith apples (about 1¾ pounds), peeled, cored, and cut into ¼-inch slices
   1 dry pint (2 cups) fresh blueberries, washed and picked over
   ½ cup lightly packed light brown sugar
   2 teaspoons ground cinnamon (optional)
   2 tablespoons all-purpose flour or 1½

   tablespoons cornstarch
Granola Topping
   ½ cup all-purpose flour
   ½ cup lightly packed light brown sugar
   6 tablespoons cold unsalted butter, cut into pieces
   1½ cups Kellogg's Healthy Choice Low Fat Granola without Raisins

1. Preheat the oven to 375°F. Have an 8- or 9-inch baking dish ready.
2. To make the filling, combine all of the ingredients in a large bowl and mix until well blended. Transfer the filling to the baking dish and set aside.
3. To make the granola topping, combine the flour and brown sugar in a bowl. Add the butter and, using your fingers, rub the mixture until it resembles coarse meal. Add the granola and continue to mix until the granola is incorporated and the topping holds together in small clumps.
4. Distribute the topping evenly over the filling. Bake for about 45 minutes, or until the apples are tender when pierced with the tip of a knife and the juices are bubbling. Remove the crisp from the oven and allow to cool slightly before serving. (Refrigerate leftovers.)

▶ *Timesaving Tip:* Use frozen blueberries instead of fresh.
▶ *Cooking Tip:* Other good baking apple varieties include Stayman, Cortland, Golden Delicious, Winesap, and Rome Beauty.

APPROXIMATE NUTRITIONAL INFORMATION: Serving size: one-eighth apple-blueberry granola crisp; Calories: 366 cals; Protein: 3 g; Carbohydrates: 68 g; Fat: 11 g; Fiber: 5 g; Sodium: 59 mg; Folic Acid: 168 mcg

bed rest

Every woman's dream of a normal and pleasant pregnancy doesn't always come true. Some conditions in pregnancy lead to activity restrictions, which can be as simple as elevating your legs or as strict as conservative bed rest with no bathroom privileges. Bed-rest restrictions cause added stress for the entire family, and can make meal planning and food preparation difficult. Often the husband or partner, other family members, and friends will need to help with the cooking, household chores, and care of small children.

TIPS FOR COPING WITH MEALS WHILE ON BED REST

► Keep a cooler at your bedside stocked with milk, cheese, fruit, fruit juices, yogurt, and your other favorite foods. Make sure that your cooler is properly chilled (the danger zone is temperatures between 40° and 140°F) and remains cold throughout the day.

► If possible, set up a microwave oven or toaster oven at your bedside to reheat precooked, frozen, or semi-prepared meals and to cook vegetables and other simple dishes.

► Keep a thermos of soup, pasta, or any other food that can be kept warm for a few hours at your bedside.

► Keep cut-up fresh fruits and vegetables, raisins, peanut butter, granola bars, whole grain bread, whole wheat crackers, nuts, individual fruit cups, fruit juices, and other snack items within easy reach.

► Keep two to three sport bottles filled with water within reach. Most bed rest situations also mean an increase in fluid requirements.

► Freeze water bottles so they stay cold all day.

► Keep plastic utensils, napkins, paper cups, and wipes by your bedside.

► Discuss your prenatal meal plan with your caretaker (your husband or partner, mother, friend, or hired help) and share recipes with family and friends who may be bringing meals to you.

strawberry whole wheat shortcake

What's in this for baby and me? Vitamin C.

THESE SHORTCAKE BISCUITS are so good you'll have trouble keeping little hands (or big hands) from eating the shortcake before the dessert is assembled. Rich in **vitamin C**, and a good source of calcium, folic acid, and fiber, this dessert is a true summer treat. The strawberries should be allowed to sit for at least two hours before serving for their juices to release. If you need to speed thing up, sauté half of the berries with the sugar, combine with the uncooked berries, and serve. This recipe can be halved.

serves 6

Strawberry Filling
    1½ pounds (about 6 cups) fresh strawber-
       ries, washed and hulled; half of the
       strawberries cut into quarters, or
       eighths if they are large
    ⅓ cup sugar, or to taste
Shortcake
    ½ cup all-purpose flour

½ cup whole wheat flour
1½ teaspoons baking powder
¼ cup sugar
3 tablespoons unsalted butter, cut into
   pieces
½ cup whole milk or reduced-fat 2% milk
Whipped cream, for topping (optional)

1. To make the filling, 2 hours before serving, combine the sliced strawberries and sugar in a bowl, mix and set aside. Place the whole strawberries in the bowl of a food processor and pulse until they are chopped into small pieces; do *not* puree. Add the chopped strawberries to the the sliced strawberries, stir, cover, and refrigerate until ready to serve.
2. Preheat the oven to 450°F. Line a baking sheet with parchment paper or lightly grease with canola oil cooking spray.
3. To make the shortcake dough, combine the all-purpose and whole wheat flour, baking powder, and sugar in a large bowl and mix. Add the butter and, using your fingers, rub the mixture until it resembles coarse meal. Add the milk and stir until just combined; do not overmix.
4. Measure scant ¼-cupfuls of the shortcake dough and arrange on the baking sheet. You should have 6 shortcakes. Bake for 10 minutes, or until light golden brown. Immediately remove the shortcake biscuits from the baking sheet and cool them on a plate or cooling rack.
5. To serve, slice each shortcake biscuit in half. Put the bottoms of the biscuits on the dessert plates, and cover each with some strawberry filling (and juices). Top with whipped cream if desired, cover with the tops of the biscuits, and serve. (Refrigerate leftovers.)

▶ *Cooking Tip:* An equal amount of all-purpose flour can be substituted for the whole wheat flour.

▶ *Variation:* Use fat-free nondairy whipped topping instead of whipped cream.

APPROXIMATE NUTRITIONAL INFORMATION: Serving size: one strawberry shortcake; Calories: 239 cals; Protein: 4 g; Carbohydrates: 42 g; Fat: 7 g; Fiber: 4 g; Sodium: 113 mg; Vitamin C: 65 mg

no-bake fresh
strawberry-raspberry pie

~

What's in this for baby and me? Vitamin C.

Topped with a dollop of whipped cream, this is one of the best-tasting and healthiest desserts you'll ever eat. The strawberries and raspberries are an excellent source of **vitamin C** and a good source of fiber. Don't substitute frozen fruit in this recipe.

makes one 9-inch pie; serves 8

1 pound fresh strawberries (about 5 cups), washed and hulled, large berries halved or quartered

12 ounces fresh raspberries (about 1½ cups), rinsed quickly

¾ cup sugar

¼ cup cornstarch

½ cup water

2 tablespoons freshly squeezed lemon juice

2 tablespoons unsalted butter

One 9-ounce store-bought graham cracker crust "with 2 extra servings" or one 9-inch store-bought piecrust (preferably whole wheat, prebaked according to the package directions)

1. In a large bowl, combine the strawberries and raspberries. Puree 2 cups of the strawberries and raspberries in a food processor or blender until smooth. (*Note:* The pureed berries should equal about 1⅓ cups.) Set aside the remaining berries.
2. Combine the strawberry-raspberry puree, sugar, cornstarch, water, lemon juice, and butter in a saucepan, bring to a simmer over medium heat, stirring constantly, and simmer, stirring, for 2 minutes, or until the mixture becomes thick and shiny. Remove from the heat.
3. Place half of the reserved strawberries and raspberries in the pie shell and pour half of the hot berry mixture over them. Add the remaining strawberries and raspberries and top with the remaining hot berry mixture. Using a spoon, gently move the strawberries until all of them are covered with sauce and the sauce touches the sides of the pie crust.
4. Cover tightly with plastic and refrigerate for at least 4 hours, or until the filling is set. Serve chilled. (Refrigerate leftovers.)

▶ *Variation:* A total of about 6 cups of either fresh strawberries or raspberries can be used instead of a mixture of both.

APPROXIMATE NUTRITIONAL INFORMATION: Serving size: one-eighth of the strawberry-raspberry pie; Calories: 232 cals; Protein: 2 g; Carbohydrates: 43 g; Fat: 7 g; Fiber: 3 g; Sodium: 88 mg; Vitamin C: 40 mg

low-fat frozen raspberry pie

～

What's in this for baby and me? It's practically fat-free!

THIS DESSERT IS light, cool, and perfect for a hot summer night. Chunks of meringue cookies give the pie a bright-pink-and-white marbled look. When making this recipe, factor in the defrosting time for the frozen nondairy whipped topping, about 5 hours in the refrigerator. Also, be sure to use a 9-ounce store-bought graham cracker crust "with 2 extra servings" to hold all the filling. Or, if you don't want to use a pie crust, simply freeze this dessert in individual (or one large) freezer-proof serving dishes. The raspberries are a good source of vitamin C.

makes one 9-inch pie; serves 10

8 vanilla or plain meringue cookies (such as Miss Meringue)

Two 6-ounce containers fresh raspberries (about 1½ cups raspberries), rinsed quickly

⅓ cup sugar

One 12-ounce container frozen fat-free nondairy whipped topping, defrosted

One 9-ounce store-bought graham cracker crust "with 2 extra servings"

1. Place the meringue cookies in the bowl of a food processor and pulse until they are crushed into small pieces about the size of peas. Transfer to a large bowl and set aside. (Set the food processor bowl aside.) Alternatively, place the meringues in a gallon-size zip-lock bag and crush them with a rolling pin or bottle, or use your hands to crush the cookies into a large bowl.
2. Puree the raspberries and sugar in the food processor or a blender. Add the puree to the crushed meringues. Add the nondairy whipped topping and mix with a rubber spatula until well combined. Spoon into the graham cracker crust, cover with plastic wrap, and freeze until firm.
3. To serve, slice the pie while it is still frozen, but, if possible, let stand at room temperature for 10 minutes to soften slightly before serving. (Freeze leftovers.)

▶ *Variation:* Use one 12-ounce bag frozen raspberries. Thaw slightly, but don't drain unless there is a lot of juice.

APPROXIMATE NUTRITIONAL INFORMATION: Serving size: one-tenth of the frozen raspberry pie: Calories: 261 cals; Protein: 2 g; Carbohydrates: 48 g; Fat: 5 g; Fiber: 2 g; Sodium: 173 g

pumpkin pie

What's in this for baby and me? Vitamin A.

Packed with **vitamin A** and a good source of protein and calcium, pumpkin pie isn't just for Thanksgiving anymore! A store-bought frozen crust, preferably of the whole wheat variety, can be substituted for the graham cracker crust (be sure to use the 9-ounce crust with 2 extra servings to hold all the filling). Ideally, either crust should be prebaked to prevent the bottom from getting soggy. If you feel like making a crust from scratch, the Homemade Whole Wheat Pie Crust on page 175 works well. Notes for a **Calcium Boost** follow the recipe.

makes one 9-inch pie; serves 10

One 9-ounce store-bought graham cracker crust "with 2 extra servings" or one 9-inch store-bought piecrust (preferably whole wheat)

One 15-ounce can solid-pack pumpkin (not pumpkin pie mix)

One 12-ounce can light evaporated skim milk

2 large eggs

½ cup light or dark brown sugar

2 tablespoons mild molasses (optional)

½ teaspoon salt

2 teaspoons pumpkin pie spice mix

1. Preheat the oven to 350°F.
2. Place the graham cracker crust on a baking sheet lined with foil and bake for 7 minutes, or until the crust feels crisp. (Prebake any other store-bought crust according to package directions.) Remove from the oven and set aside. (Leave the oven on.)
3. To prepare the filling, combine the remaining ingredients in a large bowl and whisk until well blended.
4. Pour the filling into the prepared crust. Bake for 50 minutes, or until a knife inserted into the center comes out clean. Cool completely before slicing. (Refrigerate leftovers.)

▶ *Calcium Boost:* In a measuring cup, combine the evaporated milk with 1/3 cup pasteurized instant nonfat dry milk. Mix until the powder has dissolved, then proceed as directed in Step 3.

▶ *Cooking Tip:* Two teaspoons mixed ground cinnamon, ginger, and cloves, or just one of these spices, can be substituted for the pumpkin pie spice mix.

APPROXIMATE NUTRITIONAL INFORMATION: Serving size: one-tenth of the pumpkin pie; Calories: 183 cals; Protein: 6 g; Carbohydrates: 25 g; Fat: 6 g; Fiber: 2 g; Sodium: 312 mg; Vitamin A: 11,021 IU; Diabetic Exchange: Bread/Starch 1.5, Fat 1

leg cramps: a common annoyance

Some pregnant women experience leg cramps, usually during the last three months of pregnancy. These often occur while sleeping, but they can hit anytime. Following are some tips to help relieve leg cramps:

- ▶ Stretch your legs (especially your calf muscles) before going to bed.
- ▶ Avoid pointing your toes while stretching or exercising.
- ▶ Drink plenty of water.
- ▶ Try to have three or four servings of calcium-rich food every day.
- ▶ Apply heat to or massage your calves to relieve cramping.

carrot cake with cream cheese frosting

~

What's in this for baby and me? Vitamin A.

FROST THIS CARROT cake for a celebration, or keep it simple for a family dessert or snack. Some grocery stores have salad bars that carry coarsely grated (*not* shredded) carrots, which makes the cake a cinch to make. Rich in **vitamin A** and a good source of protein, this carrot cake is a worthy staple.

makes one 13 x 9-inch cake; serves 12

Canola oil cooking spray and flour, for the baking pan
¾ cup all-purpose flour
¾ cup whole wheat flour
2 teaspoons baking soda
1½ teaspoons baking powder
2 teaspoons ground cinnamon
½ teaspoon salt
¾ cup canola oil

4 large eggs
1 cup sugar
2 cups grated carrots (about 4 large carrots)
One 8-ounce can crushed pineapple, drained (optional)
½ cup chopped walnuts or pecans (optional)
Cream cheese frosting (recipe follows) (optional)

1. Preheat the oven to 350°F. Lightly grease and flour a 13 x 9 x 12-inch baking pan.
2. In a large bowl, combine the all-purpose and whole wheat flours, baking soda, baking powder, cinnamon, and salt, stir and set aside.
3. In a large bowl, combine the canola oil and eggs and beat with an electric mixer on medium speed for 3 minutes. Add the sugar and beat for another 3 minutes. Add the dry ingredients in 3 batches, beating on low speed and scraping the sides of the bowl after each addition. Mix just until the flour is absorbed. With a rubber spatula, fold in the carrots and optional pineapple and walnuts until evenly distributed.
4. Fill the baking pan with the batter and tap gently to release any air bubbles. Bake for about 45 minutes, or until a toothpick inserted into the center comes out clean. Remove from the oven and let stand for 5 minutes, then invert onto a cooling rack. Cool completely.
5. Frost the cake if desired. (Refrigerate leftovers.)

▶ **Storage Tip:** Slice this cake into individual-size portions and freeze to satisfy your sweet-tooth at any time of day.

▶ **Cooking Tip:** An equal amount of all-purpose flour can be substituted for the whole wheat flour.

APPROXIMATE NUTRITIONAL INFORMATION: Serving size: one-twelfth of the carrot cake; Calories: 308 cals; Protein: 5 g; Carbohydrates: 32 g; Fat: 18 g; Fiber: 2 g; Sodium: 386 mg; Vitamin A: 5,844 IU

cream cheese frosting

makes about 2½ cups

One 8-ounce package reduced-fat cream
    cheese or Neufchâtel, slightly softened
4 tablespoons unsalted butter, softened

1 tablespoon pure vanilla extract
3 cups confectioners' sugar

Combine the cream cheese and butter in a large bowl and beat with an electric mixer on medium speed for 2 minutes, or until creamy and most of the lumps have disappeared. Add the vanilla and half of the confectioners' sugar and beat for 1 minute, scraping down the sides of the bowl as necessary. Add the remaining sugar and beat until the frosting is smooth. Cover and refrigerate for 1 to 2 hours, or until thickened enough to spread. Use on a completely cooled cake.

APPROXIMATE NUTRITIONAL INFORMATION: Serving size: about 3 tablespoons of the cream cheese frosting; Calories: 178 cals; Protein: 2 g; Carbohydrates: 26 g; Fat: 7 g; Fiber: 0 g; Sodium: 57 mg

angel food cake with lemon drizzle

~

What's in this for baby and me? A fat-free dessert!

THERE IS NO comparison between package-mix and homemade angel food cake. The key to getting good height on this cake is to bake the cake on the lowest oven rack. Also, it is essential to use cake flour—other flours are too heavy. The optional lemon drizzle adds a nice finish. Fresh berries tossed with a bit of sugar, the Diabetic-Friendly Strawberry-Raspberry Syrup (page 38), or the Rhubarb Sauce (page 287) make wonderful accompaniments. By the way, don't feel guilty about throwing out the yolks—a dozen eggs costs less than two dollars, and it is not worth the time and energy it would take to create something with 12 yolks.

makes one 9- or 10-inch tube cake; serves 8

1 cup cake flour	**1 tablespoon freshly squeezed lemon juice**
1⅓ cups sugar	**1 teaspoon cream of tartar**
½ teaspoon salt	**2 teaspoons pure vanilla extract**
1½ cups egg whites (from about 12 large eggs)	**Lemon drizzle (recipe follows)**

1. Adjust an oven rack to the lowest position and preheat the oven to 350°F. Have an ungreased 9- or 10-inch angel food cake tube pan ready.
2. Sift the flour, ⅔ cup of the sugar, and the salt into a medium bowl or onto a piece of parchment or wax paper; set aside.
3. In a large bowl (make sure the bowl is very clean), combine the egg whites, lemon juice, cream of tartar, and vanilla extract. Beat with an electric mixer on low speed for 30 seconds. Increase the speed to medium and beat for about 30 seconds, until frothy bubbles begin to appear. Gradually add the remaining ⅔ cup sugar, increase the speed to high, and continue beating just until soft, glossy peaks form, about 3 minutes.
4. With a rubber spatula, gradually fold in the flour mixture about ¼ cup at a time. Work with a slicing and lifting motion, and make sure to bring up the egg whites from the bottom of the bowl. All of the flour needs to be absorbed, but try not to overmix—that can deflate the whites.
5. Spoon the batter into the tube pan. Bake for 40 minutes, or until the top is golden and springs back when lightly touched.
6. Remove from the oven and allow to cool for 5 minutes. If the pan sides have "feet" to keep them elevated, simply invert the pan onto a cake rack. If not, set the inverted pan on three upside-down mugs or similar objects to keep it suspended.

7. Once cooled, run a long thin knife around the sides of the pan and the center tube and invert the cake onto a serving plate. Cover leftovers with aluminum foil and store in a cool, dry place.

8. Slowly pour the lemon drizzle over the cooled cake.

▶ *Cooking Tip:* Cake flour is a very fine chemically bleached wheat flour. Because its high starch content allows it to support the high proportion of sugar in this recipe, it produces a high-rising cake. Unbleached all-purpose flour is more nutritious, but it produces a cake that will not rise as high. Both flours taste the same.

APPROXIMATE NUTRITIONAL INFORMATION: Serving size: one-eighth of the angel food cake; Calories: 201 cals; Protein: 6 g; Carbohydrates: 43 g; Fat: 0 g; Fiber: .2 g; Sodium: 228 mg; Diabetic Exchange: Bread/Starch 3

lemon drizzle

makes about ¾ cup

1½ cups confectioners' sugar	3½ tablespoons freshly squeezed lemon juice
1 tablespoon grated lemon zest	1½ teaspoons hot water

Mix all of the ingredients in a bowl until smooth.

▶ *Diabetic Tip:* Omit lemon drizzle.

APPROXIMATE NUTRITIONAL INFORMATION: Serving size: one-eighth of the lemon drizzle; Calories: 75 cals; Protein: 0 g; Carbohydrates: 19 g; Fat: 0 g; Fiber: 0 g; Sodium: 0 mg

vanilla flan with fresh berries

~

What's in this for baby and me? Calcium and vitamin C.

BECAUSE THE CUSTARD needs to sit overnight to absorb as much of the caramel flavor as possible, plan to make this fabulous vanilla flan *a day in advance*. The flan is an excellent source of **calcium** and a good source of protein, and the berries are high in **vitamin C**. A word of advice: because bending is not always easy during pregnancy, have someone help you get this flan (which is baked in a water bath) in and out of the oven.

serves 8

One 14-ounce can nonfat sweetened condensed milk

1½ cups whole or reduced-fat 2% milk

2 teaspoon pure vanilla extract

3 large eggs

¾ cup sugar

4 cups fresh raspberries, sliced strawberries, blueberries, or a mixture, for garnish (optional)

1. Preheat the oven to 325°F. Put a kettle of water on to boil. Have a 2-quart soufflé dish and a baking pan large enough to hold the soufflé dish ready.
2. In a bowl, combine the sweetened condensed milk, regular milk, and eggs, whisk thoroughly, and set aside.
3. Place the sugar in a small nonstick saucepan. Cook, over medium-high heat, stirring with a wooden spoon, until it reaches a rich caramel color. Carefully pour the caramel into the bottom of the soufflé dish, then swirl the soufflé dish to allow some of the caramel to coat 1 inch up the sides of the dish. (*Note:* The caramel will be extremely hot, so be *very careful*.) Place the hot saucepan in the sink and immediately fill with water for easier cleanup.
4. Pour the egg mixture through a fine-mesh strainer into the caramel-coated soufflé dish. Add enough boiling water to the baking pan to reach 1½ inches up the sides of the soufflé dish. Bake for 1½ hours: the middle will still be a little jiggly but will harden as it cools. Remove the soufflé dish from the baking pan and let cool to room temperature, then refrigerate for at least 8 hours, or overnight.
5. To serve, fill a baking pan with boiling water. Place the soufflé dish in it for at least 5 minutes to allow the caramel to melt and create a sauce. Loosen the sides of the flan by running a sharp knife around the inside of the soufflé dish. Carefully invert the flan onto a large serving platter with sides to catch the caramel sauce. Serve with fresh berries, if desired. (Refrigerate leftovers.)

APPROXIMATE NUTRITIONAL INFORMATION: Serving size: one-eighth of the vanilla flan; Calories: 285 cals; Protein: 8 g; Carbohydrates: 56 g; Fat: 3 g; Fiber: 2 g; Sodium: 98 mg; Calcium: 202 mg

orange, blueberry, and date salad with frozen yogurt

What's in this for baby and me? Vitamin C and fiber.

THIS FRUIT SALAD is loaded with **vitamin C** and **fiber**, and the frozen yogurt is a good source of protein and calcium. Vary the ingredients to suit your family's taste—raspberries, bananas, and peaches are great additions. Omit the mint leaves, and possibly the cinnamon, for kids. Topped with plain yogurt, this salad is wonderful for breakfast or as a snack.

serves 3 (makes about 2 cups fruit salad)

2 large navel oranges, peeled and cut into segments (see Cooking Tip 1 below)
¾ cup fresh blueberries, washed and picked over
10 pitted dates, thinly sliced (optional)

Dash of ground cinnamon (optional)
About 12 fresh mint leaves, finely sliced (optional)
1½ cups vanilla frozen yogurt (optional)

Combine all of the ingredients except the frozen yogurt in a bowl. Toss gently. Accompany the fruit salad with the frozen yogurt if desired.

▶ *Timesaving Tip:* Use one 15-ounce can mandarin orange segments, drained, instead of the fresh oranges.

▶ *Cooking Tip 1:* To slice the oranges into segments: Slice the peel and white pith off the top and bottom of each orange. Then stand each orange on a cutting board and, using a sharp thin knife, working from the top of the orange to the base, slice the peel from the orange. (Use the first slice as your guide to know how deep to slice.) Working over a bowl to catch the juices, hold the orange in one hand and slice the orange segments from the membranes, getting the knife as close to the membranes as possible and allowing the segments to drop into the bowl. Once all of the segments have been removed, squeeze the membranes to extract as much juice as possible.

▶ *Cooking Tip 2:* To prevent sticking, oil your knife before slicing the dates.

APPROXIMATE NUTRITIONAL INFORMATION: Serving size: one-third of othe fruit salad and ½ cup vanilla frozen yogurt; Calories: 220 cals; Protein: 6 g; Carbohydrates: 52 g; Fat: .3 g; Fiber: 5 g; Sodium: 55 mg; Vitamin C: 52 mg; Diabetic Exchange: Bread/Starch 3.5, Fat 1

fruit-filled granola

～

What's in this for baby and me? Fiber.

IF YOU FEEL a sudden urge to get crunchy during pregnancy, this recipe is for you. Home-made granola goes way beyond the call of duty to get **fiber** into your diet, and this version is also a good source of protein and iron. Those who make their own granola are a rare breed, dedicated to leading a healthy, fiber-filled life. For those not so dedicated, there are endless varieties of granola on the shelves and in the bins of grocery and whole food stores. Read labels for the one that best suits your family's tastes and dietary needs.

Use this surprisingly easy and fun recipe as a blueprint—change it according to the availability of ingredients in your area and new items as you discover them. Some common healthy additions include: sunflower seeds, unsweetened coconut flakes, unsalted sesame seeds, shelled pumpkin seeds, raisins and other dried fruits, and wheat germ. Freeze-dried fruits are a sweet touch and add a burst of color, not to mention vitamins. Granola will keep in a zip-lock bag or airtight container for weeks. It's great as a topping on anything from yogurt, cottage cheese, or ice cream to applesauce and oatmeal, or solo as a snack. Mix your kids' favorite fruits (dried bananas, raisins, dried dates, or dried cherries) and nuts (pecans or walnuts) into the granola and watch them gobble it up. This recipe can easily be doubled—use two baking sheets.

makes about 5 cups

Canola oil or canola oil cooking spray for greasing the baking sheet
½ cup honey, molasses, or maple syrup, or a mixture
¼ cup canola oil
2 cups "old-fashioned" rolled oats (not quick-cooking oats) (see Variation below)
½ cup sliced almonds
⅓ cup dried cherries
⅓ cup chopped dried apricots
⅓ cup dried banana slices

1. Preheat the oven to 250°F. Lightly grease a large baking sheet with sides; set aside.
2. Combine the honey and oil in a small saucepan and heat just until hot (or use the microwave). Place the rolled oats and sliced almonds in a bowl and mix. Add the honey-oil mixture and mix until well combined.
3. Spread the granola mixture evenly on the baking sheet. Bake for about 40 minutes, or until light golden. It will still be soft when it comes out of the oven, but it will harden as it cools. Do not overbake, or the granola will have a bitter, burnt taste. Allow the granola to cool completely.

4. Add the optional dried fruit to the granola and mix well. Store in an airtight container or a zip-lock bag.

▶ *Cooking Tip:* Measure the canola oil first, swirl it around the measuring cup to coat the sides, then measure the honey, which will easily slide out of the measuring cup.

▶ *Variation:* You can use 2 cups of barley, rye, or wheat flakes in place of the oats, or mix and match all four types.

▶ *Diabetic Tip:* Reduce serving size to ¼ cup.

APPROXIMATE NUTRITIONAL INFORMATION: Serving size: ½ cup of the fruit-filled granola; Calories: 357 cals; Protein: 7 g; Carbohydrates: 55 g; Fat: 14 g; Fiber: 5 g; Sodium: 2 mg; Diabetic Exchange (values per ¼ cup serving): Bread/Starch 1, Fat 1, Fruit 1

patricia terry's pumpkin bread

What's in this for baby and me? Vitamin A.

YOU'LL KEEP COMING back to this recipe for pumpkin bread. Add your favorite ingredients, such as walnuts or mini chocolate chips, to get little ones to try a bite. The pumpkin is a good source of **vitamin A**. This recipe can be cut in half.

makes two 8½ x 4½-inch loaves or five 5¾ x 3-inch loaves
(each large loaf serves 12 and each small loaf serves 5)

Canola oil cooking spray for greasing the baking pan

2 cups all-purpose flour

1½ cups whole wheat flour

2½ cups sugar

½ teaspoon baking powder

2 teaspoons baking soda

½ teaspoon salt

2 teaspoons ground cinnamon

1 teaspoon ground nutmeg (optional)

½ teaspoon ground ginger (optional)

½ cup canola oil

½ cup applesauce

2 large eggs plus 2 large egg whites

⅔ cup water

2 cups solid pack pumpkin (*not* pumpkin pie mix)

1 cup dark or light raisins (optional)

1. Preheat the oven to 350°F. Spray two 8½ x 4½ x 2½-inch loaf pans or three 5¾ x 3 x 2⅛-inch loaf pans with canola oil cooking spray.
2. In a large bowl, combine the dry ingredients and mix until well blended; set aside.
3. In another large bowl, combine the canola oil, applesauce, eggs, egg whites, and water and whisk to mix. Add this mixture to the dry ingredients and whisk just until combined. Add the pumpkin and raisins, if using and mix until well blended.
4. Divide the batter among the prepared loaf pans. Bake until a toothpick inserted into the center of each loaf comes out clean, about 70 minutes for large loaves, about 40 minutes for smaller loaves. Let sit for 5 minutes, then remove from the pans and cool completely before slicing.

▶ *Variation:* An equal amount of all-purpose flour can be substituted for the whole wheat flour.

▶ *Storage Tip:* To freeze, wrap the cooled loaves in aluminum foil and freeze. Wrap leftovers in aluminum foil and store in a cool dry place.

APPROXIMATE NUTRITIONAL INFORMATION: Serving size: one-twelfth of one large loaf of pumpkin bread; Calories: 131 cals; Protein: 2 g; Carbohydrates: 25 g; Fat: 3 g; Fiber: 1 g; Sodium: 104 mg; Vitamin A: 2,718 IU; Diabetic Exchange: Bread/Starch: 1.5, Fat 1

rhubarb sauce

~

What's in this for baby and me? Vitamin C and calcium.

Hᴵɢʜ ɪɴ **vitamin C** and **calcium**, and a good source of fiber, this sauce is irresistible if you like rhubarb. It's the perfect way to jazz up any snack or dessert, including yogurt, frozen yogurt, or ice cream.

makes about 1 cup

1 pound rhubarb, any leaves trimmed, washed, and cut into ½-inch pieces

½ cup sugar

2 tablespoons water

In a small saucepan, combine all of the ingredients and bring to a boil. Reduce the heat and simmer for 15 to 20 minutes, or until the rhubarb is soft and falling apart. Serve hot or cold. Refrigerate leftovers for up to 3 days. This sauce can also be frozen for up to 1 month.

APPROXIMATE NUTRITIONAL INFORMATION: Serving size: ½ cup rhubarb sauce; Calories: 233 cals; Protein: 2 g; Carbohydrates: 58 g; Fat: .4 g; Fiber: 4 g; Sodium: 10 g; Vitamin C: 18 mg; Calcium: 196 mg

exercise tips:
fitness for two

Exercise in moderation is a good thing during pregnancy. It promotes general physical health, good muscle tone, and a stronger respiratory system. Exercise helps reduce stress, combat fatigue, relieve backaches, improve posture, combat varicose veins, improve self-image, and keep your digestion on track. Better fitness can also make delivery easier and will probably help with postpartum recovery. Throughout your pregnancy, keep in mind that you are exercising to stay fit, healthy, and relaxed, not to lose weight. Discuss the exercise routine that is appropriate for you at different stages of your pregnancy with your doctor.

All of the following information regarding exercise during pregnancy comes from the March of Dimes.[41] To start, here is a list of women who should *not* exercise during pregnancy without the consent of their doctor.

WOMEN WHO SHOULD NOT EXERCISE WITHOUT THEIR DOCTOR'S PERMISSION

▶ Women with a history of miscarriage
▶ Women who have experienced preterm labor in this or a previous pregnancy
▶ Women who have obstetrical complications, including an incompetent cervix, ruptured membranes (broken bag of water), or vaginal bleeding
▶ Women with diabetes
▶ Women with preeclampsia or pregnancy-induced high blood pressure
▶ Women whose fetus is not growing as rapidly as it should be
▶ Women carrying multiples
▶ Women with *any* other pregnancy complication

There are a couple of things to keep in mind while exercising during pregnancy. First, it is more difficult for you to breathe when exercising because oxygen must be supplied to your additional body mass (including your baby) and to your increased volume of red blood cells. Second, as your belly gets bigger, breathing becomes even more difficult, because your uterus increasingly crowds your diaphragm, the large muscle between your chest and abdomen. Third, your increased hormone levels soften your connective tissues, making your joints more susceptible to injury. And fourth, your balance shifts as your abdomen and chest enlarge, which can cause clumsiness and possibly falls.

Two of the two best exercises for pregnant women are brisk walking and swimming (but not diving). Swimming is particularly good because it uses many muscle groups while the water supports your extra weight. Another option might be to join a prenatal exercise class. Many prenatal classes offer support group discussions on a range of pregnancy-related topics, including how to stretch your pregnancy wardrobe, how to choose a name for the baby, and tips for breastfeeding.

Following are some exercise guidelines recommended by the American College of Obstetricians and Gynecologists (ACOG).

- Regular exercise (three to five days per week) is preferable to occasional activity.
- Swimming, stationary cycling, and brisk walking are highly recommended.
- Exercises that require jumping, jarring motions, or rapid changes in direction should be avoided. These can cause damage to connective tissue.
- Exercises done lying flat on the back or right side should be avoided. These positions can allow a woman's expanding uterus to compress the vein that carries blood to the heart, which could interfere with blood flow to the uterus.
- Exercise sessions should be preceded by a five-minute period of muscle warm-up (for example, slow walking or stationary cycling at low resistance).
- Exercise should be done on a safe surface, such as a wooden floor or a tightly carpeted or outdoor surface, to reduce the risk of injury.
- Strenuous exercise should not be performed in hot, humid weather or during illness accompanied by fever.
- Moderate or intense aerobic activities should be limited to periods of fifteen to twenty minutes. Lower-intensity activities may be conducted continuously over a longer period of time, but should not exceed forty-five minutes.
- Heart rate should be measured at times of peak activity and should not exceed 140 beats per minute.
- A pregnant woman's temperature should not exceed 100.4°F while exercising. She should drink plenty of water before and after exercise to prevent dehydration and hyperthermia and take a break during exercise if more water is needed or she is tired.
- Care should be taken to rise from the floor gradually to avoid an abrupt drop in blood pressure, and to continue some form of activity involving the legs for a brief period.
- Exercise sessions should be followed by a brief cool-down period of gradually declining activity that includes gentle stationary stretching. Stretches should not be taken to the maximum of resistance.
- A pregnant woman should consume enough calories to meet the needs of her pregnancy (300 extra calories per day) as well as her exercise program. Women should not try to lose weight by exercising during pregnancy.

WARNING SIGNS TO STOP EXERCISING
Pain

Dizziness

Shortness of breath

Palpitations (pounding, racing, or irregular heartbeat)

Faintness

Tachycardia (rapid heartbeat)

Pubic pain

Uterine contractions

Vaginal bleeding/fluid loss

Absence of fetal movement

RECOMMENDED WEIGHT GAIN FOR
PREGNANT WOMEN USING THE BODY MASS INDEX[42]

PREPREGNANCY WEIGHT CLASSIFICATION	OPTIMAL WEIGHT GAIN (LBS)	
	BMI (KG/M²)	POUNDS
Underweight	< 19.8	28–40
Normal	19.8–26	25–35
Overweight	26.1–29	15–25
Obese	>29	< or equal to 15

CALORIE AND PROTEIN REQUIREMENTS
FOR PREGNANT WOMEN WITH A NORMAL BODY MASS INDEX

HEIGHT	PREGNANCY WEIGHT (LBS)	AVERAGE PREGNANCY WEIGHT (LBS)	CALORIE REQUIREMENT	AVERAGE CALORIE REQUIREMENT	MINIMUM PROTEIN (G) REQUIREMENT
5'0"	102–128	112	1,800–2,000	1,900	60
5'1"	106–132	116	1,800–2,300	2,000	60
5'2"	109–136	120	1,800–2,300	2,100	60
5'3"	113–141	124	1,900–2,400	2,100	60–65
5'4"	116–145	128	2,000–2,400	2,200	60–65
5'5"	120–150	132	2,000–2,500	2,300	60–65
5'6"	124–155	137	2,100–2,600	2,300	60–65
5'7"	127–159	140	2,100–2,700	2,400	60–70
5'8"	131–164	145	2,200–2,700	2,500	60–70
5'9"	135–169	149	2,200–2,700	2,500	60–70
5'10"	139–174	153	2,300–3,000	2,600	60–75
5'11"	143–179	158	2,300–3,000	2,600	65–75
6'0"	147–184	162	2,400–3,000	2,700	65–80

Body Mass Index Table

BMI	Normal						Overweight					Obese										Extreme Obesity															
	19	20	21	22	23	24	25	26	27	28	29	30	31	32	33	34	35	36	37	38	39	40	41	42	43	44	45	46	47	48	49	50	51	52	53	54
Height (inches)												**Body Weight (pounds)**																								
58	91	96	100	105	110	115	119	124	129	134	138	143	148	153	158	162	167	172	177	181	186	191	196	201	205	210	215	220	224	229	234	239	244	248	253	258
59	94	99	104	109	114	119	124	128	133	138	143	148	153	158	163	168	173	178	183	188	193	198	203	208	212	217	222	227	232	237	242	247	252	257	262	267
60	97	102	107	112	118	123	128	133	138	143	148	153	158	163	168	174	179	184	189	194	199	204	209	215	220	225	230	235	240	245	250	255	261	266	271	276
61	100	106	111	116	122	127	132	137	143	148	153	158	164	169	174	180	185	190	195	201	206	211	217	222	227	232	238	243	248	254	259	264	269	275	280	285
62	104	109	115	120	126	131	136	142	147	153	158	164	169	175	180	186	191	196	202	207	213	218	224	229	235	240	246	251	256	262	267	273	278	284	289	295
63	107	113	118	124	130	135	141	146	152	158	163	169	175	180	186	191	197	203	208	214	220	225	231	237	242	248	254	259	265	270	278	282	287	293	299	304
64	110	116	122	128	134	140	145	151	157	163	169	174	180	186	192	197	204	209	215	221	227	232	238	244	250	256	262	267	273	279	285	291	296	302	308	314
65	114	120	126	132	138	144	150	156	162	168	174	180	186	192	198	204	210	216	222	228	234	240	246	252	258	264	270	276	282	288	294	300	306	312	318	324
66	118	124	130	136	142	148	155	161	167	173	179	186	192	198	204	210	216	223	229	235	241	247	253	260	266	272	278	284	291	297	303	309	315	322	328	334
67	121	127	134	140	146	153	159	166	172	178	185	191	198	204	211	217	223	230	236	242	249	255	261	268	274	280	287	293	299	306	312	319	325	331	338	344
68	125	131	138	144	151	158	164	171	177	184	190	197	203	210	216	223	230	236	243	249	256	262	269	276	282	289	295	302	308	315	322	328	335	341	348	354
69	128	135	142	149	155	162	169	176	182	189	196	203	209	216	223	230	236	243	250	257	263	270	277	284	291	297	304	311	318	324	331	338	345	351	358	365
70	132	139	146	153	160	167	174	181	188	195	202	209	216	222	229	236	243	250	257	264	271	278	285	292	299	306	313	320	327	334	341	348	355	362	369	376
71	136	143	150	157	165	172	179	186	193	200	208	215	222	229	236	243	250	257	265	272	279	286	293	301	308	315	322	329	338	343	351	358	365	372	379	386
72	140	147	154	162	169	177	184	191	199	206	213	221	228	235	242	250	258	265	272	279	287	294	302	309	316	324	331	338	346	353	361	368	375	383	390	397
73	144	151	159	166	174	182	189	197	204	212	219	227	235	242	250	257	265	272	280	288	295	302	310	318	325	333	340	348	355	363	371	378	386	393	401	408
74	148	155	163	171	179	186	194	202	210	218	225	233	241	249	256	264	272	280	287	295	303	311	319	326	334	342	350	358	365	373	381	389	396	404	412	420
75	152	160	168	176	184	192	200	208	216	224	232	240	248	256	264	272	279	287	295	303	311	319	327	335	343	351	359	367	375	383	391	399	407	415	423	431
76	156	164	172	180	189	197	205	213	221	230	238	246	254	263	271	279	287	295	304	312	320	328	336	344	353	361	369	377	385	394	402	410	418	426	435	443

Source: Adapted from *Clinical Guidelines on the Identification, Evaluation, and Treatment of Overweight and Obesity in Adults: The Evidence Report.*

IMPORTANT NOTE

IF YOU DO not fit into the normal range of the Body Mass Index Table, if you are carrying multiples, or if you are a teenager, use the following variations for determining calorie requirements during pregnancy. You should consult your doctor or dietitian for your individual protein needs.

▶ **If underweight (90 percent below your IBW):**
  40 cals x Ideal Body Weight in kilograms

▶ **If overweight (20% above your IBW):**
  25 cals x Current Body Weight in kilograms

▶ **If obese (50% above your IBW):**
  12 cals x Current Body Weight in kilograms

▶ **For twins:**
  Add 300 cals to your requirements

▶ **For triplets:**
  Add 600 cals to your requirements

▶ **For teenagers:**
  40 cals x Ideal Body Weight in kilograms

FORMULA FOR DETERMINING YOUR CURRENT BODY WEIGHT AND IDEAL BODY WEIGHT IN KILOGRAMS

To determine your ideal body weight (IBW):
  The first 5 feet of your total height = 100 pounds
  For every inch over the first 5 feet add 5 pounds
  Your IBW should be within a plus/minus 10-pound range

For example: A woman who is 5'4":
  5 feet = 100 pounds
  4" x 5 pounds per inch = 20 pounds
  100 + 20 = 120 pounds
  Plus or minus 10-pound range: 110 to 130 pounds (Average = 120 pounds)

To convert pounds to kilograms, divide by 2.2:
For example: 120 pounds ÷ 2.2 = 55 kilograms
Plus or minus 10-pound range: 50 to 59 kilograms

FOOD GROUPS AND SERVING SIZES
FOR PREGNANT WOMEN

▶ *Whole Grains (6 to 11 servings per day)*
  1 slice bread (preferably whole wheat or bran)
  ½ bagel or English muffin (preferably whole wheat)
  1 tortilla
  ½ cup cooked oatmeal or Cream of Wheat
  ⅓ cup cooked rice, bulgur wheat, or barley
  ½ cup bran or wheat flakes or ¾ cup unsweetened cereal
  ¼ cup wheat germ
  6 whole wheat crackers
  ½ cup cooked enriched pasta or couscous

▶ *Fruits and Vegetables*
  (Fruits: 2 to 4 servings per day, Vegetables: 3 to 5 servings per day)
  Choose at least one serving rich in vitamin A and one rich in vitamin C.
  (See Vitamin A and C Sources, page 294.)

▶ *Meat and Meat Substitutes (2 to 3 servings per day)*
  3 ounces lean beef, poultry, veal, or pork
  3 ounces fish (see Limitations on Certain Fish Consumption, page 247)
  6 ounces shellfish (shrimp)
  ¾ cup canned tuna
  4 ounces tofu = 1 ounce meat
  1 large Grade A egg = 1 ounce meat
  2 tablespoon peanut butter = 1 ounce meat
  1 cup cooked dried beans or peas = 1 ounce meat

▶ *Milk and Dairy (3 to 4 servings per day)*
  1 cup reduced-fat 2% milk
  ¾ cup low-fat or nonfat yogurt
  1 cup low-fat cottage cheese
  1¼ ounces low-fat pasteurized hard cheese or 2 ounces processed cheese
  ½ cup frozen yogurt or ice milk
  1 cup enriched soy beverage
  ⅓ cup pasteurized instant nonfat dry milk

▶ *Fats and Oils (use sparingly)*
  1 teaspoon margarine or butter
  1 teaspoon mayonnaise (1 tablespoon reduced-fat or light mayonnaise)
  ¼ large avocado
  1 teaspoon vegetable or plant oil
  1 tablespoon cream cheese (2 tablespoons low-fat cream cheese)
  2 tablespoons nuts
  2 tablespoons sour cream
  1 tablespoon salad dressing

vitamin a and c fruit and vegetable sources

VITAMIN A

Vegetables

1 cup broccoli
1 cup Brussels sprouts
⅔ cup cooked spinach, mustard greens, collard greens, kale, bok choy, or Swiss chard
1 cup packed sliced romaine or loose leaf lettuce
½ cup sliced asparagus
8 baby carrots
½ cup chopped or pureed cooked pumpkin
½ cup chopped or pureed cooked butternut squash
½ cooked sweet potato
½ large red bell pepper

Fruits

¾ cup cantaloupe
5 dried apricots
½ mango
2 tangerines

VITAMIN C

Vegetables

¾ cup cauliflower florets
1 cup Brussels sprouts
1 cup broccoli florets
½ cooked bok choy
½ cup cooked mustard greens
½ cup cooked kale
1 cup raw cabbage
1 baked potato
½ large red bell pepper
½ tomato

Fruits

½ cup orange or grapefruit juice
½ grapefruit
1 orange or other citrus fruit
1 cup diced cantaloupe
1 cup diced papaya
1 mango
1 cup berries (any kind)
½ cup cooked rhubarb
1 cup pineapple
1 kiwi

PROTEIN SOURCES

FOOD	SERVING SIZE	PROTEIN (G)
Cooked chicken	3 ounces	26
Cooked beef	3 ounces	23
Cooked shrimp	4 ounces	23
Canned tuna fish	3 ounces	22
Cooked salmon	3 ounces	19
Low-fat cottage cheese	½ cup	16
Tempeh	½ cup	15
Cheddar cheese	1 cup	14
Low-fat yogurt	1 cup	13
Hard-boiled egg	1 egg	13
Extra-firm tofu	2 ounces	11
Peanut butter	2 tablespoons	8
Reduced-fat 2% milk	1 cup	8
Kidney beans	½ cup	7

DAIRY CALCIUM SOURCES

FOOD	SERVING SIZE	CALCIUM (MG)
Swiss cheese	2 ounces	545
Nonfat plain yogurt	1 cup	488
Low-fat plain yogurt	1 cup	448
Monterey Jack cheese	2 ounces	423
Part-skim low-moisture mozzarella cheese	2 ounces	414
Cheddar cheese	2 ounces	409
Processed cheese	2 ounces	325
Fontina cheese	2 ounces	312
Nonfat milk	8 ounces	301
Reduced-fat 1% milk	8 ounces	300
Reduced-fat 2% milk	8 ounces	298
Whole (3.3%) milk	8 ounces	290
Nonfat dry milk	⅓ cup	283
Pasteurized feta cheese	2 ounces	280
Pasteurized goat cheese	1 ounce	253
Part-skim ricotta cheese	¼ cup	167
Reduced-fat buttermilk	½ cup	142
Parmesan cheese	2 tablespoons	138
Frozen yogurt	½ cup	138
Vanilla ice cream	½ cup	87
Low-fat 2% cottage cheese	½ cup	78

NONDAIRY CALCIUM SOURCES

FOOD	SERVING SIZE	CALCIUM (MG)
Calcium-fortified orange juice	8 ounces	350
Blackstrap molasses	2 tablespoons	344
Enriched soy beverage	8 ounces	300
Calcium fortified bread	2 slices	160
All-Bran cereal	½ cup	150
Cooked spinach	½ cup	122
Canned salmon (bone-in)	2 ounces	121
Cooked turnip greens	½ cup	99
Tempeh	½ cup	92
Almonds, dry roasted	¼ cup	92
Corn tortillas	2 tortillas	91
Cooked soybeans	½ cup	88
Almond butter	2 tablespoons	86
Molasses	2 tablespoons	82
Flour tortillas	2 tortillas	80
Cooked bok choy	½ cup	79
Tofu (not fortified)	4 ounces	75
Dried figs	¼ cup	72
Vegetarian baked beans	½ cup	64
Plain bagel	1 bagel	53
Cooked mustard greens	½ cup	52
Cooked okra	½ cup	50
Cooked kale	½ cup	47
Baked acorn squash	½ cup	45
Baked butternut squash	½ cup	42
Fresh orange	1 medium	42
Cooked pinto beans	½ cup	41
Cooked chickpeas	½ cup	40
Collard greens	½ cup	40

IRON SOURCES

FOOD	SERVING SIZE	IRON (MG)
Blackstrap molasses	2 tablespoons	7.0
All-Bran cereal	½ cup	4.5
Cooked soybeans	½ cup	4.4
Cooked spinach	½ cup	3.2
Cooked lentils	½ cup	3.2
Baked potato with skin	1 potato	2.7
Cooked split peas	½ cup	2.5
Beef (short loin)	3 ounces	2.3
Cooked chickpeas	½ cup	2.3
Tempeh	½ cup	2.2
Green soybeans	½ cup	2.2
Cooked pinto beans	½ cup	2.2
Flour tortillas	2 tortillas	2.1
Cooked lima beans	½ cup	2.0
Molasses	2 tablespoons	1.8
Cooked black beans	½ cup	1.8
Ground beef patty	3 ounces	1.7
Tofu	4 ounces	1.7
Whole wheat bread	2 slices	1.6
Almonds, dry roasted	¼ cup	1.5
Canned kidney beans	½ cup	1.5
Quick-cooked oatmeal (prepared with water)	1 cup	1.5
Lamb loin	3 ounces	1.5
Prune juice	4 ounces	1.5
Romaine lettuce	2 cups	1.2
Sunflower seeds	¼ cup	1.2
Turkey breast	3 ounces	1.1
Dried figs	¼ cup	1.1
Dried apricots	5 halves	1.0
Wheat germ	2 tablespoons	1.0
Avocado	½ avocado	1.0

FIBER SOURCES

FOOD	SERVING SIZE	FIBER (G)
General Mills Fiber One cereal	½ cup	14
Kellogg's All Bran cereal	½ cup	10
Raspberries	1 cup	8
Cooked lentils	½ cup	8
Cooked black beans	½ cup	7
Cooked chickpeas	½ cup	5
Potato with skin	1 potato	5
Canned kidney beans	½ cup	5
Cooked green peas	⅛ cup	4
Kellogg's Raisin Bran cereal	½ cup	4
Quick-cooked oatmeal (prepared with water)	1 cup	4
Blueberries	1 cup	4
Apple with skin	1 medium	4
Whole wheat bread	2 slices	3
Strawberries	1 cup	3
Orange	1 medium	3
Wheat germ	¼ cup	3
Dried dates	5 dates	3
Broccoli	½ cup	2
Whole wheat crackers	5 items	2
Brussels sprouts	½ cup	2

FOLIC ACID SOURCES

FOOD	SERVING SIZE	FOLIC ACID (MCG)
All Bran cereal	½ cup	400
Cooked lentils	½ cup	179
Romaine lettuce	2 cups	152
Chickpeas	½ cup	141
Asparagus	½ cup	131
Cooked black beans	½ cup	128
Cooked spinach	½ cup	131
Brewer's yeast	1 teaspoon	104
Sunflower seeds	¼ cup	76
Orange juice	1 cup	74
Canned kidney beans	½ cup	64
Avocado	½ medium	56
Wheat germ	2 tablespoons	51
Tomato juice	1 cup	49
Calcium-fortified white bread	2 slices	48
Brussels sprouts	½ cup	47
Roasted peanuts	¼ cup	45
Orange	1 medium	39
Cooked broccoli	½ cup	39

BREAKFAST CEREALS THAT CONTAIN 100 PERCENT OF THE DAILY VALUE OF FOLIC ACID[43]

FOLLOWING IS A list of some cereals that are enriched with 100 percent of the Daily Value (DV) of folic acid based on a 2,000-calorie diet for *nonpregnant women*.

- General Mills Harmony
- General Mills Multi-Grain Cheerios
- General Mills Multi-Grain Cheerios Plus
- General Mills Total Brown Sugar and Oat
- General Mills Total Corn Flakes
- General Mills Raisin Bran
- General Mills Whole Grain
- Kellogg's All-Bran Original
- Kellogg's All-Bran with Extra Fiber
- Kellogg's All-Bran Bran Buds
- Kellogg's Complete Oat Bran Flakes
- Kellogg's Complete Wheat Bran Flakes
- Kellogg's Crispix
- Kellogg's Healthy Choice Almond Crunch with Raisins
- Kellogg's Healthy Choice Low Fat Granola with Raisins
- Kellogg's Healthy Choice Low Fat Granola without Raisins
- Kellogg's Healthy Choice Müeslix
- Kellogg's Healthy Choice Toasted Brown Sugar Squares
- Kellogg's Just Right Fruit and Nut
- Kellogg's Product 19
- Kellogg's Smart Start
- Kellogg's Special K
- Kellogg's Special K Plus

CEREALS THAT CONTAIN 100 PERCENT OF THE DAILY VALUE OF VITAMIN B$_{12}$

FOLLOWING IS A list of some cereals that are enriched with 100 percent of the Daily Value (DV) of vitamin B$_{12}$ based on a 2,000-calorie diet for *nonpregnant women*.

- Kellogg's Product 19
- Kellogg's Complete Wheat Bran Flakes
- Kellogg's Just Right Fruit and Nut
- Kellogg's Müeslix
- Kellogg's Low-Fat Granola with or without Raisins
- Kellogg's All Bran Original, Bran Buds, and Extra Fiber
- General Mills Total Corn Flakes
- General Mills Total Whole Grain
- General Mills Total Raisin Bran
- General Mills Total Brown Sugar and Oats

WELL-DONE TEMPERATURE GUIDE[44]

Beef	170°F
Pork (fresh)	170°F
Lamb	170°F
Veal	170°F
Chicken and Turkey (whole)	180°F
Breast	170°F
Thigh	170°F
Ground	165°F
Stuffing (cooked alone or in the bird)	165°F
Duck and Goose	180°F
Ground Beef, Veal, Lamb, and Pork	160°F
Fish	130°F

FOOD SAFETY TIPS ON
MEAT, POULTRY, AND SEAFOOD

▶ *Buying, Storing, and Thawing Meat, Poultry, and Seafood*[45]

- Read expiration dates on all meat, poultry, and seafood and give the food a visual and smell test before purchasing. For meats and poultry, an inspection sticker from the U.S. Department of Agriculture (USDA) and grade mark should be displayed. Avoid any foods that look old, dehydrated, or freezer burnt and any that have an offensive odor.

- Judge the freshness of seafood by its appearance and odor. Fresh fish has full, clear (not murky or opaque), bright-red gills, and shiny skin with glistening color. The flesh should spring back when pressed, and the fish should have a mild odor. If fresh seafood will not be used within one to two days, it should be frozen. (See *Seafood Storage Chart* below.)

- Store live shellfish (such as mussels, oysters, and clams) in a shallow dish covered with a damp dish towel. Never store them in water or in an airtight container or plastic bag—they need air to breathe. Live shellfish should have closed shells; if they do not, discard them. Other shellfish, such as shrimp, lobster and scallops, should be stored in their original packaging in the coldest part of the refrigerator. Eat all types of fresh shellfish as soon as possible.

- After shopping, get fresh or frozen meat, poultry, or seafood into the freezer or refrigerator as soon as possible. (If you are not going home immediately, ask the fishmonger to store your seafood on ice in a plastic bag.) Do not leave these perishable foods out of the refrigerator for more than two hours. Ideally, the temperature of your refrigerator should be below 40°F and your freezer should be 0°F. Use a thermometer to check these temperatures if you have any doubts.

- Make sure that the packing is not leaking, then store fresh meat, poultry or seafood in the coldest part of your refrigerator (your meat bin or the back of the bottom shelf). If packages are leaking, leave the original packaging on the food, and place the item in a zip-lock plastic bag or on a plate; refrigerate immediately. This will prevent a big mess down the road.

- Regardless of the expiration or "sell by" date, freeze any fresh meat, poultry or seafood if you are not going to use it within two days. The "sell by" date indicates the last day the item can be sold, *not* the last date it can be stored in your refrigerator. Almost all meats and poultry are "chill packed" and kept in the meat department's refrigerator at 28° to 32°F, versus the 40°F temperature of the home refrigerator. This increase in temperature in your own refrigerator creates the need to consume or freeze the product within two days.

- Before freezing, break down large quantities of meat, poultry, or seafood into appropriate serving sizes and place them in freezer bags. This will avoid having to defrost an entire 5-pound package of chicken parts to broil two breasts for dinner.

- Label and date all items in the freezer.
- Don't thaw frozen meat, poultry, or seafood on a kitchen counter at room temperature. Room temperature will promote the growth of bacteria on the outer surface of the product even while the product remains frozen inside. Allow extra time to thaw foods on a plate (to catch the juices) in your refrigerator. If you are short on time, use the defrost setting of your microwave (use the manufacturer's guidelines); or thaw the unopened meat, poultry or fish in a sink or large container filled with cold (not warm) water. Change the water about every 30 minutes to keep it cold.
- If it has been frozen and partially thawed, do not refreeze any meat, poultry, or seafood *unless* there are still ice crystals in the meat.
- Do not thaw pre-stuffed or precooked poultry, meat, or seafood dishes before cooking or reheating. Follow the manufacturer's instructions.

poultry freezer storage chart[46]

PRODUCT		MAXIMUM STORAGE AT 0°F (MONTHS)
Uncooked Poultry		
Chicken	cut up	9
	giblets	3
	livers	3
	whole	12
	ground	3–4
Duck	whole	6
Goose	whole	6
Turkey	cut up	6
	whole	12
Cooked Poultry		
Chicken/turkey dinners (sliced meat and gravy)		6
Chicken/turkey pies		6
Chicken/turkey (without broth or gravy)		1
Cooked poultry dishes		4–6
Fried chicken		4
Poultry gravy or broth		2–3
Processed Meat Products		
Chicken frankfurters		1
Luncheon meat		Do not freeze
Turkey ham (cured turkey thigh meat)		Do not freeze

meat storage chart

PRODUCT	STORAGE PERIOD	
	Refrigerator *35–40°F (days)*	*Freezer* *0°F (months)*
Fresh Meat		
Chops:		
Pork	3–5	4–6
Veal/lamb	3–5	6–9
Roasts:		
Pork/veal	3–5	4–6
Lamb	3–5	6–9
Beef	3–5	6–12
Steaks:		
Beef/veal	3–5	6–12
Stew meats	1–2	3–4
Ground meats	1–2	3–4
Variety meats	1–2	3–4
Sausage	1–2	1–2
Cooked Meats		
Cooked meat Dishes	3–4	2–3
Gravy and meat broth	1–2	2–3
Commercially Frozen Meats		
Ground meat	3	3
Thin steaks	3	3
Meat dinners	3	3
Meat pies	3	3

seafood storage chart[47]

PRODUCT	STORAGE PERIOD	
	Refrigerator 34–40°F (hours)	Freezer 0°F (months)
Lean Fish		
Cod, flounder, haddock, halibut	36	6–8
Pollock, ocean perch, sea trout, rockfish	36	4
Fat Fish		
Rainbow trout, salmon, shad, smelt	36	4

HANDLING AND PREPARATION OF
MEAT, POULTRY, AND SEAFOOD

- Wash your hands thoroughly with hot, soapy water before handling any raw meat, seafood, or poultry.
- Do not use a dish towel or sponge to clean up meat, poultry, or seafood juices–use a paper towel. Sponges and damp dish towels are bacteria heaven, so keep them clean and replace them frequently. If you cannot afford to replace your sponges as often as you would like, boil them for 10 minutes to sterilize them.
- After handling raw meat, poultry, or seafood, wash all surfaces (countertops, sink surface, and cutting boards) and utensils (knives, dishes, etc.) with hot soapy water or place them in the dishwasher. (Be sure your plastic cutting boards are dishwasher safe.) Nonporous, plastic cutting boards are recommended over wooden ones, which absorb juices from raw products.
- Do not use the plate that held raw products for cooked products. Raw juices can contaminate the cooked foods. For example, when grilling outdoors, use two separate plates—one for the raw foods and another for the cooked foods. Also, discard any marinades or sauces (such as barbecue sauce) that came in contact with the raw product. Do *not* serve them as a sauce and do *not* recycle them.
- Keep all marinating meat, poultry, or seafood covered and refrigerated. Do *not* marinate at room temperature.

COOKING AND STORING LEFTOVERS

- Poultry can go straight from the freezer to the oven if you allow one and a half times the normal cooking period. Frozen pre-stuffed poultry and frozen poultry dishes should never be thawed before cooking.
- Rinse (with cold water) and dry all meat, poultry, and seafood before cooking. Trim any excess fat from meat and poultry.
- Cook all meat, poultry, and seafood thoroughly, or to the well-done stage—this is especially important when you are pregnant. When pierced, juices from cooked meat and poultry should run clear and slightly yellow with no traces of pink. You can test fish and other seafood by cutting into it to make sure that the flesh is cooked through. Whether baking, broiling, or microwaving, use an instant-read thermometer to judge doneness of meat and poultry.
- Do *not* interrupt the cooking time (unless specified in a recipe). Partial cooking may promote bacterial growth.
- After cooking, transfer foods to shallow containers and refrigerate or freeze immediately. You do not have to let the food cool before refrigerating or freezing.
- Reheat leftovers thoroughly, to at least 165°F. Bring gravies and soups to a boil for 1 minute before serving.

■ Stuffed poultry needs special attention because bacteria from raw poultry can grow in the stuffing. Ideally, the stuffing should be cooked in a separate dish, but that takes the fun out of it. To prevent bacterial growth, stuff the bird *just before* cooking. Stuff loosely (most stuffings will expand during cooking) to ensure uniform heating, and remove all of the stuffing from the cavity *immediately* after cooking.

BARBECUE FOOD SAFETY TIPS

BARBECUING CAN BE great fun, not to mention delicious! Here are a few things to remember when the warm weather hits and grills get going.[48]

- When shopping, select your meats, poultry, and fish just before checking out. Refrigerate them as soon as possible—if you are driving a long distance (more than thirty minutes) try to place them in a cooler with ice. If these items are not intended to be used right away, freeze them as soon as possible.
- Completely defrost meat, poultry, or fish before grilling it.
- Marinate foods in the refrigerator, not at room temperature. If some of the marinade is to be used as a sauce, remove that portion of it before adding the raw meat, poultry, or fish to the marinade.
- Keep food cold until ready to grill.
- Do not use the same platter or utensils for raw and cooked foods.
- Precooking food, partially or completely, in the kitchen is a good way to reduce grilling time, especially for foods that require a lot of cooking, such as bone-in chicken. Any precooked foods should be immediately transferred to the grill.
- Cook foods to a safe internal temperature to destroy all harmful bacteria. Because the temperatures of grills, smokers, and pit barbecues can vary, always use an instant-read thermometer to check doneness. Refer to the Well-Done Temperature Guide on page 303.
- Never partially grill foods to finish cooking later.
- Keep hot foods hot. In hot weather (outside temperature 90°F and above), no food should sit out for more than 1 hour.

SLOW COOKER SAFETY TIPS

COOKING IN A slow cooker is a convenient way to prepare meals, especially if you are at work or on the go all day. The temperatures of slow cookers usually range from 170° to 280°F, which is high enough to avoid bacteria growth. Here are a few basic points to keep in mind when using a slow cooker.[49]

- Always begin with a clean cooker, clean utensils, and a clean work area.
- Do not use the slow cooker for thawing, storing, or reheating food.
- Keep all food refrigerated until it is ready to be placed in the slow cooker. This reduces the chance of bacteria developing during the first few hours of cooking.
- Always completely defrost meat and poultry before placing it in the slow cooker.
- Cut foods into small pieces to ensure thorough cooking. Do not use the slow cooker for large pieces of meat or poultry, such as roasts or whole chickens, because the food will cook so slowly it could remain in the bacterial "danger zone" (temperatures between 40° and 140°F) for too long.
- Fill your cooker no less than half-full and no more than two-thirds full. Vegetables cook more slowly than meat and poultry in a slow cooker, so, if using them, put the vegetables in first, on the bottom and around the sides of the pot, then add the remaining ingredients.
- Keep the lid in place. Remove it only to check doneness or to stir.
- Ideally, turn the cooker on the highest setting for the first hour of cooking time, and then turn it to low, or to the setting called for in your recipe. It is perfectly safe to cook foods on the low setting the entire time.
- In case of power outage, throw away the food, even if it looks done. Or, if you are at home during the outage, immediately cook the food by some other nonelectrical means.
- Always use hot pads when removing the stoneware from the slow cooker.

SAFE COOKING IN THE MICROWAVE OVEN

MOST OF US could not live without our microwave ovens, and for good reason. However, microwave ovens can cook unevenly, leaving cold spots where harmful bacteria can survive. Here are a few tips to keep in mind.[50]

- Arrange foods evenly in a microwave-safe container. Add a little liquid if needed, then loosely cover with a lid or microwave-safe plastic wrap. Cooking bags also provide safe and even cooking.
- Do not cook large cuts of meat on high power (100 percent). They should be cooked on medium power (50 percent) for longer periods. This allows the heat to reach the center without overcooking the outer areas.
- Stir or rotate food midway through the microwaving process to eliminate cold spots.
- After defrosting or partially cooking food in a microwave oven, immediately transfer it to the next heat source to finish the cooking process.
- Because the temperatures of microwave ovens can vary, always use an instant-read thermometer to check doneness. Refer to the Well-Done Temperature Guide on page 303.
- Cooking whole stuffed poultry in a microwave oven is not recommended.
- Heat ready-to-eat foods, such as hot dogs, luncheon meats, fully cooked ham, and leftovers until steaming hot. An instant-read thermometer should read 165°F.
- Never use thin plastic storage bags, brown paper or plastic grocery bags, newspaper, or aluminum foil in the microwave oven.

TIPS FOR CLEANING FRESH PRODUCE

ARE THE FRUITS and vegetables you eat really clean? Probably not. Depending on the surface of the fruit or vegetable, washing with plain water is an effective means of removing particles of dust and dirt, and possibly some bacteria. Following are a few tips to help get your produce a bit cleaner.

- Wash produce under cool running water. Soaking can lead to cross-contamination, or bacteria floating from one item to another. The exception is leafy greens (such as spinach, Swiss chard, lettuce, and fresh herbs), which are best washed by plunging them into a sink or tub of water. Be sure to lift the greens out of the water, leaving the dirt behind—do not pour them into a colander to drain, which would throw the dirt right back on them. Repeat the procedure until no dirt or sand remains in the sink or tub. Dry with a salad spinner.
- Scrub produce with a vegetable brush if possible, as it causes friction and gets into hard-to-reach nooks and crannies.
- Always wash or scrub fruits and vegetables *before* they are peeled or sliced, as the blade of the knife or peeler can move bacteria from the skin to the interior. Large fruits such as melons or pineapples and vegetables such as winter squash should always be scrubbed before slicing.
- Produce-washing liquid solutions can be effective in removing more bacteria than plain water, but exactly how much more is unknown.
- Disinfecting fruits and vegetables with chlorine or iodine is not necessary unless the drinking water has been deemed unsafe, as in underdeveloped countries or after natural disasters.

TIPS FOR WASHING AND STORING GREENS

HAVING PREPARED SALADS on hand can save time, energy, and frustration. A handful of greens can jazz up a sandwich and is perfect for throwing together a quick salad any time of day. It is important to wash all greens as thoroughly as possible to remove all dirt and any harmful bacteria. Wash greens under running water while rubbing gently with your fingertips to remove any particles. If you prefer to use a tub or sink filled with water, rub the leaves while washing them, then lift them out of the water and rinse them under running water. The following instructions should help to maximize the shelf-life of salad greens and fresh herbs.

- *Large-leaf lettuce* (romaine, red and green leaf, Boston, curly escarole, collard greens, kale, and mustard greens): Wash the leaves, discarding any badly bruised ones. Tear the leafy part of the lettuce into bite-size pieces, discarding the thick stems. Spin-dry the lettuce and, if not using immediately, place it in a zip-lock bag and store it in the vegetable bin of the refrigerator. Greens washed and stored this way will keep for three to five days.
- *Small-leaf lettuce* (watercress, Belgian endive, arugula, chicory, and radicchio): Wash the lettuce leaves, discarding any badly bruised ones, then spin-dry. Discard the thick stems of the watercress and break the leafy tops into bite-size pieces. Stack the endive or radicchio leaves and slice them just before adding them to the salad, or tear them into bite-size pieces. Store lettuce in a zip-lock bag in the vegetable bin of the refrigerator.
- *Prepackaged baby greens and boxed lettuce* (including mesclun or mixed baby greens): Wash and thoroughly spin-dry. These delicate greens tend to deteriorate quickly if a lot of moisture is left on them. Store in a zip-lock bag in the vegetable bin of the refrigerator.
- *Prepackaged lettuce labeled "prewashed"*: Wash it anyway if you have the time.
- *Prepackaged spinach*: Always wash spinach, even if the package says that the spinach has already been washed three times (it can still be sandy).
- *Fresh leafy herbs* (such as parsley, cilantro, dill, basil, and chervil): Wash according to directions for prepackaged baby greens or boxed lettuce. Once washed, remove the leaves from the stems and store then in a zip-lock bag in the vegetable bin of the refrigerator.
- *Woody-stemmed herbs* (such as rosemary and thyme): These do not require immediate washing. Keep woody-stemmed herbs refrigerated in their containers and rinse them just before using.

TIPS TO HELP KEEP YOUR
KITCHEN WORKSPACE CLEAN

- Place a piece of plastic wrap over the top of your food processor or blender before you put the lid on. You may not even need to wash the lid after using it.
- When grating slightly moist soft cheese, such as cheddar or mozzarella, lightly spray the grater with canola oil cooking spray to prevent sticking. Do the same for the grater attachment of a food processor.
- Spray canola oil cooking spray on measuring spoons and cups before measuring sticky substances such as molasses or honey.
- When grating lemon zest or Parmesan cheese, place a piece of plastic wrap or parchment paper under the grater to catch the zest.
- Use parchment paper to line baking sheets.
- Use foil to line baking sheets and baking dishes.
- Use a splatter lid when sautéing things that tend to splatter.
- Rinse a strainer or colander immediately after using it. This will prevent the starch from pasta or potatoes from drying on it.
- Keep a separate scrub brush for fruits and vegetables.
- Keep a separate plastic (not wood) chopping board for preparing raw poultry and meats.
- Line the container of your kitchen scale with plastic wrap, a paper towel, or parchment paper (depending on what you are weighing) to reduce cleanup.
- Choose one day a week to clean out your refrigerator—the day before you go grocery shopping or the day of trash pickup usually works well. This will help you keep track of your shopping needs and eliminate expired items.
- Store all opened packages and boxes of dry goods in zip-lock bags to avoid spills.
- Store all opened packages (especially hot dogs and luncheon meats) in zip-lock bags to avoid spills.

■ ENDNOTES ■

► **Introduction**

1 *The American Dietetic Association Manual*, Fifth Edition, "Nutrition Management During Pregnancy," Chicago, 1996, page 73.

2 ACOG (The American College of Obstetricians and Gynecologists), "Food, Pregnancy, and Health," January 1982 (revised September 1986).

3 The American Dietetic Association, "Blue Ribbon Babies: Eating Well During Pregnancy," Revised edition, 1998, CAT: 9015.

4 *Dietary Reference Intakes: Applications in Dietary Assessment*. National Academy Press, Washington, D.C., 2000, page 287.

5 *Recommended Dietary Allowances*, Tenth Edition, National Academy Press, Washington, D.C., 1989.

6 March of Dimes, Health Library [Internet]. Fact Sheet, "Should A Pregnant Woman Eat Liver?" [cited November 25, 2001]. Available from: www.modimes.org/HealthLibrary/334_543.htm.

7 March of Dimes Resource Center, March of Dimes Birth Defects Foundation, "Folic Acid," 09-1144-98, January 1999.

8 The National Heart, Lung, and Blood Institute, NIH (National Institutes of Health) [Internet]. "High Blood Pressure in Pregnancy," January 2001 [cited November15, 2002]. Available from: www.nhlbi.nih.gov/health/public/heart/hbp/hpb/_preg.htm.

9 March of Dimes Birth Defects Foundation, Public Health Information Sheet, "Diabetes in Pregnancy," 09-601-00, 1993.

10 *Diabetes and Pregnancy: What to Expect, Your Guide to a Healthy Pregnancy and a Happy, Healthy Baby*, Fourth Edition, The American Diabetes Association, Inc., Alexandria, VA, 2000.

11 The American Dietetic Association Manual, Fifth Edition, "Nutrition Management During Pregnancy," Chicago, 1996, page 89.

12 CDC (Centers for Disease Control) Media Relations: Press Release [Internet]. "Neural Tube Birth Defects Down by 19 Percent Since Food Fortification," June 19, 2001 [cited November 15, 2001]. Available from: www.cdc.gov/od/oc/media/pressrel/r010619.htm.

► **Chapter One**

14 FSIS (Food Safety and Inspection Service) U.S. Department of Agriculture [Internet]. Food Safety Facts, Information for Consumers, "Egg and Egg Product Safety," April 2001, [cited June 11, 2002]. Available from: www.fsis.usda.gov/OA/pubs/eggfact.htm.

13 NIDDK, National Diabetes Information Clearinghouse, NIH (National Institutes of Health) [Internet]. "Hypoglycemia," Publication No. 95-3926, May 1995 [last updated October 1999; cited March 27, 2002]. Available from: www.niddk.nih.gov/health/diabetes/pubs/hypo/hypo.htm.

15 CDC, Centers for Disease Control and Prevention, Division of Bacterial and Mycotic Diseases [Internet]. Disease Information, "*Salmonella Enteritidis*" [last reviewed April 25, 2001; cited June 11, 2002]. Available from: www.cdc.gov/ncidod/dbmd/dideaseinfo/salment_g.htm.

[16] CFSAN FDA, Center for Food Safety and Applied Nutrition, U.S. Food and Drug Administration [Internet]. Food Service Safety Facts, Information for Retail Food Stores and Food Service Operations, "Assuring the Safety of Eggs and Menu and Deli Items Made from Raw, Shell Eggs," April 2002 [cited June 11, 2002]. Available from: www.cfsan.fda.gov/~dms/fs-eggs2.html.

[17] CERHR [Internet]. Caffeine, "Caffeine Levels in Foods and Drinks," March 12, 1999 [last updated October 4, 2000; cited March 1, 2002]. Available from: http://cerhr.niehs.nih.gov/genpub/topics/caffeine-ccae.html.

[18] *The American Dietetic Association Manual*, Fifth Edition, "Nutrition Management During Pregnancy," Chicago, 1996, page 77.

▶ Chapter Two

[19] FSIS (Food Safety and Inspection Service) U.S. Department of Agriculture [Internet]. Food Safety Facts, Information for Consumers, "Keeping 'Bag' Lunches Safe," August 2001 [cited June 11, 2002]. Available from: www.fsis.usda.gov/OA/pubs/facts_lunches.htm.

[20] CERHR [Internet]. "*Listeria* and Food Poisoning," March 11, 1999 [last updated October 4, 2000; cited March 1, 2002]. Available from: http://cerhr.niehs.nih.gov/genpub/topics/listeria-ccae.html.

[21] CDC, Centers for Disease Control and Prevention, Division of Bacterial and Mycotic Diseases [Internet]. Disease Information, "Listeriosis" [last reviewed March 6, 2001; cited June 11, 2002]. Available from: www.cdc.gov/ncidod/dbmd/diseaseinfo/listeriosis_g.htm.

[22] "Listeriosis and Pregnancy: What is Your Risk? Safe Food Handling for a Healthy Pregnancy" [Internet]. Information provided by Association of Women's Health, Obstetric and Neonatal Nurses (AWHONN), International Food Information Council Foundation (IFIC), U.S. Department of Agriculture (USDA), and U.S. Department of Health and Human Services (DHHS) [cited March 1, 2002]. Available from: www.fsis.usda.gov/oa/pubs/lm_tearsheet.htm.

[23] FDA CFSAN, U.S. Food and Drug Administration, Center for Food Safety and Applied Nutrition [Internet]. FDA Brochure: June 1996 [updated July 1997; cited June 11, 2002]. "Keep Your Baby Safe: Eat Hard Cheeses Instead of Soft Cheeses During Pregnancy." Available from: http://vm.cfsan.fda.gov/~dms/listeren.html.

[24] FSIS (Food Safety and Inspection Service) U.S. Department of Agriculture [Internet]. Consumer Information from USDA, "Listeriosis and Food Safety Tips," May 1999 [cited June 11, 2002]. Available from: www.fsis.usda.gov/OA/pubs/lmtips.htm.

[25] FDA CFSAN, U.S. Food and Drug Administration, Center for Food Safety and Applied Nutrition [Internet]. *FDA Consumer*: "All About Eating for Two," By Judith Levine Willis, March 1984 [revised April 1990; cited June 11, 2002]. Available from: www.cfsan.fda.gov/~dms/wh-preg1.html.

[26] Medline Plus Health Information, A Service of the U.S. National Library of Medicine [Internet]. Medical Encyclopedia, "Pica," June 6, 2001 [updated January 2, 2002; cited March 27, 2002]. Available from: www.nim.nih.gov/medlineplus/ency/article/001538.htm.

▶ Chapter Three

[27] ACOG News Release (American College of Obstetricians and Gynecologists) [Internet]. "ACOG Addresses Air Travel During Pregnancy," December 12, 2002 [cited March 1, 2002]. Available from: www.acog.org/from_home/publications/press_releases/nr12-12-01-3.htm.

▶ Chapter Four

[28] Yale-New Haven Hospital, New Haven, CT.

[29] The calcium availability from some fruits and vegetables depends upon the oxalic acid they contain. Oxalic acid combines in the digestive tract with calcium to form an insoluble compound, calcium

oxalate. This calcium is not absorbed. Rhubarb, spinach, chard, and beet greens contain oxalic acid in appreciable amounts.

[30] Phytic acid, a phosphorous-containing compound found principally in the outer husks of cereal grains (especially oatmeal), combines with calcium to form calcium phytate which is insoluble and is not absorbed by the intestines.

[31] Marie V. Krasue, B.S., M.S., R.D., and L. Kathleen Mahan, M.S., R.D., *Food, Nutrition and Diet Therapy*, Sixth Edition, W.B. Saunders Company, Philadelphia, 1979 [source for definitions of oxalic acid and phytic acid above].

[32] Srimathi, Kannan, Ph.D., Factors in Vegetarian Diets Influencing Iron and Zinc Bioavailability, A Continuing Education Article, Andrews University Nutrition Department [Internet]. Article last edited March 12, 20002 [cited April 26, 2002]. Available from: www.andrews.edu/NUFS/FeZn-bioavail.htm.

[33] Ibid.

▶ Chapter Five

[34] March of Dimes [Internet]. Health Library: Fact Sheet, "Which Fish Are Unsafe to Eat in Pregnancy?" [cited May 6, 2002]. Available from: www.modimes.org/HealthLibrary/334_543.htm.

[35] March of Dimes, Public Health Education Information Sheet, "Toxoplasmosis," 09-408-00, October, 1993.

[36] FSIS (Food Safety and Inspection Service) U.S. Department of Agriculture [Internet]. Food Safety Focus, "Parasites and Food-Borne Illness," May 2001 [cited June 11, 2002]. Available from: www.fsis.usda.gov/OA/pubs/parasite.htm.

[37] March of Dimes, Public Health Education Information Sheet, "Toxoplasmosis," 09-408-00, October, 1993.

[38] CDC, Centers for Disease Control and Prevention [Internet]. Division of Bacterial and Mycotic Diseases, Disease Information, "*Escherichia coli O157:H7*" [cited June 11, 2002]. Available from: www.cdc.gov/ncidod/dbmd/diseaseinfo/escherichiacoli_g.htm.

[39] *eMedine Journal* [Internet]. "Salmonella Infection," Article by Robert Barrali, M.D., Volume 2, Number 10, October 4, 2001 [cited July 11, 2002]. Available from: www.emedicine.com/EMERG/topic515.htm.

▶ Chapter Six

[40] *Diabetes and Pregnancy: What to Expect, Your Guide to a Healthy Pregnancy and a Happy, Healthy Baby*, Fourth Edition, The American Diabetes Association, Inc., Alexandria, VA, 2000, page 30–31.

[41] March of Dimes Birth Defects Foundation, Public Health Education Information Sheet, "Fitness for Two," 09-406-00, January 1992.

▶ Appendix

[42] *Journal of Obstetric, Gynecologic, and Neonatal Nursing (JOGNN) in Review*, "Nutrition for the Childbearing Years," Elizabeth Reifsnider, R.N., C., Ph.D., WHNP, and Sara L. Gill, R.N., Ph.D., IBCLC, Volume 29, Number 1, January/February 2000, page 46.

[43] CDC, Centers for Disease Control and Prevention, Division of Birth Defects and Pediatric Genetics [Internet]. National Center for Birth Defects and Developmental Disabilities, "Folic Acid Now," [last updated March 5, 2002; cited June 11, 2002]. Available from: www.cdc.gov/ncbddd/folicacid/cereal.htm.

[44] Excerpt from *U.S. Department of Agriculture Food Safety and Inspection Service, Home and Garden Bulletin No. 248*, August 1995.

⁴⁵ *U.S. Department of Agriculture Home and Garden Bulletin No. 110.*

⁴⁶ *U.S. Department of Agriculture Home and Garden Bulletin No. 248.*

⁴⁷ National Fisheries Institute, Washington, D.C.

⁴⁸ FSIS (Food Safety and Inspection Service) U.S. Department of Agriculture [Internet]. Food Safety Facts, Information for Consumers, "Barbecue Food Safety," May 2001 [cited June 11, 2002]. Available from: www.fsis.usda.gov/OA/pubs/facts_barbecue.htm.

⁴⁹ FSIS (Food Safety and Inspection Service) U.S. Department of Agriculture [Internet]. Consumer Education and Information, "Focus On: Slow Cooker Safety," [slightly revised July 2000; cited June 11, 2002]. Available from: www.fsis.usda.gov/OA/pubs/slocookr.htm.

⁵⁰ FSIS (Food Safety and Inspection Service) U.S. Department of Agriculture, Food Safety Facts, "Cooking Safely in the Microwave Oven," [revised November 2000; cited June 11, 2002]. Available from: www.fsis.usda.gov/OA/pubs/fact_microwave.htm.

■ ACKNOWLEDGMENTS ■

Finding Rose Ann Hudson to co-author this book is a striking example of life working out the way it should. I could not have asked for a more knowledgeable, patient, sensitive, optimistic, and pleasant person with whom to work. Lisa Ekus, my agent, is another example. She has always believed in this book and eventually found it the perfect home. Matthew Lore, my talented editor and publisher at Marlowe & Company, is yet a third example. Matthew helped shape this book inside and out, and also offered continuous words of encouragement and support for which both Rose Ann and I are truly grateful.

I thank my mother, Mary Abernethy, a fabulous cook and mother of five, who taught me the importance of taking the time to sit down to family meals no matter how busy I am. Her cooking is always fresh, simple, and tasty and many of the recipes in this book are adaptations of her originals. I am forever indebted to my team of recipe testers whose enthusiasm, energy, and valuable comments made the recipes what they are. Martha Grove (my sister-in-law), Nan Wood Mosher, and Mary Mulard led the pack of testers, feeding their families recipes from this book for months at a time. My other recipe-testing heroes include Mary Fortino, Laura Wright, Melissa Alshab, Patricia Terry, Peggy Terry, Lynn Rudolf, Lisa Natanson, Annie Mozer, Margaret Jones, Paul Grove (my brother), Carol Scheangold, Mari Webel, and Jan Greenburg.

My friend and editor Shari Bistransky, who reviewed the book soon after giving birth to her second child, offered insightful comments and valuable suggestions for which I am grateful. Words of encouragement from fellow writers Kathleen Luft and Judith Sutton fueled my creative energy over the years. In addition, Judith Sutton, the best cookbook copy-editor in the business, polished my recipes as only she can do. Sue McCloskey and Peter Jacoby, Matthew Lore's assistants, worked hard to make this manuscript as perfect as possible—thank you.

I am grateful for the support of my father, Brandon Grove, and his wife, Mariana, my step-father Robert Abernethy, my mother-in-law Evelyn Jones, my brothers Jack (and his wife Hannah), Paul, and Mark, and my sister, Elizabeth. My deepest gratitude goes to my husband, Paul, for his love, friendship, and support, and for his willingness to edit anything I put in front of him. My children, Aleksandra and Hale, give meaning to my world and bring me more joy than they will ever know.

—Catherine Jones

I WOULD LIKE to thank my parents, Thomas and Lilian Angotti, who have always given me the love, guidance, and support I needed to achieve my goals. They have my deepest gratitude. Other members of my family have given a part of themselves to this project and I thank them: my wonderful husband, Mark, and beautiful daughters, Emily and Rachel, who gave me love and encouragement throughout; my sisters, Angela Angotti Morris and Antoinette Angotti, who have always been there for me; and my sister, Alma Angotti, who helped me organize my thoughts for this book on paper.

I thank my good friend Julian Safran, M.D., for sharing his expertise, and always offering words of encouragement; my colleagues, Mary Ellen Sabatella, R.D. and Martha Betts, R.D., for their careful review of the material. My gratitude also goes to my close friend, Laura Wright, for her unwavering enthusiasm for this project since its conception. Finally, I would like to thank Catherine Jones for her hard work and tremendous dedication, and for giving me the opportunity to be a part of this special book, which I hope will help pregnant women everywhere for years to come.

—Rose Ann Hudson

■ INDEX ■